英漢實用中醫藥大全

趙樸初題

6

THERAPEUTICS OF
ACUPUNCTURE
AND MOXIBUSTION

針灸治療學

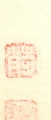

THE ENGLISH–CHINESE ENCYCLOPEDIA OF PRACTICAL TRADITIONAL CHINESE MEDICINE

Chief Editor   Xu Xiangcai

Assistants   You Ke   Kang Kai

     Bao Xuequan   Lu Yubin

英汉实用中医药大全

主 编 徐象才

主编助理 尤 可 康 凯

鲍学全 路玉滨

Higher Education Press
高等教育出版社

6

针 灸 治 疗 学

	中文	英文	
主　编	刘玉檀	俞昌正	
副主编	吴富东	朱海洪	张　峰
编　者	刘国真	解培萍	寻建英
	单秋华	张灵泉	
	崇桂琴		
审　校		尤本林	
		J·布莱克	

THERAPEUTICS OF ACUPUNCTURE AND MOXIBUSTION

	English	Chinese
Chief Editor	Yu Changzheng	Liu Yutan
Deputy Chief Editors	Zhu Haiheng	Wu Fudong
	Zhang Feng	
Editors	Xie Peiping	Liu Guozhen
	Xun Jianying	Shan Qiuhua
	Zhang Lingquan	Chong Guiqin
Revisers	You Benling	
	John Black(New Zealand)	

The Leading Commission of Compilation and Translation
编译领导委员会

Honorary Director 名誉主任委员	Hu Ximing 胡熙明		
Honorary Deputy Directors 名誉副主任委员	Zhang Qiwen 张奇文	Wang Lei 王 镭	
Director 主任委员	Zou Jilong 邹积隆		
Deputy Director 副主任委员	Wei Jiwu 隗继武		
Members 委员 (以姓氏笔划为序)	Wan Deguang 万德光	Wang Yongyan 王永炎	Wang Maoze 王懋泽
	Wei Guikang 韦贵康	Cong Chunyu 丛春雨	Liu Zhongben 刘中本
	Sun Guojie 孙国杰	Yan Shiyun 严世芸	Qiu Dewen 邱德文
	Shang Chichang 尚炽昌	Xiang Ping 项 平	Zhao Yisen 赵以森
	Gao Jinliang 高金亮	Cheng Yichun 程益春	Ge Linyi 葛琳仪
	Cai Jianqian 蔡剑前	Zhai Weimin 翟维敏	
Advisers 顾问	Dong Jianhua 董建华	Huang Xiaokai 黄孝楷	Geng Jianting 耿鉴庭
	Zhou Fengwu 周凤梧	Zhou Ciqing 周次清	Chen Keji 陈可冀

The Commission of Compilation and Translation
编译委员会

Director 主任委员	Xu Xiangcai 徐象才

Deputy Directors 副主任委员	Zhang Zhigang 张志刚	Zhang Wengao 张文高	Jiang Zhaojun 姜兆俊
	Qi Xiuheng 秀恒	Xuan Jiasheng 宣家声	Sun Xiangxie 孙祥燮
Members 委员 (以姓氏笔划为序)	Yu Wenping 于文平	Wang Zhengzhong 王正忠	Wang Chenying 王陈应
	Wang Guocai 王国才	Fang Tingyu 方廷钰	Fang Xuwu 方续武
	Tian Jingzhen 田景振	Bi Yongsheng 毕永升	Liu Yutan 刘玉檀
	Liu Chengcai 刘承才	Liu Jiaqi 刘家起	Liu Xiaojuan 刘晓娟
	Zhu Zhongbao 朱忠宝	Zhu Zhenduo 朱振铎	Xun Jianying 寻建英
	Li Lei 李磊	Li Zhulan 李竹兰	Xin Shoupu 辛守璞
	Shao Nianfang 邵念方	Chen Shaomin 陈绍民	Zou Jilong 邹积隆
	Lu Shengnian 陆胜年	Zhou Xing 周行	Zhou Ciqing 周次清
	Zhang Sufang 张素芳	Yang Chongfeng 杨崇峰	Zhao Chunxiu 赵纯修
	Yu Changzheng 俞昌正	Hu Zunda 胡遵达	Xu Heying 须鹤瑛
	Yuan Jiurong 袁久荣	Huang Naijian 黄乃健	Huang Kuiming 黄奎铭
	Huang Jialing 黄嘉陵	Cao Yixun 曹贻训	Lei Xilian 雷希濂
	Cai Huasong 蔡华松	Cai Jianqian 蔡剑前	

Preface

I am delighted to learn that THE ENGLISH—CHINESE ENCYCLOPEDIA OF PRACTICAL TRADITIONAL CHINESE MEDICINE will soon come into the world.

TCM has experienced many vicissitudes of times but has remained evergreen. It has made great contributions not only to the power and prosperity of our Chinese nation but to the enrichment and improvement of world medicine. Unfortunately, differences in nations, states and languages have slowed down its spreading and flowing outside China. At present, however, an upsurge in learning, researching and applying Traditional Chinese Medicine (TCM) is unfolding. In order to maximize the effect of this upsurge and to lead TCM, one of the brilliant cultural heritages of the Chinese nation, to the world for it to expand and bring benefit to the people of all nations, Mr. Xu Xiangcai called intellectuals of noble aspirations and high intelligence together from Shandong and many other provinces in China and took charge of the work of both compilation and translation of THE ENGLISH—CHINESE ENCYCLOPEDIA OF PRACTICAL TRADITIONAL CHINESE MEDICINE. With great pleasure, the medical staff both at home and abroad will hail the appearance of this encyclopedia.

I believe that the day when the world's medicine is fully

developed will be the day when TCM has spread throughout the world.

I am pleased to give it my preface.

Prof. Dr. Hu Ximing

 Deputy Ministerof the Ministry of Public Health of the People's Republic of China,

 Director General of the State Administrative Bureau of Traditional Chinese Medicine and Pharmacology,

 President of the World Federation of Acupuncture —Moxibustion Societies,

 Member of China Association of Science & Technology,

 Deputy President of All—China Association of Traditional Chinese Medicine,

 President of China Acupuncture & Moxibustion Society.

December, 1989

Preface

The Chinese nation has been through a long, arduous course of struggling against diseases and has developed its own traditional medicine—Traditional Chinese Medicine and Pharmacology (TCMP). TCMP has a unique, comprehensive, scientific system including both theories and clinical practice. Some thousand years since ito—beginnings, not only has it been well preserved but also continuously developed. It has special advantages, such as remarkable curative effects and few side effects. Hence it is an effective means by which people prevent and treat diseases and keep themselves strong and healthy.

All achievements attained by any nation in the development of medicine are the public wealth of all mankind. They should not be confined within a single country. What is more, the need to set them free to flow throughout the world as quickly and precisely as possible is greater than that of any other kind of science. During my more than thirty years of being engaged in Traditional Chinese Medicine(TCM), I have been looking forward to the day when TCMP will have spread all over the world and made its contributions to the elimination of diseases of all mankind. However it is to be deeply regretted that the pace of TCMP in extending outside China has been unsatisfactory due to the major difficulties in expressing its concepts in foreign languages.

Mr. Xu Xiangcai, a teacher of Shandong College of TCM, has sponsored and taken charge of the work of compilation and translation of The English—Chinese Encyclopedia of Practical Traditional Chinese Medicine—an extensive series. This work is a great project, a large—scale scientific research, a courageous effort and a novel creation. I deeply esteem Mr. Xu Xiangcai and his compilers and translators, who have been working day and night for such a long time, for their hard labor and for their firm and indomitable will displayed in overcoming one difficulty after another, and for their great success achieved in this way. As a leader in the circles of TCM, I am duty—bound to do my best to support them.

I believe this encyclopedia will be certain to find its position both in the history of Chinese medicine and in the history of world science and technology.

Mr. Zhang Qiwen

Member of the Standing Committee of
All—China Association of TCM,
Deputy Head of the Health Department
of Shandong Province.

March, 1990

Publisher's Preface

Traditional Chinese Medicine(TCM) is one of China's great cultural heritages. Since the founding of the People's Republic of China in 1949, guided by the farsighted TCM policy of the Chinese Communist Party and the Chinese government, the treasure house of the theories of TCM has been continuously explored and the plentiful literature researched and compiled. As a result, great success has been achieved. Today there has appeared a world—wide upsurge in the studying and researching of TCM. To promote even more vigorous development of this trend in order that TCM may better serve all mankind, efforts are required to further it throughout the world. To bring this about, the language barriers must be overcome as soon as possible in order that TCM can be accurately expressed in foreign languages.

Thus the compilation and translation of a series of English—Chinese books of basic knowledge of TCM has become of great urgency to serve the needs of medical and educational circles both inside and outside China.

In recent years, at the request of the health departments, satisfactory achievements have been made in researching the expression of TCM in English. Based on the investigation into the history and current state of the research work mentioned above, the English—Chinese Encyclopedia of Practical TCM has been published to meet the needs of extending the knowledge of TCM around the world.

The encyclopedia consists of twenty—one volumes, each dealing with a particular branch of TCM. In the process of compilation, the distinguishing features of TCM have been given close attention and great efforts have been made to ensure that the content is scientific, practical, comprehensive and concise. The chief writers of the Chinese manuscripts include professors or associate professors with at least twenty years of practical clinical and / or teaching experience in TCM. The Chinese manuscript of each volume has been checked and approved by a specialist of the relevant branch of TCM. The team of the translators and revisers of the English versions consists of TCM specialists with a good command of English professional medical translators, and teachers of English from TCM colleges or universities. At a symposium to standardize the English versions, scholars from twenty—two colleges or universities, research institutes of TCM or other health institutes probed the question of how to express TCM in English more comprehensively, systematically and accurately, and discussed and deliberated in detail the English versions of some volumes in order to upgrade the English versions of the whole series. The English version of each volume has been re—examined and then given a final checking.

Obviously this encyclopedia will provide extensive reading material of TCM English for senior students in colleges of TCM in China and will also greatly benefit foreigners studying TCM.

The assiduous efforts of compiling and translating this encyclopedia have been supported by the responsible leaders of the State Education Commission of the People's Republic of China, the State Administrative Bureau of TCM and Pharmacy, and the Education Commission and Health Department of Shandong

Province. Under the direction of the Higher Education Department of the State Education Commission, the leading board of compilation and translation of this encyclopedia was set up. The leaders of many colleges of TCM and pharmaceutical factories of TCM have also given assistance.

We hope that this encyclopedia will bring about a good effect on enhancing the teaching of TCM English at the colleges of TCM in China, on cultivating skills in medical circles in exchanging ideas of TCM with patients in English, and on giving an impetus to the study of TCM outside China.

Higher Education Press
March, 1990

Foreword

The English—Chinese Encyclopedia of Practical Traditional Chinese Medicine is an extensive series of twenty—one volumes. Based on the fundamental theories of traditional Chinese medicine(TCM) and with emphasis on the clinical practice of TCM, it is a semi—advanced English—Chinese academic works which is quite comprehensive, systematic, concise, practical and easy to read. It caters mainly to the following readers: senior students of colleges of TCM, young and middle—aged teachers of colleges of TCM, young and middle—aged physicians of hospitals of TCM, personnel of scientific research institutions of TCM, teachers giving correspondence courses in TCM to foreigners, TCM personnel going abroad in the capacity of lecturers or physicians, those trained in Western medicine but wishing to study TCM, and foreigners coming to China to learn TCM or to take refresher courses in TCM.

Because Traditional Chinese Medicine and Pharmacology is unique to our Chinese nation, putting TCM into English has been the crux of the compilation and translation of this encyclopedia. Owing to the fact that no one can be proficient both in the theories of Traditional Chinese Medicine and Pharmacology and the clinical practice of every branch of TCM, as well as in English, to ensure that the English versions express accurately the inherent meanings of TCM, collective translation measures have been taken. That is, teachers of English familiar with TCM, professional medical translators, teachers or physicians of TCM and even teachers of palaeography with a strong command of English were all invited together to co—translate the Chinese manuscripts and, then, to co—deliberate and discuss the English versions. Finally English—speaking foreigners studying TCM or teaching English in China were asked to polish the English versions. In this way, the skills of the above translators and foreigners were merged to ensure the quality of the English versions. However, even using this method, the uncertainty that the English versions will be wholly accepted still remains. As for the Chinese manuscripts, they do reflect the essence, and give a general picture, of traditional Chinese medicine and pharmacology. It is not asserted, though, that they are perfect, I whole—heartedly look forward to any criticisms or opinions from readers in order to make improvements to future editions.

More than 200 people have taken part in the activities of compiling, translating and revising this encyclopedia. They come from twenty—eight institutions in all parts of China. Among these institutions, there are fifteen colleges of TCM:Shandong, Beijing, Shanghai, Tianjin, Nanjing, Zhejiang, Anhui, Henan, Hubei, Guangxi, Guiyang, Gansu, Chengdu, Shanxi and Changchun, and scientific research centers of TCM such as China Academy of TCM and Shandong Scientific Research Institute of TCM.

The Education Commission of Shandong province has included the compilation and translation of this encyclopedia in its scientific research projects and allocated funds accordingly. The Health Department of Shandong Province has also given financial aid together with a number of pharmaceutical factories of TCM. The subsidization from Jinan Pharmaceutical Factory of

TCM provided the impetus for the work of compilation and translation to get under way.

The success of compiling and translating this encyclopedia is not only the fruit of the collective labor of all the compilers, translators and revisers but also the result of the support of the responsible leaders of the relevant leading institutions. As the encyclopedia is going to be published, I express my heartfelt thanks to all the compilers. translators and revisers for their sincere cooperation, and to the specialists, professors, leaders at all levels and pharmaceutical factories of TCM for their warm support.

It is my most profound wish that the publication of this encyclopedia will take its role in cultivating talented persons of TCM having a very good command of TCM English and in extending, rapidly, comprehensive knowledge of TCM to all corners of the globe.

Chief Editor Xu Xiangcai

Shandong College of TCM

March, 1990

Contents

Notes

THERAPEUTICS OF ACUPUNCTURE AND MOXIBUSTION is the sixth volume of THE ENGLISH–CHINESE ENCYCLOPEDIA OF PRACTICAL TCM an extensive series.

This volume consists of the following seven chapters: Diseases of Internal Medicine, Diseases of Surgery, Diseases of Gynecology, Diseases of Pediatrics, Diseases of Eyes. Ears. Nose and Throat, Emergency Cases and Miscellaneous Conditions. It deals with in detail the acupuncture and moxibustion therapy of 135 disorders common in the clinic. Each disorder is stated by features, cause and mechanism, types, treatment of each type, and alternative treatment for every type. "Treatment of each type" involves treatment principle, prescription, explanation (brief introduction to the curative effect of the selected points), point modification and acupuncture; while "alternative treatment for every type", the prescriptions and manupulations of other methods such as moxibustion, ear needling, embedding of ear seeds, scalp needling, puncturing with a heated needle, cataneous acupuncture (plum–blossom needle), point electric stimulation, blood–letting puncturing and cupping, pricking therapy, laser therapy, etc.

This volume, therefore, will prove to be a novel clinical reference book on acupuncture and moxibustion fit for the readers both in and outside China.

The Chinese edition has been checked and approved by Pro.

Cheng Shennong, deputy chairman of Chinese Acupuncture Association and deputy director of Beijing International Acupuncture Training Center; the English edition by Mr. You Benlin from Nanjing International Acupuncture Training Center and Mr. John Black, a foreign friend from New Zealand. Pro. Fang Tingyu from Beijing College of TCM has also helped to refresh the English edition.

The location of acupuncture points in this book is the standard one promulgated in 1990 by the State Bureau of Technic Supervision and Pharmacy of the People's Republic of China. It is to be put into effect from Jan 1, 1991.

Editor

1　Diseases of Internal Medicine

1.1　Common Cold

Common cold, also known as catching cold, is a common exogenous disease in the clinic characterized by nasal obstruction and discharge, cough, headache, chills, fever and superficial pulse. It may occur around the year, but more often in autumn and winter. This condition includes the upper respiratory tract inflammation due to viral or bacterial infection as well as influenza in modern medicine.

Cause and Mechanism

Common cold involves mainly the invasion of exogenous pathogenic wind. Pathogenic wind however often mingles with other pathogenic factors such as cold, heat, summer—heat and dampness to cause the onset of disease. Invasion of exogenous pathogenic wind—cold often takes place in autumn and winter, that of wind—heat often in spring and summer, and that of damp—heat in mid—summer. Invasion of exogenous pathogenic wind—cold affects the body superficies, leading to closed pores and dysfunction of lung in dispersing. Invasion of exogenous pathogenic wind—heat attacks the lung, leading to dysfunction of lung in descending and abnormal opening and closing of pores. Exogenous pathogenic invasion involving summer—heat and dampness which is often lingering and difficult to be eliminated brings about obstruction to the lucid *Yang*.

Differentiation

1. Wind-cold Type

The chief manifestations include a mild fever without sweating but more aversion to cold, headache, running nose, itching throat, cough with thin whitish sputum, general aching, thin white tongue coating, and rapid superficial pulse.

2. Wind-heat Type

The chief manifestations include a high fever with slight chills, spontaneous sweating with aversion to wind, headache, stuffy nose with yellowish discharge, sore throat, dry mouth with desire for drinking, cough with yellowish thick sputum, thin yellow tongue coating, and rapid superficial pulse.

3. Damp-heat Type

The chief manifestations include high fever without sweating, distending headache as if the head is tightly bound, general heavy sensation, lassitude, fullness sensation in the chest, nausea, anorexia, abdominal distention, loose stools, slight cough with sticky whitish sputum, thick greasy or yellow greasy tongue coating, and soft rapid pulse.

Treatment

1. Wind-cold Type

Principle: Eliminate wind, disperse cold from the body surface and promote the function of the lung in dispersing by puncturing points mainly from The Lung Channel of Hand-*Taiyin*, The Large Intestine Channel of Hand-*Yangming* and The Bladder Channel of Foot-*Taiyang*.

Prescription: Lieque(LU 7)   Fengmen(BL12)

Fengchi(GB20)   Hegu(LI 4)

Explanation: Lieque(LU 7), the *Luo*-connecting point of the Lung channel, has the effect of promoting the lung to disperse and arresting cough. Fengmen(BL12) is chosen to promote the *Qi* circulation of the lung channel and disperse the pathogenic wind—cold from the body surface since the *Taiyang* channel dominates the superficial portion of the body. Fengchi (GB20), the intersecting point of The Gallbladder Channel of Foot—*Shaoyang* and The *Yangwei* Channel, which dominates the exterior *Yang* of the body, is used to eliminate exogenous pathogenic factors from the exterior of the body. The *Taiyin* and *Yangming* channels of the hand are internally—externally related. Therefore, Hegu (LI 4), the *Yuan*—source point of The Large Intestine Channel of Hand—*Yangming*, is selected to enhance the function of relieving the exogenous pathogenic factors from the body surface in order to achieve a better therapeutic effect.

Point Modification: Add Yintang (EX—HN3) and Taiyang (EX—HN5) for headache; and Yingxiang (LI20) for nasal obstruction.

Method: Use filiform needles with reducing method and retain the needles for 15—20 minutes, manipulating them 2—3 times. Even method is applied instead for patients with poor body constitution. Moxibustion is also applicable to Fengmen (BL12) and Fengchi (GB20) after being needled.

2. Wind— heat Type

Principle: Eliminate wind, disperse heat and promote the circulation of lung *Qi* by needling points mainly from The *Du* Channel, The Lung Channel of Hand—*Taiyin* and The Large Intestine Channel of Hand—*Yangming*.

Prescription: Dazhui(DU14) Quchi(LI11)

　　　　　　　Hegu(LI 4) Yuji(LU10) Chize(LU 5)

Explanation: Dazhui (DU14), the point converging all the

Yang channels, is used to expel superficial wind−heat and relieve high fever. Hegu(LI 4) and Quchi(LI11), being respectively the *Yuan*−source and *He*−sea points of The Large Intestine Channel of Hand−*Yangming* which forms an internal−external relationship with The Lung Channel of Hand−*Taiyin,* may clear the lung and reduce heat when they are *treat punctured* with reducing method. Yuji(LU10), the *Xing*−spring point of the lung channel in combination with Chize(LU 5), the *He*−sea point of the lung channel, eliminates the pathogenic heat from the lung, clears the throat, resolves phlegm and ceases cough. The joint use of these five points may fulfil the function of eliminating pathogenic wind−heat and promoting the lung in descending *Qi*.

Point Modification: Add Shaoshang(LU11)for sore throat; and Shixuan(EX−UE11)to be pricked with a three−edged needle to cause bleeding for high fever and convulsions.

Method: Apply filiform needles with reducing method and retain the needles for 15−20 minutes, manipulating them two to three times. Prick Dazhui(DU14), Shaoshang(LU11) and Shixuan(EX−UE11)with the three−edged needle to cause bleeding.

3. Damp−heat Type

Principle: Expel superficial summer−heat and resolve dampness by puncturing points mainly from The Lung Channel of Hand−*Taiyin,* The Large Intestine Channel of Hand−*Yangming* and The *Sanjiao* Channel of Hand−*Shaoyang*.

Prescription: Kongzui(LU 6)   Hegu(LI 4)

　　　　　　　Zhongwan(RN12)   Zusanli(ST36)

　　　　　　　Waiguan(SJ 5)

Explanation: Kongzui(LU 6)and Hegu(LI 4)have the effect of promoting the dispersing function of the lung, relieving summer—heat and resolving dampness from the superficial portion of the body. Zhongwan(RN12)and Zusanli(ST36)resolve phlegm, descend the turbid phlegm, pacify the stomach and arrest vomiting. Waiguan(SJ 5), the *Luo*—connecting point of the *Sanjiao* channel, can promote the *Qi* mechanism of the *Sanjiao,* eliminate the summer—heat and resolve the dampness together with the rest of the points.

Point Modification: Add Dazhui(DU14)and Weizhong(BL40) for high fever; Yinlingquan(SP 9)for excessive dampness; and Tianshu(ST 25)for abdominal distention and loose stools.

Method: Use filiform needles with reducing method and retain the needles for 15—20 minutes, manipulating them two to three times. Prick Dazhui(DU14)and Weizhong(BL40)with a three—edged needle to cause bleeding.

Alternative Treatment

1. Auricular Acupuncture

Prescription: Lung Internal nose Trachea Throat Ear
　　　　　　　apex *Sanjiao* Stomach Subcortex Adrenal gland Spleen

Method: Use filiform needles with strong stimulation and retain the needles for 10—20 minutes. Select three to five points for each treatment. Embedding of ear seeds of subcutaneous needles is also applicable.

2. Moxibustion Therapy

During the epidemic season of common cold, apply moxibustion to Dazhui (DU14), Fengmen (BL12) and Zusanli (ST36) for 15—20 minutes both in the morning and in the evening. This is an effective method for preventing common cold because it has the effect to strengthen the defensive *Qi,* promote the function of the spleen and stomach, and strengthen the immune function against the common cold.

1.2 Cough

Cough refers to an abrupt air expelling with production of sputum due to upward attack of lung *Qi*. It is a symptom indicating the impaired function of the lung in its normal descending and dispersing caused by either invasion of exogenous pathogenic factors or dysfunction of *Zangfu* organs. In traditional Chinese medicine, cough is further classified as *Ke,* cough loud and without sputum, *Sou,* cough feeble and with sputum and *Kesou,* cough loud and with sputum, with the last one usually seen in pair in the clinic. According to different causative factors, cough consists of two major types, the exopathogenic cough and endopathogenic cough.

In modern medicine, cough is commonly seen in upper respiratory tract infection, acute and chronic bronchitis, bronchiectasis, pneumonia and tuberculosis.

Cause and Mechanism

Exopathogenic cough is mostly due to invasion of wind—cold or wind—heat affecting the lung and defensive *Qi* of the body, leading to the dysfunction of the lung in descending and dispersing.

Endopathogenic cough is mostly due to repeated attacks of cough, leading to chronic damage of lung *Qi*. The deficiency of lung *Qi* affects the spleen while the deficiency of the spleen gives rise to internal dampness whose excessive accumulation produces phlegm. Phlegmdamp in return may go up into the lung, causing the dysfunction in descending. Furthermore, stagnation of liver

Qi turning into heat may also result in the endopathogenic cough because the heat simply dries up the fluid of the lung.

Differentiation

1. Exopathogenic Cough

(1) Wind—cold Type

This type of cough is characterized by itching sensation in the throat and thin whitish sputum which is difficult to be expectorated. It is accompanied by fever without sweating, but aversion to cold, headache, stuffy running nose, soreness of joints, thin white tongue coating, and superficial tense pulse.

(2) Wind—heat Type

The cough is frequent and severe with coarse breathing, sore throat, dry mouth and sticky yellowish sputum which is difficult to be expectorated. It is accompanied by headache, feverish sensation with aversion to wind, some but obstructed sweating, yellowish nasal discharge, thin yellow tongue coating, and rapid superficial pulse.

2. Endopathogenic Cough

(1) Turbid Phlegm Obstructing the Lung

The chief manifestations include cough with profuse sputum of white colour and sticky quality, fullness sensation in the chest and epigastric region, general lassitude, poor appetite, white greasy tongue coating, and slippery pulse.

(2) *Yin* Deficiency with Dryness of the Lung

The cough is dry without sputum or with a little sputum that is difficult to be expectorated. It also causes pain in the chest and epigastric region. Other symptoms and signs include dry throat, thirst, feverish palms and soles, tidal fever, red tongue proper with thin yellow coating that lacks fluid distribution, thready rapid or thin rapid pulse.

Treatment

1. Exopathogenic Cough

(1) Wind−cold Type

Principle: Eliminate pathogenic wind and cold, promote the lung in dispersing and stop cough by needling points mainly from The Lung Channel of Hand−*Taiyin* and The Large Intestine Channel of Hand−*Yangming*.

Prescription: Lieque(LU 7)　Feishu(BL13)　Hegu(LI 4)
　　　　　　　 Waiguan(SJ 5)

Explanation: Lieque(LU 7), the *Luo*−connecting point of the lung channel, is used in combination with Feishu(BL13)to promote the dispersing function of the lung and stop cough. Hegu (LI 4)is used in combination with Waiguan(SJ 5)to relieve the pathogenic factors from the body surface by causing sweating. The joint use of the four points can achieve the effect of expelling the pathogenic wind−cold, promoting the lung in dispersing and ceasing cough.

Point Modification: Add Fengchi(GB20)and Shangxing(DU23)for headache; Fenglong(ST40)for profuse sputum; and Kunlun(BL60)and Wenliu(LI 7)for general soreness.

Method: Apply filiform needles with reducing method and retain the needles for 15−20 minutes, manipulating them two to three times. Moxibustion is applicable to Feishu(UB 13)for 15−20 minutes after needling.

(2) Wind−heat Type

Principle: Eliminate wind−heat, resolve phlegm and cease cough by needling points mainly from The Lung Channel of Hand−*Taiyin*, The Large Intestine Channel of Hand−*Yangming* and The *DU* Channel.

Prescription: Chize(LU 5)　Feishu(BL13)

Dazhui(DU14)　Quchi(LI11)

Explanation: Chize(LU 5), the *He*—sea point of the lung and also the water point of the channel, is used in combination with Feishu(BL13)to eliminate heat from the lung and resolve phlegm and cease cough. Dazhui(DU14), the important point of The *Du* Channel where all *Yang* merges, is used to promote *Yang Qi* in order to relieve exterior syndrome. It is also applied in combination with Quchi(LI11)to clear up wind—heat. The combined use of these points can eliminate wind—heat from the body surface, sedate phlegm—fire, soothe the affected lung *Qi* and relieve cough.

Point Modification: Add Shaoshang(LU11)for sore throat; Hegu(LI 4)for difficult sweating; and Tiantu(RN22)and Fenglong(ST 40)for cough with profuse sputum.

Method: Apply filiform needles with reducing method and retain the needles for 15—20 minutes, manipulating them two to three times. Dazhui(DU14)and Shaoshang(LU11)are usually pricked with a three—edged needle to cause bleeding.

2. Endopathogenic Cough

(1) Turbid Phlegm Obstructing the Lung

Principle: Reinforce the lung *Qi*, strengthen the spleen and resolve phlegm by puncturing points mainly from The Spleen Channel of Foot—*Taiyin* and The Stomach Channel of Foot—*Yangming*, plus some Back—*Shu* points.

Prescription: Feishu(BL13)　Pishu(BL20)　Taiyuan(LU 9)

Taibai(SP 3)　Fenglong(ST40)

Explanation: The spleen is considered as the source for producing phlegm while the lung as the organ to contain the phlegm.

Taiyuan(LU 9)and Taibai(SP 3), being respectively the *Yuan*—source points of the lung and spleen channels, are selected in combination with Feishu(BL13) and Pishu(BL20) to cope with both the superficial manifestations and the root cause of the condition. It is a principal method for treating patients with turbid phlegm obstructing the lung. Fenglong(ST40), the *Luo*—connecting point of the stomach channel, may invigorate the *Qi* of the middle—*Jiao*. Therefore, the *Qi* circulation promotes body fluid distribution so that the lung returns to its normal physiological status.

Point Modification: Add Dingchuan(EX—B1) for cough with asthmatic breathing; Zusanli (ST36) and Neiguan (PC 6) for fullness sensation in the chest and epigastric region.

Method: Use filiform needles with either the reinforcing or even method and retain the needles for 15—20 minutes, manipulating them two to three times. Moxibustion is also applicable to Pishu (BL20) and Feishu (BL13) for 10—15 minutes each time.

(2) Deficiency of *Yin* with Dryness of the Lung

Principle: Nourish *Yin,* moisten dryness, clear the lung and cease cough by puncturing points mainly from The Lung channel of Hand—*Taiyin* and The Liver Channel of Foot—*Jueyin*.

Prescription: Feishu(BL13) Zhongfu(LU 1)

Lieque(LU 7) Zhaohai(KI 6) Taichong(LR 3)

Explanation: The combined use of Zhongfu(LU 1) and Feishu(BL13), being respectively the Front—*Mu* point and Back—*Shu* point of the lung, also known as the combination of Front—*Mu* and the Back—*Shu* points of the lung, may regulate the *Qi* passage of the lung and promote the lung in descending and dispersing. Lieque(LU 7) in combination with Zhaohai(KI 6), known as one of the combinations of the Eight Confluent Points, may nourish *Yin*, moisten the dryness, clear the throat and promote the lung in descending. Taichong(LR 3), the *Yuan*—source point of the liver channel, can sedate the liver fire. The above points may jointly nourish *Yin*, moisten dryness, sedate fire, clear lung, resolve phlegm and cease cough.

Point Modification: Add Kongzui(LU 6) and Geshu(BL 17) for hemoptysis.

Method: Apply filiform needles with even method to all these points except Taichong(LR 3) which is done with reducing method. Retain the needles for 15—20 minutes, manipulating them two to three times.

Alternative Treatment: **Auricular Acupuncture**

Prescription: Lung Bronchea Ear—shenmen Occipit Adrenal gland Spleen Sympathetic Kidney

Method: Select two to three points each time and use filiform needles with moderate stimulation and retain the needles for 10—20 minutes. Embedding of ear seeds is also applicable.

1.3 Asthma

Asthma is a common illness mainly characterized by prolonged attacks of dyspnea with wheezing, prolonged expiration and difficulty lying down during the attack. It consists of two disease conditions in the perception of traditional Chinese medicine, i.e. sounding asthma and soundless asthma. The former is marked by asthmatic breathing with wheezing sound in the throat, and the latter by hasty shallow breathing or even with opening mouth and raising shoulders in the severe cases. Since both may appear at the same time and be actually inseparable, the two are normally called asthma. Their etiology and treatment principle are more or less the same.

Asthma may oocur in any of the four seasons, especially in cold seasons because of the inclement changes of the weather. It includes bronchial asthma and asthmatic bronchitis in modern medicine.

Cause and Mechanism

Numerous factors may result in asthma, but it is mainly ascribed to either exogenous or endogenous pathogenic factors. Exogenous pathogenic wind—cold invading the lung causes the poor function of the lung in dispersing *Qi*. Improper diet may cause dysfunction of the spleen in transforming and transporting, leading to subsequent accumulation of dampness which further produces phlegm. Prolonged accumulation of dampness may turn into heat. Internal retention of phlegm—heat can cause obstruction of *Qi* passage. Asthma can also be caused by impairment of the lung *Qi* due to prolonged illness and protracted cough. Internal damage of kidney essence and deficiency of kidney *Qi* due to over strain or sexual indulgence may result in the failure of kidney to receive *Qi*, which also leads to the asthmatic attacks.

Differentiation

1. Asthma during Attacks

(1) Dormant Cold in the Lung

The chief manifestations include difficult respiration, cough with shortness of breath and wheezing sound in the throat, dilute sputum of white colour, cold limbs without sweating, greyish facial complexion, white or white greasy tongue coating, and super ficial tense or superficial slippery pulse. This type of asthma may also be accompanied by headache and general pain.

(2) Phlegm—heat Retention in the Lung

The chief manifestations include shallow breathing in hast with high breathing sound, fever, flushed face, thick yellow sputum that is difficult to be expectorated, stuffy sensation in the chest and epigastric region, thirst with desire for cold drinking, straw urination, constipation, yellow greasy tongue coating, and rapid slippery pulse.

2. Asthma in the Remission Stage

(1) *Qi* Deficiency of the Spleen and Lung

The chief manifestations include reluctant speech, shortness of breath, cough in low sound, sweating by exertion, pallor complexion, poor appetite, swelling of the face and limbs, pale tongue with white coating, and soft weak pulse.

(2) Deficiency of the Spleen and Kidney

The chief manifestations include cough and shortness of breath aggravated by exertion that is gestured by opening mouth and raising shoulders, lassitude, weakness and soreness of the lumbar region and knees, vertigo with tinnitus, night sweating, nocturnal emission, cold limbs, darkened complexion, pale tongue and deep thready pulse.

Treatment

1. Asthma in Attack

(1) Dormant Cold in the Lung

Principle: Dispel pathogenic cold from the lung, eliminate phlegm and relieve asthma by puncturing points mainly from The Lung Channel of Hand—*Taiyin* and The Bladder Channel of Foot—*Taiyang*.

Prescription: Lieque (LU 7)   Feishu (BL13)

Fengmen (BL12)   Renying (ST 9)

Dingchuan (EX−B1)

Explanation: Lieque (LU 7), the *Luo*−connecting point of the lung channel, has the function to disperse the lung *Qi* and relieve superficial cold from the body surface. Feishu (BL13) and Fengmen (BL12), points of the urinary bladder channel anatomically located adjacent to the lung, have the effect of clearing the lung and eliminating pathogenic cold. Renying (ST 9), point of the stomach channel beside the Adam's apple, is used in combination with Dingchuan (EX−B1), meaning asthma−relief, to eliminate phlegm and stop asthma.

Method: Use filiform needles with reducing method or even method and retain the needles for 15−20 minutes, manipulating them two to three times. Feishu (BL13) and Fengmen (BL12) are more often applied with moxibustion for 10−15 minutes. These two points may also be applied with both acupuncture and moxibustion, or with cupping after needling.

(2) Phlegm−heat Retention in the Lung

Prinicple: Disperse the heat from the lung, eliminate phlegm and promote the circulation of *Qi* by needling points mainly from The Lung channel of Hand−*Taiyin* and The Large Intestine Channel of Hand−*Yangming*.

Prescription: Chize(LU 5)   Kongzui(LU 6)

Dazhui(DU14)   Fenglong(ST40)

Danzhong(RN17)   Hegu(LI 4)

Explanation: Chize (LU 5), the *He*−sea point of the lung channel, also the water point of the channel, is used in combination with Kongzui (LU 6), the *Xi*−cleft point of the lung channel, to promote the dispersing function of the lung and to dispel the pathogenic heat. Fenglong (ST40), the *Luo*–connecting point of the stomach channel, is combined with Danzhong (RN17), the Influential Point of *Qi,* to eliminate phlegm and promote the circulation of *Qi.* The joint use of the above points have the function of clearing up pathogenic heat, promoting the dispersing function of the lung, eliminating phlegm and stopping asthma.

Point Modification: Add Feishu (BL13) and Zhongfu (LU 1) for severe asthma.

Method: Apply filiform needles with reducing method and retain the needles for 15–20 minutes, manipulating them two to three times.

2. Asthma in the Remission Stage

(1) *Qi* Deficiency of the Spleen and Lung

Principle: Strengthen the spleen *Qi* in order to replenish the lung by puncturing points mainly from The Spleen Channel of Foot–*Taiyin* and The Stomach Channel of Foot–*Yangming,* plus some Back–points.

Prescription:　Taiyuan(LU 9)　Feishu(BL13)
　　　　　　　　Zusanli(ST36)　Taibai(SP 3)
　　　　　　　　Gaohuangshu(BL43)

Explanation: Taiyuan (LU 9), the *Yuan*–source as well as the earth point of the lung channel, is combined with Feishu (BL13) to replenish the *Qi* of the lung. Zusanli (ST36) is the earth point of the stomach channel and Taibai (SP 3), the *Yuan*–source point of the spleen channel. In the light of the five element theory, the lung pertains to metal and the spleen and stomach pertain to earth. Earth can promote metal, meaning that the mother promotes the son. Therefore, points from both the spleen and stomach channels are used to reinforce the mother in order to promote the son, the lung on the basis of the prinicple that tonify the mother in case of deficiency. Gaohuangshu (BL43) is effective in the treatment of deficient type of cough and asthma. The joint use of the above points may achieve the effect of strengthening the anti–pathogenic Qi by reinforcing the middle–*Jiao*, resolving phlegm and relieving the asthma.

Method: Use filiform needles with reinforcing method and retain the needles for 20–30 minutes, manipulating them two to three times. Moxibustion is also applicable to Feishu (BL13) and Gaohuangshu (BL43) for 10–15 minutes.

(2) Deficiency of the Lung and Kidney

Principle: Tonify the Qi of the lung and kidney and stop asthma by needling points mainly from the Kidney Channel of Foot–*Shaoyin* and The *Ren* Channel.

Prescription: Taixi(KI 3) Shenshu(BL23) Feishu(BL13)
　　　　　　 Danzhong(RN17) Guanyuan(RN 4)

Explanation: Taixi (KI 3), the *Yuan*–source point of the kidney channel in combination with Shenshu (BL23), is effective to invigorate the vital energy of the kidney. Danzhong (RN17), the Influential Point of the Qi, is used together with Feishu (BL13) to reinforce Qi and stop asthma. Guanyuan (RN 4) may regulate the Qi passage of the *Sanjiao* and reinforce Qi of the general body. The joint use of the above five points can strengthen the function of kidney in receiving Qi, reinforce Qi and stop asthma.

Point Modification: Add Neiguan (PC 6) for palpitation and asthma due to deficiency of heart Qi in order to strengthen the heart and stop asthma.

Method: Apply filiform needles with reinforcing method and

retain the needles for 20—30 minutes. Moxibustion is applicable to shenmen (BL23), Feishu (BL13) and Guanyuan(RN 4) for 10 —15 minutes.

Alternative Treatment

1. Auricular Acupuncture

Prescription: Asthma—relief   Adrenal gland   Lung Trachea
        subcortex   Sympathetic   Ear—shenmen   End—
        ocrine

Method: Apply filiform needles at three to four points each time with strong stimulation and retain the needles for 10—15 minutes. Besides, embedding of ear seeds of sub—cutaneous needles is applicable.

2. Mid—summer Moxibustion Therapy

Prescription: Feishu(BL13)   Gaohuangshu(BL43)
        Pishu(BL20)   Shenshu(BL23)

Method: Apply ignited moxa cones similar to the size of date nuts on slices of ginger at points proposed. Each point is heated with three to five moxa cones to make the local skin turn red without causing any blisters. The treatment is given once daily commencing from the mid—summer dog—days to the arrival of autumn season.

1.4   Hemoptysis

Hemoptysis, a condition with bleeding originated from the lung caused by impairment of the pulmonary collaterals, is manifested by cough with blood—strained sputum, bloody sputum or cough with fresh blood involving occasional foams. It is commonly seen in the diseases as bronchiectasis, pulmonary abscess, pulmonary tuberculosis, pulmonary cancer in modern medicine.

Cause and Mechanism

Hemoptysis is often caused by constitutional *Yin* deficiency of the lung with repeated invasions of exogenous pathogenic wind—heat affecting the lung portion. Such invasions usually lead to the poor function of the lung in descending and dispersing as well as the subsequent impairment of the lung collaterals. Excessive emotional disturbance with flaring—up of liver fire may cause the fire to burn the pulmonary collaterals, resulting in hemoptysis. *Yin* defieiency of both the lung and kidney with hyperactive deficient fire in prolonged illness can also give rise to the consequence of hemoptysis because of the upward ascending of deficient fire affecting the pulmonary collaterals.

Differentiation

1. Wind—heat Affecting the Lung

The chief manifestations include cough with itching sensation in the throat, fresh bloody sputum, thirst and sore throat which may be accompanied by fever with aversion to cold, headache, thin yellowish tongue coating and rapid superficial pulse.

2. Liver Fire Attacking the Lung

The chief manifestations include cough, bloody sputum or expectoration of pure fresh blood, restlessness, irritability, pain in the chest and hypochondriac region, dry mouth, bitter taste in the mouth, constipation, scanty urine, red tongue proper with thin yellow coating, and thready rapid pulse.

3. Flaring Fire due to *Yin* Deficiency

The chief manifestations include dry cough with little sputum, bloody sputum, or constant cough with fresh blood, tidal fever, night sweating, dry mouth and throat, emaciation, dizziness, tinnitus, red tongue proper with less coating, and rapid thready pulse.

Treatment

1. Wind—heat Affecting the Lung

Principle: Clear up the exogenous pathogenic heat, moisten the lung, ease the collaterals and arrest bleeding by needling points mainly from The Lung Channel of Hand—*Taiyin* and The Large Intestine Channel of Hand—*Yangming*.

Prescription: Lieque(LU 7) Yuji(LU 10)
            Kongzui(LU 6) Hegu(LI 4)

Explanation: Lieque(LU 7), the *Luo*—connecting point of the lung channel, is used in combination with Yuji (LU10), the *Ying*—spring point of the same channel, and Hegu(LI 4), the *Yuan*—source point of the large intestine channel, to dispel the wind—heat, moisten the lung and cool the blood. Kongzui (LU 6), the *Xi*—cleft point of the lung channel, serves as the principal point in the treatment of hemoptysis because of its effect in eliminating pulmonary heat and stopping bleeding. The joint use of these four points ease the lung collaterals and stop bleeding.

Point Modification: Add Dazhui (DU14) and Quchi (LI11) for fever with aversion to cold.

Method: Use filiform needles with reducing method and retain the needles for 15—20 minutes, manipulating them two to three times.

2. Liver Fire Attacking the Lung

Principle: Eliminate fire from the liver and lung, pacify the pulmonary collaterals and stop bleeding by puncturing points mainly from The Lung Channel of Hand—*Taiyin* and The liver Channel of Foot—*Jueyin*.

Prescription: Feishu(BL13)   Yuji(LU10)
              Kongzui(LU 6)   Xingjian(LR 2)
              Laogong(PC 8)

Explanation: Feishu (BL 13) in combination with Yuji (LU 10) and Kongzui (LU 6) may eliminate heat from the lung, pacify the collaterals and stop bleeding. Xingjian (LR 2) reduces the liver fire and descends the adverse rise of *Qi* so that the liver regains its function in storing blood. Laogong (PC 8) clears up blood heat, and restricts the abnormal blood circulation. These five points used together can soothe the liver, eliminate heat, pacify the collaterals and stop bleeding.

Point Modification: Add Shenmen(HT 7) and Taichong (LR 3) for restlessness and irritability; and Zhigou(SJ 6) for constipation.

Method: Apply filiform needles with reducing method and retain the needles for 15—20 minutes, manipulating them two to three times.

3. Flaring Fire due to *Yin* Deficiency

Principle: Nourish pulmonary *Yin,* eliminate heat and stop bleeding by needling points mainly from The Lung Channel of Hand—*Taiyin* and The Kidney Channel of Foot—*Shaoyin.*

Prescription: Chize(LU 5)   Yuji(LU10)
              Kongzui(LU 6)   Taixi(KI 3)   Rangu(KI 2)

Explanation: Chize(LU 5) is the *He*—sea point of the lung channel, pertaining to water according to the five elements theory, while Yuji(LU10), the *Ying*—spring point from the same channel pertaining to fire. Applying reinforcing method to Chize(LU 5) and reducing method to Yuji(LU10), may therefore moisten the *Yin* of the lung, eliminate heat from the lung and stop bleeding. Kongzui(LU 6), the *Xi*—cleft point of the lung channel, is used to stop bleeding. Taixi(KI 3) and Rangu(KI 2), respectively the *Yuan*-source and *Ying*-spring points of the kidney channel, are used to nourish *Yin* and clear up heat. The joint use of the above points have the function of nourishing *Yin*, quenching fire, eliminating heat and arresting bleeding.

Point Modification: Add Yinxi (HT 6) and Dazhui (DU14) for tidal fever and night sweating.

Method: Use filiform needles with both reinforcing and reducing methods in the same treatment, i. e. reinforcment for Chize (LU 5), Taixi (KI 3) and Rangu (KI 2), and reduction for Yuji (LU10) and Kongzui (LU 6). Retain the needles for 15—20 minutes, manipulating them two to three times.

Alternative Treatment: Auricular Acupuncture

Prescription: Lung Trachea Heart Kidney Endocrine
                          Subcortex Ear—Shenmen Adrenal gland

Method: Select three to four points each time for treatment with the use of filiform needles. Apply moderate stimulation and retain the needles for 10—15 minutes. Embedding of ear seeds is also applicable.

1.5 Aphonia

Aphonia is characterized by an abrupt or slow onset of husky voice or even loss of voice. Since such a condition often results from laryngeal or glottal diseases, it should be distinguished from loss of voice with stiff tongue and dysphasia due to apoplepxy and gestational aphonia. The TCM concept of aphonia broadly includes laryngeal tuberculosis, laryngitis, vocal cord injury, vocal nodules and hysteric aphonia in modern medicine. For their treatment, the differentiation and treatment in this section can be referred to.

Cause and Mechanism

There are numerous factors that can cause aphonia although these factors are generally divided into the external and internal types. Invasion of exogenous pathogenic wind—cold into the lung with subsequent poor dispersing and descending of lung Qi and impaired Qi mechanism, or invasion of exogenous pathogenic wind—heat into the lung causing phlegm retention in the lung due to heat steaming the fluid, can both lead to a sudden onset of aphonia, known as the excess type of aphonia resulted from exogenous pathogenic invasion. However, abrupt aphonia due to Qi stagnation turning into fire accounts for another excess type of aphonia. A gradual hoarseness of voice with over consumption of vital energy and poor moistening of the throat due to the lack of lung fluid or $Yang$ deficiency of both lung and kidney in patients with prolonged illness or poor constitution is known as the endogenous deficient type of aphonia.

Differentiation

1. Excess Type

(1) Wind—cold Type: The sudden hoarseness of voice is accompanied by difficult cough, fullness in the chest, stuffy nose, headache, chills, fever, thin white tongue coating and superficial pulse.

(2) Phlegm—heat Type: The sudden low voice or husky voice is accompanied by cough, yellow sputum, sore—throat, dry nose, fever, thirst, thin yellow tongue coating and rapid superficial pulse.

(3) Qi Stagnation Type: The sudden aphonia that is often induced by emotional upset such as sorrow, grief, depression or an-

ger appears paroxysmal. It is accompanied by restlessness, irritability, suffocating sensation in the chest, or a foreign body sensation in the throat, thin yellow tongue coating and thready pulse.

2. Deficient Type: The progressive aphonia is accompanied by dry throat, thirst, tidal fever, night sweating, dry cough, palpitation, dizziness, tinnitus, red tongue with less coating, and thin rapid pulse.

Treatment

1. Excess Type

(1) Wind–cold type

Principle: Expel pathogenic wind–cold and promote lung Qi circulation by needling points mainly from The Lung Channel of Hand–*Taiyin* and The Large Intestine Channel of Hand–*Yangming*.

Prescription: Lieque(LU 7)   Hegu(LI 4)

Renying(ST 9)   Tianding(LI17)

Explanation: Lieque (LU 7), the *Luo*–connecting point of the lung channel, also one of the Eight Confluent Points communicating with The *Ren* Channel, is combined with Hegu (LI 4), the *Yuan*–source point of the large intestine channel, to eliminate wind–heat, promote lung Qi circulation and ease sore–throat. Renying (ST 9) and Tianding (LI17), the points of the *Yangming* channels of hand and foot, are used to directly promote the circulation of Qi and blood in the affected area and reinforce the functional activities of Qi. The joint use of the above points can relieve aphonia by expelling wind–cold, promoting the lung Qi and restoring the normal Qi mechanism.

Method: Apply filiform needles with reducing method and

retain the needles for 15—20 minutes, manipulating them two to three times. In order to avoid injurying the arteries, no strong lifting or thrusting of the needles is performed when puncturing Renying (ST 9) or Tianding (LI17).

(2) Phlegm—heat Type

Principle: Eliminate the pathogenic phlegm—heat and clear up the lung by puncturing points mainly from The Lung Channel of Hand—*Taiyin* and The Stomach Channel of Foot—*Yangming*.

Prescription: Yuji(LU10)   Fenglong(ST 40)

Renying(ST 9)   Tianding(LI 17)

Tiantu(RN 22)

Explanation: Yuji (LU10), the *Xing*—spring point of the lung channel, has the effect of clearing up heat, moistening the lung and relieving sore—throat. Fenglong (ST40), the *Luo*—connecting point of the stomach channel, may eliminate heat and resolve sputum. Renying (ST 9), Tianding (LI 17) and Tiantu (RN 22) many promote the circulation of *Qi* in the affected area and clear sore—throat. The combineduse of the above points can restore normal voice by eliminating phlegm—heat from the lung and clear the throat.

Point Modifications: Add Hegu (LI 4) for fever; and Erjian (ST 2) and Shaoshang (LU 11) for sore—throat.

Method: Apply filiform needles with reducing method and retain the needles for 15—20 minutes manipulating them two to three times.

(3) *Qi* Stagnation Type

Principle: Soothe the depressed liver *Qi* and clear the throat by needling points mainly from The Liver Channel of Foot—*Jueyin,* The *Sanjiao* Channel of Hand—*Shaoyang* and The

Stomach Channel of Foot—*Yangming*.

Prescription: Taichong(LR 3)   Zhigou(SJ 6)
　　　　　　Guanchong(SJ 1)   Hegu(LI 4)
　　　　　　Renying(ST 9)

Explanation: Taichong (LR 3), the *Yuan*—source point of the liver channel, may relieve the depression of the liver *Qi*. Zhigou (SJ 6), a point of the *Sanjiao* channel, that has the effect of regulating *Qi* and helping to relieve depression, is combined with Guanchong (SJ 1) to eliminate pathogenic heat from the *Sanjiao* channel for the purpose of regaining voice. Hegu (LI 4) and Renying (ST 9) are chosen to clear up the throat. The joint use of the above points have the function of soothing the depressed liver *Qi* and restoring normal voice.

Method: Apply filiform needles with reinforcing method and retain the needles for 15—20 minutes, manipulating them two to three times.

2. Deficiency Type

Principle: Nourish *Yin,* quench fire, moisten dryness and clear up the lung by needling points mainly from The Lung Channel of Hand—*Taiyin* and The Kidney Channel of Foot—*Shaoyin*.

Prescription: Yuji (LU10)   Lieque (LU 7)   Zhaohai (KI 6)
　　　　　　Taixi (KI 3)   Renying (ST 9)

Explanation: Yuji (LU10), the *Xing*—spring point of the lung channel, in combination with Lieque (LU 7), the *Luo*—connecting point of the same channel, may clear up the lung and reduce fire. Taixi (KI 3), the *Yuan*—source point of the kidney channel, and Zhaohai (KI 6), one of the Eight Confluent Points, can nourish the kidney *Yin*. Renying (ST 9) can promote the circulation of *Qi* in the affected channels. The above points in combination have the function to nourish *Yin,* sedate fire, clear up heat and dryness from the lung, benefit the throat and restore the voice.

Method: Apply filiform needles with reinforcing method and retain the needles for 15—20 minutes, manipulating them two to three times.

Alternative Treatment: Auricular Acupuncture

Prescription: Large Intestine Lung Kidney Throat Trochea

Method: Use filiform needles at three to four points with mild stimulation and retain the needles for 10—15 minutes. Embedding of subcutaneous needles is also applicable.

1.6 Hiccup

Hiccup is a clinical symptom referring to the adverse rise of stomach *Qi* manifested by an involuntary short, quick sound in the throat. It may occur alone on rare occasions or accompany other body conditions in continuous or paroxysmal attacks.

Hiccup is regarded as spasm of the diaphragm in modern medicine. The differentiation and treatment in this section can be referred to for hiccups related to the course of other acute or chronic diseases or that after abdominal operation.

Cause and Mechanism

Hiccup is mostly the result of adverse rise of stomach *Qi* caused by either the injury or blockage of the stomach *Yang* due to constitutional deficiency or overeating of raw and cold food. Sudden excessive eating of greasy or spicy food may also cause impairment of *Qi* mechanism affecting the diaphragm because such a diet makes *Qi* obstruction and retention of dryness and heat in the middle *Jiao*. Emotional disturbance with liver *Qi* stagnation can cause an impaired qi mechanism because the stagnant liver *Qi* attacks the stomach and causes the derangement of stomach *Qi*. The *Yang* deficiency of the spleen and kidney with a decline of stomach accounts for another factor of hiccup because in such a case the clear *Qi* can not be normally ascended while the turbid *Qi* is not descended.

Differentiation

1. Retention of Cold in the Stomach

The hiccup is slow, deep—sounding, forceful, but alleviated by warmth and aggravated by cold. It is accompanied by a discomfort in the chest and epigastric region, poor appetite, profuse clear urine, loose stool, white moist tongue coating, and slow pulse.

2. Ascending of Stomach Fire

The hiccup is loud and forceful in a hasty manner. It is accompanied by a foul and sour smell, fullness sensation in the epigastric region, poor appetite, straw urine, constipation, yellow tongue coating, and rapid slippery pulse.

3. Perversing of Liver *Qi* to the Stomach

The continual hiccups are accompanied by epigastric and hypochondriac distension, restlessness, belching, fullness in the chest, thin white tongue coating, and thready pulse.

4. *Yang* Deficiency of the Spleen and Kidney

The low and long hiccup is released with shortness of breath, and accompanied by pale complexion, poor appetite, lassitude, sourness and weakness in the lumbar region and knee joints, cold limbs, pale tongue proper with thin white coating, and thin weak pulse.

Treatment

Principle: Pacify the stomach, ease the adverse rise of stomach Qi and relieve the hiccup by needling points mainly from The Stomach Channel of Foot−*Yangming* and The Pericardium Channel of Hand−*Jueyin*.

Prescription: Geshu (BL17)   Danzhong (RN17)
                    Neiguan(PC 6)   Zusanli(ST36)
                    Zhongwan(RN12)

Geshu (BL17) and Danzhong (RN17), respectively the Influential Points of blood and $Qi,$ two of the Eight Influential Points, are used to regulate the flow of Qi in the chest area, relieve diaphragm spasm, and check the hiccup. Neiguan (PC 6), the *Luo*−connecting point of the percardium channel and the confluent point communicating with The *Yinwei* Channel, may pacify the middle−*Jiao* and ease hiccup. Zusanli (ST36), the *He*−sea point of the stomach channel, is combined with Zhongwan (RN12), the Front−*Mu* point of the stomach, to regulate the stomach Qi and ease the abnormal ascending of gastric Qi. The above points in combination can promote the Qi mechanism, pacify the stomach and stop hiccup.

Point Modifications: Apply moxibustion to Liangmen (ST 21) for retention of cold in the stomach; add Xiangu (ST43) for heat in the stomach; Taichong (LR 3) and Qimen (LR14) for liver Qi transversely attacking the stomach; and Pishu (BL20), Shenshu (BL23) and Qihai (RN 6) for *Yang* deficiency of spleen and kidney.

Method: Use filiform needles with reducing method, but reinforcing for *Yang* deficiency of spleen and kidney. Retain the needles for 15−30 minutes, manipulating them two to three times.

Alternative Treatment: Auricular Acupuncture

Prescription: Diaphragm Sympathetic Stomach Liver Spleen
Ear—Shenmen

Method: Apply filiform needles with strong stimulation and retain the needles for 30 minutes.

1.7 Retroaction of Stomach Qi

Retroaction of stomach Qi, also known as gastric Qi reversing, is characterized by epigastric distention with undigested food and fullness in the abdomen hours after food intake. The patient may vomit in the afternoon the food that he took in the morning, or the next morning the food that he took in the previous evening. This condition, though may be complained by patients regardless of age and sex, is more suffered by the aged.

Retroaction of stomach is seen in patients with pytorospasm, prolorochesis and gastroneurosis in terms of modern medicine.

Cause and Mechanism

Retroaction of stomach Qi is mostly caused by insufficiency of spleen $Yang$ with deficient cold in the spleen and stomach due to improper diet, overeating of cold food and emotional disturbance, leading to failure of the spleen and stomach to perform normal digestive functions and consequent vomiting. Alcoholic indulgence or impairment of the spleen due to over exertion can cause poor function of the spleen in transforming and transporting and retention of dampness to form turbid phlegm obstructing the stomach. The phlegm obstruction impairs the normal descending of gastric Qi, resulting in the retroactive stomach Qi.

Differentiation

1. Deficient Cold in the Spleen and Stomach

The retroactive stomach *Qi* is characterized by distention and fullness sensation in the epigastrium and abdomen after meals, vomiting of undigested food and gastric fluid hours after the food intake. Relief is attained with the thorough vomiting. It is accompanied by lassitude, weakness, pallor complexion, loose stools, pale tongue proper with white coating, and thin weak pulse.

2. Turbid Phlegm Obstructing the Stomach

The retroactive stomach *Qi* is characterized by epigastric and abdominal distention worse after meal, possible mass in the upper abdomen, vomiting of food retained in the stomach hours after the food intake. The vomiting may involve some watery discharge and foams. It is accompanied by dizziness, palpitation, white slippery tongue coating, and thready slippery pulse.

Treatment

1. Deficient Cold in the Spleen and Stomach

Principle: Warm up the middle *Jiao*, eliminate cold, pacify the stomach and ease the retroactive stomach *Qi* by using points mainly from The *Ren* Channel, and The Stomach Channel of Foot—*Yangming*, plus some Back—*Shu* points.

Prescription: Pishu(BL20)   Weishu(BL21)

Zhangmen(LR13)   Zhongwan(RN12)

Zusanli(ST36)   Neiguan(PC 6)

Explanation: Pishu (BL20) and Weishu (BL21) are combined with Zhangmen (LR13) and Zhongwan (RN12), respectively the Front—*Mu* points of the spleen and stomach, to strengthen the spleen, pacify the stomach, ascend the spleen *Qi* and sedate the turbid gastric *Qi*. Zusanli (ST36) and Neiguan (PC 6) regulate the

Qi of the middle—*Jiao* ease the abnormal ascending of Qi and ease nausea. The joint use of the above points may reinforce the spleen and stomach, eliminate cold in the middle—*Jiao* pacify the stomach and stop nausea.

Method: Apply filiform needles with reinforcing method and retain the needles for 20—30 minutes, manipulating them two to three times. Moxibustion is applicable to Pishu (BL20) and Weishu (BL21) for 10—15 minutes. Warming needle is also applicable.

2. Turbid Phlegm Obstructing the Stomach

Principle: Resolve the turbid phlegm, pacify the stomach and send down the adverse flow of *Qi* by puncturing points mainly from The Stomach Channel of Foot—*Yangming* and The *Ren* Channel.

Prescription: Zhongwan (RN12)   Fenglong (ST40)

Jianli(RN11)   Zusanli(ST36)

Neiguan(PC 6)

Explanation: The Front—*Mu* point of the stomach Zhongwan (RN12) is combined with Fenglong (ST40)to regulate the function of the middle—*Jiao,* strengthen stomach and eliminate the turbid phlegm. Jianli(RN11) strengthens stomach and promotes digestion. Zusanli(ST36) and Neiguan(PC 6) regulate stomach *Qi.* The joint use of these points may eliminate the turbid phlegm, pacify the stomach and send down the adverse flow of *Qi.*

Method: Apply filiform needles with reducing or even method, and retain the needles for 20—30 minutes. Needles are manipulated two to three times during the treatment.

Alternative Treatment: Auricular Acupuncture

Prescription: Stomach　　Spleen　　Ear—Shenmen　　Occipital
　　　　　　　Subcortex

Method: Apply filiform needles to three to four points with mild stimulation and retain the needles for 20 minutes. Embedding of ear seeds or subcutaneous needles is also applicable.

1.8　Dysphagia Syndrome

Dysphagia syndrome refers to a condition characterized by a feeling of obstruction during swallowing and instant vomiting after food intake. The obstructive feeling for swallowing is called *Ye* while the difficulty in swallowing food and instant vomiting is called *Ge* in Chinese language. Since the former may not only appear alone in the clinic, but also become the pretophase of the latter, these two are collectively known as the dysphagia syndrome in TCM.

The syndrome may include such diseases as pylorochesis, esophageal diverticulum, esophageal neurosis, esophagitis, esophogeal carcinoma, gastric cancer, cardiac cancer and cardiospasm in modern medicine.

Cause and Mechanism

Dysphagia syndrome is mostly caused by stagnation of due to emotional dusturbance in which the retained fluid accumulates into phlegm. On the other hand, alcoholic indulgence or hot spicy diet may cause impairment of the body fluid by accumulation of heat, resulting in dryness in the esophogus and stagnation of phlegm retention together with stagnation of *Qi* and blood obstructing the esophogus. It may also result from insufficiency *Qi* and blood, over consumption of body fluid or primordial *Qi* due to progressive decrease of food intake, leading to severe exhaustion of energy.

Differentiation

1. Stagnation of Phlegmatic *Qi*

The chief manifestations include a feeling of obstruction during swallowing, fullness in the chest and epigastrium, dull pain, belching, hiccup together with vomiting of thin mucousy sputum and food substance, severe constipation, dry mouth, progressive loss of weight, red tongue proper, and thready slippery pulse.

2. Retention of Phlegm in the Interior

The chief manifestations include dysphagia with pain in the chest and epigastrium, difficulty in swallowing food or even water, instant vomiting, vomiting of mucous sputum, and dry stools. It may also be accompanied by vomiting of reddish fluid, bloody stools, emaciation, rough dry skin and dry red tongue proper.

3. Exhaustion of *Yang Qi*

The chief manifestations include difficulty in swallowing food, pale complexion, cold limbs, shortness of breath, vomiting of frothy sputum, edema in the face and feet, abdominal distention, flabby tongue, and weak thready pulse.

Treatment

1. Stagnation of Phlegmatic *Qi*

Principle: Relieve fullness in the chest, regulate the stomach *Qi* and lower the turbid phlegm by needling points mainly from The *Ren* Channel and The Stomach Channel of Foot—*Yangming*.

Prescription: Tiantu (RN22)　Danzhong (RN17)
　　　　　　　Juque (RN14)　Neiguan (PC 6)
　　　　　　　Shangwan (RN13)　Fenglong (ST40)

Explanation: Danzhong (RN17), the Influential Point of *Qi*, is combined with Tiantu (RN22) to regulate *Qi,* relieve chest fullness, disperse accumulation of phlegm and ease sore throat. Juque (RN14), the Front—*Mu* point of the heart channel, and Neiguan (PC 6), the *Luo*—connecting point of the percardium channel, are selected to promote the *Qi* mechanism of the *Sanjiao* by adjusting *Qi* and relieving fullness sensation in the chest and diaphragm. Shangwan (RN13) and Fenglong (ST40) are used to eliminate the phlegm—damp and lower the turbid phlegm. Therefore, all these points used in combination may relieve fullness in the chest and diaphragm, lower the turbid phlegm, regulate the circulation of *Qi* and check the pain.

Point Modification: Add Geguan (BL46) for fullness in the chest and epigastrium; and Tianshu (ST25) for constipation.

Method: Apply filiform needles with reducing method and retain the needles for 20—30 minutes, maripulating them two to three times.

2. Retention of Stagnant Phlegm in the Interior

Principle: Nourish *Yin,* resolve stasis of blood and phlegm, halt reverse flow of *Qi* and ease the diaphragm by needling points mainly from The Bladder Channel of Foot—*Taiyang* and The *Ren* Channel.

Prescription: Geshu (BL17)   Geguan (BL46)

Danzhong (RN17)   Zhongwan (RN12)

Zhaohai (KI 6)   Guanchong (SJ 1)

Explanation: Since Geshu (BL17), the Back—*Shu* point of the diaphragm, and Geguan (BL46) are located near the diaphragm, they are selected to regulate *Qi* flow and promote the curculation of blood, remove blood stasis and ease the diaphragm. Danzhong (RN17), the Influential Point of *Qi,* in combination with Zhongwan (RN12) may eliminate phlegm, relieve chest fullness and lower the adverse flow of *Qi*. Guanchong (SJ 1) may clear up the asthenic—fire and benefit the body fluid. Zhaohai (KI 6) may tonify *Yin* and moisten the dryness. The combined use of these points may help nourish *Yin*, remove phlegm and blood stasis, lower the adverse flow of *Qi* and relieve diaphragm fullness.

Method: Use filiform needles with reducing method except Zhaohai (KI 6) which is needled with reinforcing one. Retain the needles for 15—20 minutes, manipulating them two to three times.

3. Exhaustion of *Yang Qi*

Principle: Warm up and tonify spleen and kidney, strengthen *Qi* and rescue patient from collapse of *Yang Qi* by needling points mainly fromThe Bladder Channel of Foot—*Taiyang* and The *Ren* Channel.

Prescription: Pishu (BL20)   Shenshu (BL23)
Weishu (BL21)   Qihai (RN 6)
Geshu (BL17)   Zusanli (ST36)

Explanation: The joint use of Pishu (BL20), Weishu (BL21) and Shenshu (BL23) is to strengthen the spleen and stomach and reinforce kidney *Yang*. Geshu (BL17) has the effect of relieving fullness in the chest and diaphragm. Qihai (RN 6) and Zusanli (ST36) can replenish *Qi* in the middle—*Jiao* and help send up the lucid *Yang*. The joint use of the above points has the function of invigorating the spleen and stomach, warming up kidney *Yang*, supplementing *Qi* and relieving fullness in the chest and diaphragm.

Method: Apply filiform needles with reinforcing method and retain the needles for 15—20 minutes, manipulating them one to two times.

Moxibustion is also applicable to the Back–*Shu* points during or after needling.

Alternative Treatment: Auricular Acupuncture

Prescription: Ear–shenmen   Stomach Esophagus Diaphragm

Method: Use filiform needles with moderate stimulation and retain the needles for 30 minutes. Implanting of ear seeds or embedding of subcutaneous needles is also applicable.

Comment: Acupuncture treatment is effective for esophagus functional diseases such as esophagitis cardiospasm, etc. It may also be applied to alleviate the symptoms appearing in esophageal carcinoma and cardiac caner such as fullness and pain in the chest, and dysphagia.

Clinically, special caution is given so as to exclude the possibility of cancer in patients with dysphagia syndrome.

1.9   Epigastric Pain

Epigastric pain, also known as gastric pain, refers to a syndrome manifested by frequent pain over the epigastric region. In the old times, this condition was mistakenly called cardiac pain because the painful area is close to the center of the chest. It may commonly be seen in acute and chronic gastritis, gastric or duodenal ulcer, gastroneurosis and gastric cancer in modern medicine.

Cause and Mechanism

Epigastric pain is mainly caused by the following factors. Melancholy or emotional disturbance may cause the stagnation of liver *Qi* and dysfunction of the liver to maintain the free flow of *Qi,* leading to the liver *Qi* attacking the stomach which results in poor descending of stomach *Qi.* Improper intake of cold or raw food or intake of unclean food may impair the spleen and stomach, resulting in poor transportation and transformation by the spleen and food retention in the middle–*Jiao.* Constitutional deficiency of the spleen and stomach plus cold invasion may give rise to accumulation of cold in the stomach and failure of the stomach *Qi* to descend, thus causing pain in the epigastrium.

Differentiation

1. Liver *Qi* Attacking the Stomach

According to the different symptoms and signs, epigastric pain caused by liver *Qi* attacking the stomach can further be divided into epigastric pain respectively due to stagnation of *Qi,* stasis of blood and heat retention.

(1) *Qi* Stagnation: Epigastric fullness, distention and wandering pain which radiates to the hypochondriac region, frequent belching, acid regurgitation, vomiting, bitter taste in the mouth, thin white tongue coating, and thready pulse.

(2) Stagnant Heat: Sudden onset of epigastric pain, restlessness, irritability, acid regurgitation, discomfort sensation in the stomach, dry mouth, bitter taste in the mouth, red tongue proper with yellow coating, and rapid thready pulse.

(3) Blood Stasis: Fixed pain aggravated by pressing or food intake, bloody vomiting, melena, dark purplish tongue proper, and uneven pulse.

2. Food Retention

The main manifestations include epigastric pain with fullness and distention, belching, acid regurgitation, poor appetite, vomiting of undigested food, pain aggravated after food intake but relieved upon vomiting, thick greasy tongue coating, and deep strong or slippery pulse.

3. Asthenic Cold in the Spleen and Stomach

The chief manifestations include dull pain in the epigastrium that is relieved by warmth and pressing, watery regurgitation, listlessness and weakness, cold limbs, loss of appetite, loose stools, pale tongue proper, and weak pulse.

Treatment

1. Liver *Qi* Attacking the Stomach

(1) Stagnation of *Qi*

Principle: Soothe the liver *Qi*, pacify the stomach and stop pain by needling points mainly from The liver Channel of Foot—*Jueyin* and The Stomach Channel of Foot—*Yangming*.

Prescription: Zhongwan (RN12)   Neiguan (PC 6)

                 Qimen (LR14)   Zusanli (ST36)

                 Taichong (LR 3)

Explanation: Zhongwan (RN12), the Front—*Mu* point of the stomach, is used together with Zusanli (ST36), the *He*—sea point of the stomach channel, to pacify the stomach and stop pain. Neiguan (PC 6), the Confluent point communicating with The Yinwei Channel, has the effect of relieving fullness sensation in the chest and depression, and stop belching and vomiting. Qimen (LR14) and Taichong (LR 3), respectively the Front—*Mu* point of the liver and the *Yuan*—source point of the liver channel, may soothe the liver *Qi*, relieve distention and stop pain. The joint use of the above points may soothe the liver, pacify the stomach and stop pain.

Method: Apply filiform needles with reducing method and retain the needles for 15—20 minutes, manipulating them two to

three times.

(2) Stagnant Heat

Principle: Sedate heat from the liver, pacify the stomach and stop pain by needling points mainly from The Liver Channel of Foot−*Jueyin* and The Stomach Channel of Foot−*Yangming*.

Prescription: Xingjian (LR 2)   Zhongwan (RN12)

Neiguan (PC 6)   Zusanli (ST36)

Taixi (KI 3)

Explanation: Xingjian (LR 2), the *Ying*−spring point of the liver channel having the effect to eliminate heat, is used in combination with Taixi (KI 3), the *Yuan*−source point of the kidney channel, to moisten kidney water, tonify liver and eliminate heat. Zhongwan (RN12), Neiguan (PC 6) and Zusanli (ST36) regulate *Qi* circulation and stop pain. The above points used in combination may soothe the liver, sedate liver fire, regulate the circulation of *Qi,* pacify stomach and stop pain.

Method: Apply filiform needles with reducing method and retain the needles for 15−20 minutes, manipulating them two to three times.

(3) Stasis of Blood

Principle: Activate blood circulation in the channels and collaterals, pacify the stomach and stop pain by needling points mainly from The Stomach Channel of Foot−*Yangming*.

Prescription: Zhongwan (RN12)   Neiguan (PC 6)

Zusanli (ST36)   Gongsun (SP 4)

Xuehai (SP10)   Geshu (BL17)

Explanation: The spleen and stomach are internally−externally related. The *Luo*−connecting point of the spleen channel Gongsun(SP 4) is used in combination with Neiguan(PC 6),

Zhongwan(RN12) and Zusanli(ST36) to regulate the circulation of *Qi*, pacify the stomach and stop pain. Geshu (BL17), the Influential point of blood, and Xuehai (SP 10) from the spleen channel may activate blood circulation and remove blood stasis from the channels and collaterals. The use of the above points may jointly regulate the circulation of *Qi*, activate blood and remove obstruction from channels and collaterals, pacify the stomach and stop pain.

Method: Apply filiform needles with reducing method and retain the needles for 15−20 minutes, manipulating them two to three times.

2. Food Retention

Principle: Relieve food retention, pacify the stomach and stop pain by needling points mainly from The Stomach Channel of Foot−*Yangming*.

Prescription: Zhongwan (RN12)   Zusanli (ST36)
　　　　　　 Liangmen (ST21)　Tianshu (ST25)

Explanation: Zhongwan (RN12) and Zusanli (ST36) may promote the circulation of stomach *Qi*, pacify the stomach and stop pain. Liangmen (ST21) regulates the middle−*Jiao*, pacifies the stomach and relieves food retention. Tianshu(ST25), the Front−*Mu* point of the large intestine, may promote the *Qi* circulation in the large intestine in order to relieve food retention. The joint use of the above four points may achieve the effect of relieving food retention and stoping pain.

Method: Apply filiform needles with reducing method and retain the needles for 20−30 minutes, manipulating them two to three times.

3. Deficient Cold in the Spleen and Stomach

Principle: Warm up the middle—*Jiao*, strengthen the spleen, eliminate cold and stop pain by needling points mainly from The Urinary Bladder Channel of Foor—*Taiyang* and The *Ren* Channel.

Prescription: Pishu (BL20)   Weishú (BL21)

Zhangmen (LR13)   Zhongwan (RN12)

Zusanli (ST36)   Neiguan (PC 6)

Explanation: Weishu (BL21) paired with Zhongwan (RN12), and Pishu (BL20) paired with Zhangmen (LR13), known as the combination of Back—*Shu* points with the Front—*Mu* points, are used to strengthen the spleen and pacify the stomach. Zusanli (ST36) and Neiguan (PC 6) are used to regulate the circulation of gastric *Qi*. The joint use of the above points can warm up the middle—*Jiao*, eliminate cold, strengthen the spleen, pacify the stomach and stop pain.

Point Modification: Add moxibustion at Qihai (RN 6) for patient with prolonged history of illness.

Method: Apply filiform needles with reinforcing method and retain the needles for 20—30 minutes, manipulating them two to three times. The Back—*Shu* points and Zusanli (ST36) are mostly treated with both acupuncture and moxibustion. 15 to 20 minutes of moxibustion or warming needle is applied at these points.

Alternative Treatment: Auricular, Acupuncture

Prescription: Spleen Stomach Sympathetic Ear—Shenmen

Liver Duodenum Subcortex Endocrine

Method: Use filiform needles at three to four points with strong stimulation for sedating the severe pain, but with mild stimulation when the pain is lessened. Needles are retained for 15—30 minutes. Embedding of ear seeds is also applicable.

1.10   Loosened Stomach

Loosened stomach is a condition manifested by distention and fullness of the epigastrium and abdomen after meal, belching, borborygmus and pain with a sinking sensation in the epigastrium. It is also characteristic that such symptoms are alleviated or relieved when the patient rests in a supine position, but aggravated in a standing posture or in physical exertion. The condition described here is similar to gastroptosia in modern medicine.

Cause and Mechanism

Loosened stomach is mostly caused by improper diet, emotional disturbances affecting the interior of the body and overstrain or stress that lead to the deficiency of spleen and stomach and sinking of *Qi* in the middle—*Jiao* in which the spleen *Qi* fails to ascend while the stomach *Qi* fails to descend.

Differentiation

Loosened stomach is mainly characterized by fullness and distention of the epigastrium and abdomen after meal, belching, pain with sinking sensation in the epigastrium which may be alleviated by resting in a supine position. The accompanying symptoms and signs include emaciation, sallow complexion, listlessness, loss of appetite, nausea, vomiting, loose stools with occasional constipation, thin greasy tongue coating, and soft weak or deep thin pulse.

Treatment

Principle: Strengthen the spleen, pacify the stomach and lift the sunken *Qi* in the middle—*Jiao* by puncturing points mainly from The *Ren* Channel and The Stomach Channel of

Foot—*Yangming*.

　　Prescription: Zhongwan (RN12)　Weishang (Extra)
　　　　　　　　　Tiwei (Extra)　Qihai (RN　6)
　　　　　　　　　Zusanli (ST36)　Baihui (DU20)

　　Explanation: Zhongwan(RN12), the Front—*Mu* point of the stomach, is used in combination with Zusanli (ST36) to strengthen the spleen, pacify the stomach and reinforce *Yang Qi*. Baihui (DU20) and Qihai (RN 6) here assist the first two points in their effect to lift the sunken *Qi* of the middle—*Jiao* Weishang (Extra) and Tiwei (Extra), both extraordinary points, are empirical points in the treatment of loosened stomach. The joint use of the above points can help lift the sunken *Qi* of the middle—*Jiao,* strengthen the spleen and pacify the stomach.

　　Point Modification: Add Neiguan (PC 6) for nausea; Pishu (BL20) and Weishu (BL21) for emaciation and sallow complexion.

　　Method: Apply filiform needles with reinforcing method and retain the needles for 20—30 minutes, manipulating them two to three times. Electric stimulation with dense—sparse wave for thirty minutes is also applicable. Moxibustion can be used at Baihui (DU20) in addition to acupuncture. An oblique insertion at 45 degree angle is done at Zhongwan (RN12), Weishang (Extra) and Tiwei (Extra) 1.5—2 *Cun* deep. The paitent is expected to rest on the bed for 15 minutes after the withdrawing of the needle.

　　Alternative Treatment: Auricular Acupuncture

　　Prescription: Stomach　Sympathetic　Ear—shenmen Spleen
　　　　　　　　　Subcortex

　　Method: Apply filiform needles at three to four points each time with mild stimulation and retain the needles for 15—20 minutes.Embedding of ear seeds is also applicable.

Comment: (1) Patient is encouraged to do physical exercises during the treatment in order to strengthen abdominal muscles. (2) Nutrition advice as well as advice for avoiding overeating are given to patient in cooperation to the treatment. (3) The patient is expected to rest on bed after meal in order to help the recovery of the loosened stomach.

1.11 Vomiting

Vomiting is a condition referring to the casting up of food substance or gastric fluid from the stomach through the mouth. The concept of vomiting in traditional Chinese medicine has a much broader context. According to record in classics, the simple term of vomiting is further divided into noisy vomiting with food substance, non—sounding vomiting with food substance, noisy nausea without food substance or gastric fluid, and simple vomiting of gastric fluid. In general, the Chinese concept of vomiting does include both vomiting and nausea. Since both may often accompany one and the other, clinically, only the word vomiting is adopted.

Vomiting may be seen in both acute and chronic gastritis, pylorospasm, pylorchesis, nervous vomiting, cholecystitis and pancreatitis in modern medicine.

Cause and Mechanism

Vomiting can be caused by various factors. Invasion of exogenous pathogenic factors such as wind, cold, summer—heat and dampness into the stomach along the stomach channel leads to derangement of stomach Qi so that the food substance and gastric fluid are cast up together with the abnormal ascending of gastric *Qi*. Over intake of cold or raw food, or intake of sour food by mistake can cause food retention in the stomach and difficulty for the descending of stomach *Qi*. Emotional depression or sudden emotional upset can cause liver *Qi* to attack the stomach so that food substance reverses along with the abnormal ascending of gastric *Qi*. Constitutional deficiency of the spleen and stomach or impairment of the spleen and stomach after illness cause the inactive *Yang* of the middle—*Jiao* and poor transformation and transportation, in which there will be retention of food and gastric fluid and abnormal ascending of gastric *Qi*. And the *Yin* deficiency of the stomach may lead to the poor moistening and descending function of the stomach.

Differentiation

1. Exogenous Pathogenic Invasion Into the Stomach

This kind of vomiting is characterized by sudden casting up of food, discomfort in the chest, and accompanied by aversion to cold, fever, headache and general pain, white tongue coating and superficial pulse.

2. Food Retention in the Stomach

This kind of vomiting is characterized by casting up of sour fluid or food substance, epigastric distention and fullness, frequent belching, abdominal pain, lessened by vomiting, either dry or loose stools, greasy tongue coating, and slippery full pulse.

3. Liver *Qi* Attacking the Stomach

The vomiting is characterized by casting up of sour fluid or food substance, frequent belching, pain and distention in the hypochondriac region, suffocating sensation, thin greasy tongue coating and wiry pulse. It is often aggravated by emotional disturbances.

4. Deficiency of the Spleen and Stomach

The vomiting involves with pallor complexion, instant vomiting in repeated attacks, lassitude, weakness, poor appetite, loose stools, pale tongue proper, and weak soft pulse.

5. *Yin* Deficiency of the Stomach

The vomiting appears in repeated attacks. It is accompanied by dryness in the mouth and throat, anorexia despite hunger, red tongue proper, lacking fluid distribution, and rapid thready pulse.

Treatment

1. Exogenous Pathogenic Invasion into the Stomach

Principle: Relieve superficial symptoms and signs, regulate *Qi* of the middle—*Jiao* and stop vomiting by needling points mainly from The Stomach Channel of Foot—*Yangming* and The *Ren* Channel.

Prescription: Dazhui(DU14) Hegu(LI 4) Neiting(ST44)
Zhongwan(RN12) Neiguan(PC 6)

Explanation: Dazhui (DU14), the merging point of all *Yang* channels, is selected to promote *Yang Qi* and expel the pathogenic factors from the body surface. Hegu(LI 4) and Neiting(ST44) clear up the pathogenic heat from the *Yangming* channels. Zhongwan(RN12), the Front—*Mu* point of the stomach channel and also the Influential Point of the *Fu* organs, helps descend gastric *Qi,* pacify the stomach and stop vomiting. Neiguan (PC 6) relieves fullness in the chest, halts abnormal ascending of *Qi* and promotes *Qi* circulation. All the above points thus used in combination have the effect of eliminating exogenous pathogenic factors and normalizing the stomach *Qi* circulation. Once the stomach *Qi* circulation is in order, vomiting stops spontaneously.

Method: Use filiform needles with reducing method and retain the needles for 15—20 minutes, manipulating them three to four times.

2. Retention of Food in the Stomach

Principle: Activate *Qi* circulation, promote digestion and remove food retention by needling points mainly from The *Ren* Channel and The Stomach Channel of Foot—*Yangming*.

Prescription: Xiawan(RN10)　Xuanji(RN21)

Zusanli(ST36)　Neiguan(PC 6)　Fujie(SP14)

Explanation: Xiawan (RN10) and Xuanji (RN21) are used to activate *Qi* circulation and promote digestion to remove retained food form the stomach. Zusanli (ST36) and Neiguan (PC 6) pacify the stomach and check vomiting. Fujie (SP14) relieves distention in the epigastrium and abdomen. The joint use of these five points have the function of activating *Qi,* stopping vomiting and promoting digestion.

Point Modification: Add Zhigou (SJ 6) for constipation; Tianshu (ST25) and Shangjuxu (ST37) for loose stools; Qihai (RN 6) for abdominal distention.

Method: Apply filiform needles with reducing method and retain the needles for 15—20 minutes, manipulating them two to three times.

3. Liver *Qi* Attacking the Stomach

Principle: Soothe the liver, pacify the stomach and check vomiting by needling points mainly from The Liver Channel of Foot—*Jueyin,* The Gallbladder Channel of Foot—*Shaoyang* and The Stomach Channel of Foot—*Yangming*.

Prescription: Shangwan (RN13)　Yanglingquan (GB34)

Taichong (LR　3)　Liangmen (ST21)

Neiguan (PC　6)　Zusanli (ST36)

Explanation: Shangwan (RN13) relieves the discomfort sensation in the chest and diaphragm. It is also combined with Liangmen (ST21) to pacify the stomach and stop vomiting. Taichong (LR 3) soothes the liver and eases abnormal *Qi* ascending. It is also used in combination with Yanglingquan (GB34) to relieve liver *Qi* stagnation. Neiguan (PC 6) and Zusanli (ST36) relieve the chest fullness and regulate the *Qi* circulation and stop vomiting.

Point Modification: Add Danzhong (RN17) for fullness in the chest with restlessness.

Method: Apply filiform needles with reducing method and retain the needles for 15—20 minutes, manipulating them two to three times.

4. Deficiency of the Spleen and Stomach

Principle: Warm up the middle—*Jiao*, strengthen the spleen and pacify the stomach by needling points mainly from The Back—*Shu*, The *Ren* Channel and The Stomach Channel of Foot—*Yangming*.

Prescription: Pishu (BL20)   Weishu (BL21)

Zhongwan (RN12)   Zhangmen (LR13)

Zusanli (ST36)   Gongsun (SP 4)

Neiguan (PC 6)

Explanation: Pishu(BL20) and Weishu(BL21) are combined with Zhangmen(LR13) and Zhongwan(RN12), respectively the Front—*Mu* points of the spleen and stomach, to invigorate the *Qi* of the spleen and stomach, adjust the function of *Qi* in ascending and descending. Zusanli(ST36) sedates the abnormal gastric *Qi* ascending. Gongsun(SP 4) in combination with Neiguan(PC 6) may regulate the function of the middle—*Jiao* and ease *Qi* ascending. The joint use of the above points have the function of strengthening the spleen and stomach, invigorating the *Qi* of the middle—*Jiao* so the spleen may resume its function in transportation and transformation and that the ascent of spleen *Qi* and the descent of gastric may return to normal.

Point Modification: Add Tianshu(ST 25) and Shangjuxu (ST 37) for loose stool.

Method: Apply filiform needles with reducing method and retain the needles for 20—30 minutes, manipulating them three to four times. Ten to twenty minutes of moxibustion at these Back—*Shu* points is also applicable together with the needling.

5. *Yin* Deficiency of the Stomach

Principle: Nourish stomach *Yin* and sedate the abnormal ascending of stomach *Qi* and check vomiting by needling points mainly from The Back *Shu* of Foot—*Taiyang,* The Spleen Channel of Foot—*Taiyin* and The Stomach Channel of Foot—*Yangming*.

Prescription: Weishu (BL21)   Yinlingquan (SP 9)
                Zusanli (ST36)   Neiguan (PC 6)
                Gongsun (SP 4)   Neiting (ST44)

Explanation: Weishu (BL21) is combined with Yinlingquan (SP 9), the *He*—sea point of the spleen channel, and Zusanli (ST 36), the *He*—sea point of the stomach channel, to nourish the stomach *Yin* and strengthen the spleen and stomach. Neiguan (PC 6) and Gongsun (SP 4) adjust the function of the middle—*Jiao,* relieve chest fullness, pacify the stomach, halt the adverse rise of *Qi* and check vomiting. Neiting (ST44), the *ying*—spring point of Stomach Channel of Foot—*Yangming,* is used to clear away heat from the stomach channel.

Point Modification: Add Jinjin (EX—HN12) and Yuye

(EX−HN13) for continuous vomiting; Zhaohai (KI 6) and Yinxi (HT 6) for dryness in the mouth and throat.

Method: Apply filiform needles with reinforcing method except Neiting (ST44) which is needled by reduction one. Retain the needles for 15−20 minutes, manipulating them two to four times. Prick Jinjin (EX−HN12) and Yuye (EX−HN13) to cause bleeding. Moxibustion is contraindicated.

Alternative Treatment: Auricular Acupuncture

Prescription: Stomach   Liver   Sympathetic   Ear−shenmen
Subcortex   Occiput

Method: Apply filiform needles at three to four points each time with strong stimulation and retain the needles for 15−30 minutes. Embedding of ear seeds or subcutaneous needles is also applicable.

1.12   Abdominal Pain

Abdominal pain refers to the pain involving the area below the epigastrium and above the suprapubic hair margin. Clinically, it is a very common symptom encountered in various *Zangfu* disorders. It can be seen in both acute and chronic enteritis, gastrointestinal spasm, intestinal neurosis and indigestion in terms of modern medicine. For the treatment of acute abdominal pain due to surgical and gynecological diseases, refer to the contents in the related sections.

Cause and Mechanism

Abdominal pain is mostly caused by overeating of cold or raw food, or invasion of exogenous pathogenic cold into the abdomen. The constraining and stagnant property of cold causes the obstruction of *Qi* mechanism which gives rise to pain.

Overeating of greasy oily food or unclean food can cause food retention which will turn into heat retained in the intestines. The intestinal heat blocks the normal circulation of intestinal *Qi* and leads to onset of abdominal pain. Constitutional *Yang* deficiency and spleen *Yang* deficiency in particular can also cause abdominal pain because of the dysfunction of both spleen and stomach.

Differentiation

1. Accumulation of Cold in the Interior

The Sudden onset of severe abdominal pain is relieved by warmth and aggravated by cold. Other manifestations include loose stools, borborygmus, profuse clear urine, poor appetite, absence of thirst, cold limbs, thin white tongue coating, and deep tense or deep slow pulse.

2. Retention of Food

The distending pain involving both the epigastrium and abdomen worsens with pressing. The pain stimulates bowel motion and lessens after the bowel movement. Other manifestations include anorexia, foul belching, sour regurgitation, nausea, vomiting, greasy tongue coating, and slippery pulse.

3. Deficiency of Spleen *Yang*

The lingering abdominal pain appears intermittently. It responds to pressing and warmth but is aggravated by cold. Other manifestations include loose stools, listlessness, weakness of the four limbs, pale tongue with teethmarks on the edge, and deep thready pulse.

Treatment

1. Accumulation of Cold in the Interior

Principle: Warm up the middle—*Jiao,* eliminate cold and stop pain by needling points mainly from The *Ren* Channel, The

Stomach Channel of Foot—*Yangming* and The Spleen Channel of Foot—*Taiyin*.

Prescription: Zhongwan (RN12) Shenque (RN 8)
          Zusanli (ST36)

Explanation: Zhongwan (RN 12), the Influential point of the *Fu* organs, is used in combination with Zusanli (ST36), the *He*—sea point of the stomach channel, to separate the turbid from the clear, regulate the *Qi* circulation of the gastrointestinal system, strengthen the middle—*Jiao* and eliminate cold. Moxibustion is applied at Shenque (RN 8) to dispel cold in the middle—*Jiao*. The joint use of these points may warm up the middle—*Jiao* eliminate cold, normalize the *Qi* mechanism and ease the abdominal pain.

Point Modification: Add Qihai(RN 6) and Sanyinjiao(SP 6) for pain in the umbilicus; Tianshu(ST25) and Dachangshu(BL25) for loose stools.

Method: Apply filiform needles with reducing method and retain the needles for 20—30 minutes, manipulating them two to three times. Moxibustion is applied at Shenque for 15—20 minutes.

2. Retention of Food

Principle: Promote digestion, relieve food retention and stop pain by needling points mainly from The *Ren* Channel and The Stomach Channel of Foot—*Yangming*.

Prescription: Xianwan (RN10) Liangmen (ST21)
          Gongsun (SP 4) Zusanli (ST36)
          Lineiting (Extra)

Explanation: Xiawan (RN10) and Liangmen (ST21) are used to strengthen the stomach and relieve food retention. Gongsun

(SP 4), the *Luo*-connecting point of the spleen channel, is used in combination with Zusanli (ST36), the *He*-sea point of the stomach channel, to strengthen the spleen, regulate *Qi* circulation and relieve food retention. Lineiting (Extra) is the empirical point for the treatment of abdominal pain due to food retention. The joint use of the above points may normalize the *Qi* mechanism, relieve food retention and ease the pain.

Point Modification: Add Yanglingquan (GB34) for belching and acid regurgitation.

Method: Apply filiform needles with reducing method and retain the needles for 15—30 minutes, manipulating them two to three times.

3. Deficiency of Spleen *Yang*

Principle: Warm up middle—*Jiao*, eliminate cold, and strengthen spleen *Qi* by needling points mainly from The Bladder Channel of Foot—*Taiyang* and The *Ren* Channel.

Prescription: Pishu (BL20) Weishu (BL21)

Zhongwan (RN12) Zhangmen (LR13)

Zusanli(ST36) Qihai(RN 6) Guanyuan(RN 4)

Explanation: Pishu (BL20) paired with Zhangmen (LR13) and Weishu (BL21) paired with Zhongwan (RN12), known as the combination of Back—*Shu* points with the Front—*Mu* points, have the effect of invigorating the *Yang* of the spleen and stomach. Qihai (RN 6) and Guanyuan (RN 4) warm up the lower—*Jiao,* consolidate the primordial *Qi* and reinforce *Yang*. It is also used in combination with Zusanli (ST 36) to strengthen the function of spleen and stomach and reinforce *Qi* of the middle—*Jiao*. The abdominal pain may be eased when the *Yang* energy in the middle *Jiao* is invigorated.

Point Modification: Add Shenque (RN 8) with moxibustion for intermittent abdominal pain.

Method: Apply filiform needles with reinforcing method and retain the needles for 15–30 minutes, manipulating them two to three times. Both needling and moxibustion are applied at Qihai (RN 6) and those Back–*Shu* points in the above prescription. Moxibustion is applied at these points for 10–15 minutes. Moxibustion with ginger in between is applied at Shenque (RN 8) for 10–20 minutes.

Alternative Treatment: Auricular Acupuncture

Prescription: Large intestine   Small intestine   Spleen abdomen   Ear–shenmen   Subcortex

Method: Apply filiform needles at three to five points each time with moderate stimulation and retain the needles for 10–20 minutes. Embedding of ear seeds is also applicable.

1.13   Abdominal Distention

Abdominal distention is characterized by a discomfort sensation and fullness in the abdomen. In severe cases, it also causes local pain, belching and vomiting. It is mostly the consequence of gastrointestinal dysfunction.

For the abdominal distention appearing as a major symptom in such diseases as gastroptosis, enteroparalysis, intestinal obstruction, gastroneurosis and acute gastrectasis, the differentiation and treatment presented in this part can be taken as reference.

Cause and Mechanism

Abdominal distention is mostly caused by impairment of the spleen and stomach due to irregular or excessive food intake, resulting in dysfunction of transportation and transformation. The food retention therefore forms an obstruction to the *Qi* mechanism, giving rise to a distending sensation in the abdomen. It may also be caused by failure of the spleen and stomach in transportation, transformation and digestion owing to constitutional deficiency of the spleen and stomach or long term illness, leading to poor circulation of *Qi* in the stomach and intestines, resulting in distention. Besides, abdominal distention may also follow some abdominal operations.

Differentiation

1. Excess Type

The persistent distention and fullness in the abdomen, which may also cause abdominal pain, is aggravated by pressing. It is accompanied by belching, foul breathing, dark yellow urine, constipation or occasional fever and vomiting, yellow thick tongue coating, and slippery rapid and forceful pulse.

2. Deficiency Type

The abdominal distention which is relieved by pressing worsens and lessens from time to time. It is accompanied by borborygmus, loose stools, poor appetite, general lassitude, poor spirit, clear urine, pale tongue proper with white coating, and feeble pulse.

Treatment

1. Excess Type

Principle: Promote the *Qi* circulation of the stomach and intestines by needling points mainly from The Stomach Channel of Foot–*Yangming* and The Large Intestine Channel of Hand–*Yang-ming*.

Prescription: Zhongwan (RN12)　Tianshu (ST25)
　　　　　　　Zusanli (ST36)　Shangjuxu (ST37)

Explanation: Zhongwan (RN12) and Tianshu (ST25),

respectively the Front–*Mu* points of the stomach and large intestine, are combined with Zusanli (ST36) and Shangjuxu (ST37), respectively *He*–sea point of the stomach channel and the lower *He*–sea point of the large intestine, may promote the *Qi* mechanism of the gastrointestines, relieve food retention and promote digestion. The unobstructed *Qi* circulation in the gastrointestines can ease the abdominal distention.

Method: Apply filiform needles with reducing method and retain the needles for 15–20 minutes, manipulating them two to three times.

2. Deficiency Type

Principle: Strengthen the spleen, pacify the stomach, regulate *Qi* circulation and relieve distention by needling points mainly from The Stomach Channel of Foot–*Yangming* and The Spleen Channel of Foot–*Taiyin*.

Prescription: Jianli(RN11) Tianshu(ST25)

Zusanli(ST36) Taibai(SP 3) Guanyuan(RN 4)

Explanation: Jianli (RN11) strengthens the stomach *Qi*. Tianshu (ST25) promotes the *Qi* circulation of the gastrointestines. Zusanli (ST36), Taibai (SP 3) and Guanyuan (RN 4) strengthen the spleen, pacify the stomach and promote digestion. The joint use of the above points can reinforce spleen and stomach, regulate the circulation of *Qi* and relieve distention.

Method: Apply filiform needles with reinforcing method and retain the needles for 15–30 minutes, manipulating them two to three times.

Alternative Treatment: Auricular Acupuncture

Prescription: Spleen Stomach Large intestine Small intestine

Sympathetic Subcortex

Method: Apply filiform needles at three to four points each time with mild stimulation and retain the needles for 15–20 minutes. Embedding of ear seeds is also applicable.

1.14 Diarrhea

Diarrhea refers to increased times of loose stools with undigested food, or even watery stools. According to the clinical manifestations and duration, it is divided into the acute and chronic types. The condition may occur in any of the four seasons, but more common in summer and autumn. Similar to that described in modern medicine, it may be seen in such diseases as acute and chronic enteritis, intestinal tuberculosis, intestinal dysfunction and irritable bowel.

Cause and Mechanism

The causative factors of diarrhea are complicated, but it is mainly caused by dysfunctions of the spleen and stomach.

Acute diarrhea is mostly due to an improper diet related to intake of cold raw food or unclean food, or due to invasion of pathogenic cold, dampness and summer heat, especially dampness. These factor can cause obstruction of the spleen *Yang* and impair the function of the spleen and stomach, leading to poor function of the spleen in transformation and transportation and nonseparation of the turbid from the clean in the intestine to form diarrhea.

Chronic diarrhea is mostly due to impairment of the spleen by over worry or constitutional deficiency of the spleen and stomach. However, the dysfunction of liver in maintaining free flow of *Qi* and stagnant liver *Qi* attacking the stomach can lead to its overacting on the spleen and stomach. *Yang* deficiency of the kidney with decline of vital gate fire after prolonged illness causes inadequate warming on the spleen and stomach to do digestion. Therefore, diarrhea is the consequence of dysfunction of the spleen and stomach.

Differentiation

1. Acute Diarrhea

Such diarrhea is characterized by a sudden onset with apparent increase of bowel movements and decrease of urinary discharge.

(1) Cold—damp Type: Loose stools or even watery stools, abdominal pain, borborygmus, general cold sensation with desire for warmth, absence of thirst, pale tongue proper with white coating, and deep slow or soft slow pulse.

(2) Damp—heat Type: Loose stools with abdominal pain, urgent bowel motion or that with difficulty, yellow stools with odour, feverish sensation in the anus, restlessness, thirst, short scanty urine, yellow greasy tongue coating, and rapid slippery or rapid soft pulse.

(3) Food Retention Type: Abdominal pain, borborygmus, fetid stools, lessened pain after releasing stools, fullness and distention in the epigastric region, belching with mouth odour, poor appetite, frequent passing of wind, sticky greasy tongue coating, and slippery pulse.

2. Chronic Diarrhea

Such a diarrhea is often resulted from the acute one with slow onset. The frequency of bowel motions is less than that of acute diarrhea. But the duration of the condition is involved with a lingering period of time.

(1) Spleen Deficiency Type: Prolonged and reccurent loose

stools with undigested food, decrease of appetite, fullness sensation in the epigastric region after food intake, apparent increase of bowel movement soon after intake of greasy or oily food, sallow complexion, white sticky tongue coating, and soft slow pulse.

(2) Liver and Spleen Derangement Type: Bowel motion stimulated by abdominal pain that still remains the same after bowel movement, reccurent diarrhea due to emotional disturbance or stress. The accompanying symptoms and signs include discomfort sensation in the hypochondriac region during diarrhea, belching, thin tongue coating, and wiry pulse.

(3) Kidney Deficiency Type: Borborygmus and diarrhea with abdominal pain just before dawn, cold limbs, soreness and weakness in the knee joint and lumbar region, white tongue coating and deep thready pulse. The patient feels comfortable after the bowel motion.

Treatment

1. Acute Diarrhea

(1) Cold−damp Type

Principle: Warm up the middle−*Jiao* and resolve the dampness by needling points mainly from The *Ren* Channel.

Prescription: Tianshu(ST25) Jianli(RN 11) Qihai(RN 6)
              Shangjuxu(ST37) Yinlingquan(SP 9)

Explanation: Tianshu(ST25), the Front−*Mu* point of the large intestine, has the effect of regulating the *Qi* mechanism of the large intestine and eliminating the cold and dampness in the abdomen. Jianli(RN11) and Qihai(RN 6), applied with both needling and moxibustion, warm up the middle−*Jiao*, regulate *Qi* circulation, eliminate cold and resolve dampness. Shangjuxu (ST37), the lower *He*−sea point of the large intestine, is used in combination with Yinlingquan (SP 9) in order to promote the functions of the intestines and stomach, help separate the turbid from the clear and dispel the damp—water. The joint use of these points can warm up the middle—*Jiao* resolve dampness and stop diarrhea.

Method: Apply filiform needles with reducing method and retain the needles for 15—20 minutes, manipulating them two to three times. Jianli(RN11), Qihai(RN 6) and Tianshu(ST25) are also applied with moxibustion for 10—15 minutes. The use of five to seven pieces of moxa cones with ginger in between at the above mentioned points is also suitable.

(2) Damp—heat Type

Principle: Eliminate heat and resolve dampness by needling points mainly from The Stomach Channel of Foot—*Yangming* and The Spleen Channel of Foot—*Taiyin*.

Prescription: Zhongwan(RN12)   Tianshu(ST25)

Yinlingquan(SP 9)   Neiting(ST44)

Quchi(LI 11)

Explanation: Zhongwan(RN12) and Tianshu(ST25) regulate the *Qi* mechanism of the stomach and intestines. Yinlingquan(SP 9) strengthens the spleen and resolves dampness. Neiting(ST44), the *Ying*—spring point of the stomach channel, is used in combination with Quchi(LI11), the *He*—sea point of the large intestine channel, to eliminate the damp—heat in the stomach and intestines. The joint use of the above points can regulate the *Qi* mechanism of the stomach and intestines, eliminate damp—heat and stop diarrhea.

Method: Apply filiform needles with reducing method and retain the needles for 15—20 minutes, manipulating them two to three times.

(3) Food Retention Type

Principle: Promote digestion, remove food retention and stop diarrhea by needling points mainly from The *Ren* Channel and The Stomach Channel of Foot—*Yangming*.

Prescription: Tianshu(ST25)   Zhongwan(RN12)
                       Xuanji(RN21)   Lineiting(Extra)
                       Zusanli(ST36)

Explanation: Tianshu(ST25),   Zhongwan(RN12)   and Zusanli (ST36), having the function of regulating the *Qi* mechanism of the stomach and intestines, are combined with Xuanji (RN21) and Lineiting (Extra) to promote digestion and remove food retention. The joint use of the above points may relieve food retention by promoting digestion, eliminate the heat accumulation, regain the harmony between the spleen and stomach and stop diarrhea.

Point Modification: Add Neiguan(PC 6) and Neiting(ST44) for belching with sour smell.

Method: Apply filiform needles with reducing method and retain the needles for 15—20 minutes, manipulating them two to three times.

2. Chronic Diarrhea

(1) Spleen Deficiency Type

Principle: Strengthen the spleen and stop diarrhea by needling points mainly from The Spleen Channel of Foot—*Taiyin* plus the related Back—*Shu* points.

Prescription: Pishu(BL20)   Zhangmen(LR13)
                       Taibai(SP 3)   Zhongwan(RN12)
                       Zusanli(ST36)   Tianshu(ST25)

Explanation: Pishu (BL20) and Zhangmen (LR13), known

as the combination of Back−*Shu* and Front−*Mu* points, have the effect of strengthening the spleen and reinforcing *Qi*. Zhongwan (RN12), Zusanli (ST36) and Tianshu (ST25) are used to regulate the *Qi* mechanism of the stomach and intestines. Taibai (SP 3), the *Yuan*−source point of the spleen, reinforces the *Qi* of the spleen. The joint use of the above points may activate spleen *Yang*, strengthen the spleen and stop diarrhea.

Method: Apply filiform needles with reinforcing method and retain the needles for 15−20 minutes, manipulating them one to two times.

Moxibustion is also applicable at Pishu (BL 20), Tianshu (ST 25), Zusanli (ST 36) for 10−15 minutes.

(2) Liver−spleen Derangement Type

Principle: Soothe the liver *Qi,* strengthen the spleen, pacify the stomach and stop diarrhea by needling points mainly from The Liver Channel of Foot−*Jueyin,* The Stomach Channel of Foot−*Yangming* and The Bladder Channel of Foot−*Taiyang*.

Prescription: Ganshu (BL18)   Taichong (LR 3)

Pishu (BL20)   Zhangmen (LR13)

Tianshu (ST25)   Zusanli (ST36)

Explanation: Ganshu (BL18) and Taichong (LR 3) soothe the liver *Qi*. Pishu (BL20) and Zhangmen (LR13) strengthen spleen *Qi*. Tianshu (ST25) and Zusanli (ST36) regulate the *Qi* mechanism of the stomach and intestines. The joint use of the above points may regain the function of the liver in maintaining free flow of *Qi,* harmonize the *Qi* mechanism of the *Zangfu* organs and stop diarrhea.

Point Modification: Add Yanglingquan(GB34) and Neiguan (PC 6)for distention in the hypochondriac region.

Method: Apply filiform needles with even method and retain the needles for 15—20 minutes, manipulating them two to three times.

(3) Kidney Deficiency Type

Principle: Warm up and tonify the spleen and kidney by needling mainly the Back—*Shu* points and points from The *Ren* Channel.

Prescription: Shenshu (BL23)   Mingmen (DU 4)
Guanyuan (RN 4)   Pishu (BL20)
Tianshu (ST25)   Shangjuxu (ST37)

Explanation: Shenshu (BL23), Mingmen (DU 4) and Guanyuan (RN 4) warm up the kidney *Yang* and eliminate cold from the abdomen. Pishu (UB20) tonifies the spleen *Qi*. Tianshu (ST25) and Shangjuxu (ST37) regulate the *Qi* mechanism of the large intestine. The joint use of the above points can warm up the spleen and kidney, promote digestion, eliminate cold and stop diarrhea.

Point Modification: Add Baihui (DU20) with moxibustion for lingering diarrhea of the deficient type and sinking of *Qi* of the middle—*Jiao*.

Method: Apply filiform needles with reinforcing method and retain the needles for 15—30 minutes, manipulating them one to two times. Moxibustion for 10—20 minutes at two to three points is also applicable.

Alternative Treatment: Auricular Acupuncture

Prescription: Large intestine Small intestine Ear—
shenmen Spleen Stomach Sympathetic
Liver Kidney

Method Apply filiform needles at three to five points with

moderate stimulation and retain the needles for 10—20 minutes. Embedding of ear seeds or subcutaneous needles is also applicable.

1.15 Dysentery

Dysentery is an intestinal epidemic disease that occurs more in the summer time. It is characterized by abdominal pain, tenesmus and frequent bowel motions containing blood and mucous. Clinically, it is divided into damp—heat dysentery, damp—cold dysentery, fasting dysentery and chronic recurrent dysentery.

The differentiation and treatment in this section can be used as reference for bacillary, toxic and amebic dysenteries, and chronic nonspecific ulerative colitis in modern medicine.

Cause and Mechanism

Dysentery in most cases is caused by impairment of the stomach and intestines due to improper intake of raw, cold or unclean food, or due to the invasion of damp—heat in summer. If the excessive damp—heat turns into fire steaming the blood and impairing the intestinal collaterals, there will be bloody stools with more blood and less pus, known as the damp—heat type of dysentery. If excessive cold—damp affects and retains in the intestines, the dysentery will involve with white mucous or with more pus but less white mucous, known as the cold—damp type dysentery. In case of pathogenic heat invading the stomach, such symptoms and signs as nausea, vomiting and complete loss of appetite will occur, known as the fasting dysentery. If the above mentioned dysenteries has undergone a long course, resulting in *Qi* deficiency in the middle—*Jiao* and weakness of body resistance against pathogenic factor invading, chronic recurrent dysentery occurs.

Differentiation

1. Damp—heat Type Dysentery

The chief manifestations include abdominal pain, tenesmus, stools with pus and mucous that run up to several or even more than ten times a day, burning sensation in the anus, scanty and dark urine, high fever in severe case, restlessness, thirst, yellow greasy tongue coating, and rapid slippery pulse.

2. Cold—damp Type of Dysentery

The chief manifestations include spasmodic pain in the abdomen, white mucous or mixed with small amount of blood in the stools, tenesmus, aversion to cold preferring warmth, fullness in the chest and epigastrium, tastelessness, absence of thirst, white greasy tongue coating, and deep slow pulse.

3. Fasting Dysentery

The chief manifestations include frequent stools containing blood and pus, total loss of appetite, nausea and vomiting, abdominal pain, or distention and fullness in the chest and abdomen, yellow greasy tongue coating, and soft rapid pulse.

4. Chronic Recurrent Dysentery

This kind of dysentery is intermittent from time to time in a lingering course. It worsens with improper diet, overstrain or invasion of exogenous pathogenic factors, general lassitude and cold limbs. It is accompanied by somnolence, poor appetite, pale tongue proper with greasy coating, and soft or full deficient pulse.

Treatment

1. Damp—heat Type Dysentery

Principle: Eliminate damp—heat. regulate *Qi* circulation and activate blood by needling points mainly from The Stomach Channel of Foot—*Yangming*.

Prescription: Tianshu(ST25)   Shangjuxu(ST37)
              Neiting (ST44)   Hegu (LI 4)

Explanation: Tianshu (ST25), the Front—*Mu* point of the large intestine, is combined with Shangjuxu (ST37), the lower *He*—sea point of the large intestine, and Hegu (LI 4), the *Yuan*—source point of the large intestine channel, to regulate the *Qi* circulation of the large intestine. Quchi (LI11), the *He*—sea point of the large intestine channel, is used in combination with Neiting (ST44), the *Ying*—spring point of the stomach channel, to eliminate damp—heat from the stomach and intestine. The joint use of the above points may eliminate heat and regulate the circulation of both *Qi* and blood. The dysentery is stopped when *Qi* is regulated and dampness is resolved.

Point Modification: Add Dazhui (DU14) for fever; and Qihai (RN 6) for tenesmus sensation.

Method: Apply filiform needles with reducing method and retain the needles for 15—20 minutes, manipulating them two to three times.

2. Cold—damp Type Dysentery

Principle: Eliminate cold by warming and resolve dampness, promote *Qi* and blood circulation by needling points mainly from The *Ren* Channel and The Stomach Channel of Foot—*Yangming*.

Prescription: Zhongwan (RN12)   Tianshu (ST25)
              Qihai (RN 6)   Shangjuxu (ST37)
              Yinlingquan (SP 9)

Explanation: Zhongwan (RN12), the Front—*Mu* point of the stomach, is used in combination with Shangjuxu (ST37), the lower *He*—sea point of the large intestine, to regulate the *Qi* mechanism of the stomach and intestines, pacify the stomach and resolves the turbid dampness. Tianshu (ST25) and Qihai (RN 6) eliminate cold from the middle—*Jiao,* promote *Qi* circulation and relieve *Qi* stagnation. Yinlingquan (SP 9), the *He*—sea point of the spleen channel, may strengthen the spleen and resolve dampness. The joint use of the above points may eliminate cold from the middle—*Jiao,* strengthen the spleen, resolve dampness, promote *Qi* circulation and benefit the blood.

Method: Apply filiform needles with even method and retain the needles for 15—20 minutes, manipulating them two to three times. Qihai (RN 6) and Tianshu (ST25) may also be applied with moxibustion for 10—15 minutes.

3. Fasting Diarrhea

Principle: Pacify the stomach and restore the appetite by needling points mainly from The *Ren* Channel, The Large Intestine Channel of Hand—*Yangming* and The Stomach Channel of Foot—*Yangming.*

Prescription: Zhongwan (RN12)   Hegu (LI 4)

Neiguan (PC 6)   Neiting (ST44)

Tianshu (ST25)

Explanation: Zhongwan (RN12), the Front—*Mu* point of the stomach, pacifies the stomach, and separates the turbid from the clean. Hegu (LI 4) and Neiting (ST44) eliminate the damp—heat accumulated in the intestines and stomach. Neiguan (PC 6) regulates the function of the *SanJiao* and sedates the abnormal ascending of *Qi* and stop vomiting. Tianshu (ST25), the Front—*Mu* point of the large intestine, is applied to adjust the flow of *Qi* in the large intestine. The joint use of these points has the effect of ascending the clear and descending the turbid, eliminating heat, resolving dampness, regulating the function of the middle—*Jiao* lowering the adverse rise of *Qi*, promoting appetite and ceasing vomiting.

Method: Apply filiform needles with reducing method and retain the needles for 15—20 minutes, manipulating them two to three times.

4. Chronic Recurrent Dysentery

Principle: Strengthen the spleen, replenish *Qi* and remove stagnation by needling points mainly from The Bladder Channel and The *Ren* Channel.

Prescription: Pishu (BL20) Weishu (BL21)

Dachangshu (BL25) Guanyuan (RN 4)

Tianshu (ST25) Zusanli (ST36)

Explanation: Pishu (BL20), Weishu (BL21) and Zusanli (ST36) strengthen the spleen and stomach, i.e. to reinforce the source for providing the acquired energy. Dachangshu (BL25) and Tianshu (ST25), known as the combination of Back—*Shu* and Front—*Mu* points, promote the *Qi* circulation of the intestines and relieve the stagnation of *Qi*. Guanyuan (RN 4), the Front—*Mu* point of the small intestine, warms up the lower *Jiao* and consolidates the *Yuan* (source) energy in order to help separate the clean from the turbid. The joint use of the above points is effective to strengthen the anti—pathogenic *Qi*, dispel the pathogenic *Qi*, reinforce the *Qi* of the middle—*Jiao* and regulate the *Qi* circulation of the intestines.

Point Modification: Add Baihui (DU20) with moxibustion for prolapse of rectum.

Method: Apply filiform needles with reinforcing method and

retain the needles for 15–30 minutes, manipulating them one to two times. Moxibustion can also be applied at Pishu (BL20), Weishu (BL21) and Guanyuan (RN 4) for 10–15 minutes.

Alternative Treatment: Auricular Acupuncture

Prescription: Large intestine   Small intestine   Stomach
Ear–shenmen   Spleen   Kidney   Lower
portion of rectum

Method: Apply filiform needles at three to five points with moderate stimulation and retain the needles for 10–15 minutes.

1.16   Constipation

Constipation is a condition manifested by prolonged intervals of dry or compacted feces from the intestines, or urgent desire for immediate bowel movement but with difficulty in defecating. It commonly includes habitual constipation, constipation due to peristalsis dysfunction and constipation due to rectum or anus disorders in modern medicine.

Cause and Mechanism

Constitutional excess of *Yang*, alcoholic indulgence, habitual intake of greasy spicy food or remnant heat after febrile disease may all cause heat accumulation in the stomach and intestine and consumption of the body fluid, leading to dryness of intestines as well as dry stools. Either emotional disturbance such as anxiety and depression, or lack of physical exertion may cause stagnation of *Qi* impairing the function of the large intestine in transmitting. As a result, the wastes are retained inside and unable to move downward, causing the constipation. Deficiency of *Qi* and blood resulted from illness or delivery causes two subsequent conditions of deficiency. Specifically, *Qi* deficiency leads to weakness of the large intestine in transmission, while blood deficiency weakens the mositening of the large intestine in descending wastes. Deficiency of *Yang Qi* in the aged causes a poor body warming by the *Yang* energy and accumulation of interior cold. The stagnant cold can not help the transformation and distribution of *Qi,* resulting in constipation.

Differentiation

1. Heat Type Constipation

The chief manifestations include an absence of bowel motions for several days, abdominal fullness and distention, abdominal pain and mass by palpating, reddish complexion, restlessness, scanty urine which may involve fever in some cases, dry mouth with foul breath, dry yellow tongue coating, and rapid slippery pulse.

2. *Qi* Stagnation Type Constipation

The chief manifestations include infrequent bowel movements, distending pain in the abdomen involving also the hypochondrium, frequent belching, bitter taste, dizziness, poor appetite, thin greasy tongue coating, and thready pulse.

3. Deficient Type Constipation

The chief manifestations include dry stools difficult to discharge, no abdominal distention nor pain but discomfort in the lower abdomen, difficulty to discharge stools despite hard efforts or profuse sweating, shortness of breath and lassitude, pale complexion, palpitation, dizziness, blurred vision, pale tongue proper with thin coating, and thin feeble pulse.

4. Cold Type Constipation

The chief manifestations include dry stool difficult to discharge or even with prolapse of rectum in severe cases, occasional pain in the abdomen, pallid complexion, cold limbs desiring for warmth, copious clear urine, pale tongue with white coating, and deep slow pulse.

Treament

1. Heat Type Constipation

Principle: Eliminate heat and moisten the intestines by needling points mainly from The Stomach Channel of Foot—*Yangming*.

Prescription: Hegu (LI 4)   Quchi(LI11)   Neiting(ST44)

Tianshu (ST25)   Fujie (SP14)

Shangjuxu (ST37)

Explanation: Hegu (LI 4), Quchi (LI11) and Neiting (ST44) may eliminate pathogenic heat from the *Yangming* channels, protect the fluid to moisten the intestines. Tianshu(ST25) and Shangjuxu (ST37), respectively the Front—*Mu* and lower *He*—sea points of the large intestine, are combined with Fujie (SP14) to promote the distribution of fluid and regulate the *Qi* of the large intestine. The joint use of the above points may eliminate heat, protect the fluid and regulate the *Qi* circulation of the intestines so that constipation can be cured.

Point Modification: Add Shaofu (HT 8) and Lianquan (RN23) for excessive heat with thirst; Chengjiang (RN24) for foul breath.

Method: Apply filiform needles with reducing method and retain the needles for 15—20 minutes, manipulating them two to three times.

2. *Qi* Stagnation Type Constipation

Principle: Descend *Qi* and promote bowel motions by needling points mainly from The *Ren* Channel, The Liver Channel of

Foot—*Jueyin* and The Gallbladder Channel of Foot—*Shaoyang*.

Prescription: Zhongwan (RN12) Tianshu (ST25)

Xingjian (LR 2) Yanglingquan (GB34)

Zhigou (SJ 6)

Explanation: Zhongwan (RN12), the Influential point of *Fu* organs, is combined with Tianshu(ST25), the Front—*Mu* point of the large intestine, to promote the *Qi* circulation of the intestines. Xingjian(LR 2), the *Ying*—spring point of the liver channel, is combined with the *He*—sea point of the gallbladder channel Yanglingquan(GB34) to soothe the stagnant liver *Qi*. Zhigou (SJ 6), the *Jing*—river point of the sanjiao channel, is used to regulate the *Qi* mechanism of the *SanJiao*. Bowel movements will be normal when the *Qi* mechanism of the intestine is regulated.

Point Modification: Add Qimen(LR14), Riyue (GB24) for severe pain in the hypochondriac region; Daheng (SP15) for severe abdominal distention.

Method: Apply filiform needles with reducing method and retain the needles for 15—20 minutes, manipulating them two to three times.

3. Deficient Type Constipation

Principle: Reinforce *Qi* and blood by needling points mainly from The Bladder Channel of Foot—*Taiyang*, The *Ren* Channel and The Stomach Channel of Foot—*Yangming*.

Prescription: Pishu (BL20) Weishu (BL21)

Guanyuan (RN 4) Qihai (RN 6)

Zusanli (ST36)

Explanation: Since spleen is the source for providing the acquired energy, Pishu(BL20) is used in combination with Weishu (BL21) and Zusanli(ST36) to strengthen the *Qi* of the middle–*Jiao* and reinforce the source for providing the acquired energy. Qihai (RN 6) and Guanyuan (RN 4) strengthen the *Yang Qi* in order to tonify the *Yuan* (source) *Qi* of the lower *Jiao* The joint use of the above points has the effect of invigorating the *Qi* of the spleen and stomach, helping manufacture *Qi* and blood so as to achieue the purpose of nourishing *Qi* and blood, moistening the intestines and promoting bowel motions.

Point Modification: Add Yinxi (HT 6) for profuse sweating; Neiguan (PC 6) for palpitation.

Method: Apply filiform needles with reinforcing method and retain the needles for 20–30 minutes, manipulating them one to two times. Qihai (RN 6), Guanyuan (RN 4) and the Back–*Shu* points may also applied with moxibustion for 10–15 minutes.

4. Cold Type Constipation

Principle: Reinforce kidney *Yang,* warm up the intestines and promote bowel motions by needling points mainly from The *Ren* Channel and The Kidney Channel of Foot–*Shaoyin.*

Prescription: Shenque (RN 8)   Qihai (RN 6)
                Zhaohai (KI 6)   Shenshu (BL23)
                Tianshu (ST25)

Explanation: Moxibustion is applied at Shenque (RN 8), Qihai (Ren 6) and Shenshu (BL23) to reinforce kidney *Qi.* Tianshu (ST 25) may promote the *Qi* circulation of the large intestine. The joint use of the above points may warm up *Yang,* eliminate cold, soften the dry stool and promote bowel motions.

Point Modification: Add Changqiang (DU 1) and Baihui (DU20) for prolapse of rectum.

Methodp Apply filiform needles with reinforcing method and retain the needles for 20–30 minutes, manipulating them one to two times. Moxibustion can also be applied at Shenque (Ren 8) and Qihai (Ren 6) for 15–20 minutes.

Alternative Treatment: Auricular Acupuncture

Prescription: Large intestine   Small intestine   lung   spleen   Su bcortex   Lower   portion of rectum

Method: Apply filiform needles at three to five points with strong stimulation and retain the needles for 15–20 minutes. Embedding of ear seeds is also applicable.

1.17   Prolapse of Rectum

Prolapse of rectum refers to the condition in which the lower portion of the rectum is lapsed out of the anus, mainly seen in aged patients, children or those with poor body constitution due to certain lingering diseases. The condition described here is similar to rectum prolapse in modern medicine.

Cause and Mechanism

Prolapse of rectum is mostly caused by sinking of *Qi* in the middle–*Jiao* and poor governing of *Qi* due to chronic diarrhea, protracted dysentery, multigravida or constitutional weakness after severe diseases. It may also be caused by pathogenic damp–heat in the spleen and lung due to improper diet, alcoholic indulgence and habitual intake of hot spicy food. The downward flowing of damp–heat results in the prolapse of rectum.

Differentiation

1. Deficiency of *Qi* in the Middle–*Jiao*

Prolapse of the rectum mostly occurs after a bowel movement. It may also occur through coughing, walking or long standing or exerting during urination. The accompanying symptoms and signs include lassitude, weakness of the limbs, sallow complexion, dizziness, palpitation, thin white tongue coating, and feeble thready pulse.

2. Damp-heat Attacking the Lower-*Jiao*

Prolapse of rectum involves with swelling and burning pain in the anus. It is accompanied by flushed face, fever, dry mouth with foul breath, chest and epigstric fullness, abdominal distention, scanty yellow urine, red tongue proper with yellow greasy coating, and soft rapid pulse.

Treatment

1. Deficiency of *Qi* in the Middle-*Jiao*

Principle: Reinforce and lift the sunken *Qi* in the middle-*Jiao* by needling points mainly from The *Du* Channel and The Bladder Channel of Foot-*Taiyang*.

Prescription: Baihui (DU20)   Changqiang (DU 1)
　　　　　　　 Dachangshu (BL25)   Qihai (RN 6)
　　　　　　　 Zusanli (ST36)

Explanation: Baihui (DU20), the meeting point of the *Du* Channel with the three *Yang* channels, is applied with moxibustion to elevate the sunken *Yang Qi* because *Qi* pertains to *Yang* subjected to The *Du* Channel. Changqiang (DU 1), the divergent collateral of The *Du* Channel near the anus, is needled to strengthen the contracting function of the large intestine. Qihai (RN 6), having the effect to tonify and regulate the *Yuan* (source) *Qi,* is combined with Zusanli(ST 36) to replenish *Qi* for elevation. Once the middle-*Jiao Qi* restores its function in elevating, prolapse of rectum can be relieved.

Method: Apply filiform needles with reinforcing method and retain the needles for 15-30 minutes manipulating them two to three times. Moxibustion is also applied at Baihui (DU20) and

Qihai (RN 6) for 15–20 minutes.

2. Damp–heat Attacking the Lower–*Jiao*

Principle: Eliminate damp–heat by needling points mainly from The *Du* Channel and The Bladder Channel of Foot–*Taiyang*.

Prescription: Baihui (DU20)   Changqiang (DU 1)
Chengshan (BL57)   Weizhong (BL40)
Fenglong (BL40)   Yinlingquan (SP 9)

Explanation: Baihui (DU20) elevates *Qi*. Changqiang(DU 1) and Chengshan (BL57) eliminate damp–heat in the rectum and anus. Weizhong (BL40) eliminates damp–heat in the intestine. Fenglong (ST40), the *Luo*–connecting point of the stomach channel, is combined with Yinlingquan (SP 9), the *He*–sea point of the spleen channel, to strengthen the spleen and resolve damp-ness and eliminate dampheat in the intestines. The joint use of the above points may regulate the *Qi* circulation in the intestines, eliminate damp–heat, elevate sunk *Qi* and help patients get re-covered from prolapse of rectum.

Point Modification: Add Tianshu(ST25) for abdominal distention; and Erbai (EX–UE2) for prolapse of rectum due to hemorrhoids.

Alternative Treatment

1. Auricular Acupuncture

Prescription: Lower portion of rectum   Subcortex
Spleen   Ear–shenmen

Method: Apply filiform needles with moderate stimulation and retain the needles for 20 minutes. Embedding of ear seeds or subcutaneous needles is also applicable.

2. Pricking

Prick any point on the longtitudinal line between the 3rd and 2nd lumbar vertebrae 1—1.5 *Cun* lateral to the spinal column.

1.18   Jaundice

Jaundice is a condition characterized by yellow pigmentation of the sclera and skin as well as dark yellow coloured urine. The yellow sclera is considered as the main sign in the clinic.

Jaundice is mostly seen in the infantile, the young and the middle aged. The condition described here is the same as that related in modern medicine, including hepatocelulor jaundice, obstructive jaundice, hemolytic jaundice, etc.

Cause and Mechanism

Jaundice may result from exogenous as well as endogenous pathogenic factors. Accumulation of exogenous pathogenic damp—heat in the liver and gallbladder with dampness retention and heat steaming impairs the liver in maintaining the free flow of *Qi* so the bile floods to cause jaundice. This is known as *Yang* type of jaundice. Impairment of the spleen and stomach and dysfunction of the spleen in transformation and transportation due to overstrain, overthinking or improper diet lead to dampness retention and *Qi* stagnation in the liver and gallbladder resulting in the unsmooth flow and excretion of bile that floods also to the superficies of the body to develop into jaundice. This is known as the *Yin* type of jaundice.

Clinically, the *Yang* type of jaundice may progress to the *Yin* type if treatment for the former appears to be inadequate or improper. On the other hand, patients with *Yin* type of jaundice may present manifestation of the *Yang* type if they are at the sametime invaded by exogenous pathogenic factors. This will result in a condition mixed with both excess and deficiency.

Differentiation

1. *Yang* Type Jaundice

The onset of jaundice is abrupt with very short duration. The symptoms and signs include yellow sclera and skin that is as apparent as orange skin, fever, thirst, short scanty urine, constipation, general heavy sensation, abdominal distention, fullness in the chest, nausea, yellow greasy tongue coating, and wiry pulse. Loss of consciousness, skin eruptions and hemorrhage will appear if the heat attacks the interior of the body. There will be less jaundice, milder fever, fullness in the epigastrium, moderate thirst, slightly yellow greasy tongue coating, and soft rapid pulse if dampness is more severe than heat as causative factor of the jaundice.

2. *Yin* Type Jaundice

The onset of the jaundice is slow over a long duration. The main symptoms and signs include yellow sclera and skin which may appear grey dark as if being smoked, general lassitude, aversion to cold, anorexia, nausea, vomiting, tastelessness in the mouth, no thirst, epigastric distention, unformed stools, pale tongue proper, greasy tongue coating, and deep slow pulse.

Treatment

1. *Yang* Type Jaundice

Principle: Soothe the *Qi* of the liver and gallbladder, eliminate heat and resolve dampness by needling points mainly from The *Du* Channel, The Bladder Channel and The Liver Channel of Foot—*Jueyin*.

Prescription: Zhiyang (DU 9)   Wangu (SI 4)

                    Ganshu (BL18)   Danshu (BL19)

Yanglingquan (GB34)   Taichong (LR 3)

Yinlingquan (SP 9)   Neiting (ST44)

Explanation: Zhiyang (DU 9), the spot where the *Qi* of The *Du* Channel infuses, may activate the *Qi* of The *Du* Channel. It is used in combination with the *Yuan* (source)point of the small intestine channel Wangu (SI 4) to promote *Qi* circulation of the *Taiyang* channel and eliminate the damp–heat from the superficial portion of the body. Ganshu (BL18) and Danshu (BL19) are combined with Yanglingquan(GB34) and Taichong (LR 3), respectively the *He*–sea point of the gall bladder channel and the *Yuan* (source) point of the liver channel, to soothe the *Qi* circulation of the liver and gall bladder, and to eliminate the damp–heat in the interior of the body. Yinlingquan (SP 9) and Neiting (ST44), respectively the *He*–sea point of the spleen channel and the *Ying*–spring point of the stomach channel, are used in combination to eliminate damp–heat from the stomach and spleen channels by means of discharging it from the urine. The joint use of the above points may eliminate heat, dispel dampness, soothe the liver and gall bladder and restore the normal bile excretion so that jaundice can be relieved.

Point Modification: Add Dazhui (DU14) for severe heat; Tianshu (ST25) and Dachangshu (BL25) for abdominal distention and constipation; Renzhong (DU26), Zhongchong (PC 9) and Shaochong (HT 9) for loss of consciousness; Zusanli (ST36) for epigastric fullness and loose stools.

Method: Apply filiform needles with reducing method and retain the needles for 20- 30 minutes, manipulating them two to four times.

2. *Yin* Type Jaundice

Principle: Strengthen the spleen, promote bile excretion, eliminate cold and resolve dampness by needling points mainly from The Stomach Channel of Foot−*Yangming*, The Spleen Channel of Foot−*Taiyin* and The Back Shu Points.

Prescription: Pishu (BL20)   Danshu (BL19)
             Zhiyang (DÜ 9)   Zhongwan (RN12)
             Zusanli (ST36)   Sanyinjiao (SP 6)

Explanation: Pishu (BL20) is combined with Zhongwan (RN12) and Zusanli (ST36), respectively the Influential point of the *Fu* organs and the *He*−sea poit of the stomach channel, to strengthen the spleen and stomach and eliminate dampness from the body. Danshu (BL19) is used to sedate the abnormal *Qi* ascending and promote the bile excretion. Zhiyang (DÜ 9) promotes the circulation of *Yang Qi*. Sanyinjiao (SP 6) reinforces the spleen and helps to descend the dampness to be discharged from the urine. The joint use of the above points can strengthen the spleen, promote bile excretion, resolve dampness and eliminate cold in order to relieve the *Yin* type jaundice.

Point Modification: Add Qihai(RN 6) and Mingmen(DU 4) for general lassitude and aversion to cold; and Tianshu (ST25) and Guanyaun (RN 4) for loose stools.

Method: Apply filiform needles with even method and retain the needles for 20−30 minutes, manipulating them two to three times.

Alternative Treatment: Auricular Acupuncture

Prescription: Liver   Gall bladder   Spleen   Stomach
             Diaphragm   Vegus nerve

Method: Apply filiform needles at three to four points with moderate stimulation and retain the needles for 15−20 minutes.

Embedding of ear seeds or subcutaneous needles is also applicable.

1.19 Hypochondriac Pain

Hypochondriac pain, a subjective symptom commonly complained of in the clinic, refers to a painful sensation either on one side or both sides of the hypochondrium. It is included in hepatopathy, biliary disorders intercostal neuralgia, etc. in modern medicine.

Cause and Mechanism

The onset of hypochondriac pain is mostly due to melancholy or violent anger that leads to the failure of the liver to spread Qi freely, thus resulting in the Qi obstruction of the channels. Invasion of exogenous pathogenic damp–heat, improper diet such as overeating or excessive alcoholic indulgence may cause accumulation of damp–heat in the liver and gallbladder and misachieved free flow of Qi. Sudden stumbling or twisting may give rise to impairment of channels and collaterals in the hypochondriac region, resulting in stagnation of Qi and blood and obstruction of channels and collaterals. Nevertheless, prolonged illness with poor constitution, overstrain and insufficiency of both Qi and blood can also be the cause of the poor nourishment of the liver.

Differentiation

1. Stagnation of Liver Qi

Distention and wandering pain in the hypochondriac region aggravated by emotional upset, accompanied by fullness sensation in the chest, poor appetite, frequent belching, irritability, poor sleep, thin white coating, and wiry pulse.

2. Damp—heat Retention in the Liver and Gallbladder

Stabbing pain with burning sensation particularly on the right hypochondriac region is accompanied by chills and fever during the acute pain, bitter taste in the mouth, irritability, nausea and vomiting, congested eyes, short scanty urine, red tongue proper with yellow coating, and wiry rapid pulse.

3. Blood Stasis Type

Localized pain with pricking sensation aggravated at night, severe pain worse by pressing with also possible hypochondriac mass, dark purplish tongue proper and deep choppy pulse.

4. Liver *Yin* Deficiency Type

Dull pain of a lingering nautre in both hypochondriac regions, dry mouth, restlessness, blurred vision, dizziness, afternoon fever, spontaneous sweating, red tongue with less coating, and thin rapid pulse.

Treatment

1. Stagnation of Liver *Qi*

Principle: Soothe the liver, regulate *Qi* circulation, and stop pain by needling points mainly from The Liver Channel of Foot—*Jueyin,* The Gallbladder Channel of Foot—*Shaoyang* and The Bladder Channel of Foot—*Taiyang*.

Prescription: Qimen (LR14) Ganshu (BL18)

Taichong (LR 3) Zhigou (SJ 6)

Yanglingquan (GB34)

Explanation: Qimen (LR14), the Front—*Mu* point of the liver, has the effect of soothing the liver and regulating *Qi* circulation in combination with Ganshu (BL18). Taichong (LR 3), the *Yuan*—source point of the liver channel, in combination with Zhigou (SJ 6) and Yanglingquan (GB34), may soothe the depressed liver *Qi* and regulate the circulation of *Qi* of the *shaoyang* channels. The joint use of the above points helps restore the function of the liver in maintaining the free flow of *Qi* and normal *Qi* mechanism, and relieve pain.

Point Modification: Add Zhongwan(RN12) and Weishu (BL21) for fullness sensation in the chest and belching; Daling (PC 7) and Shenmen (HT 7) for poor sleep.

Method: Apply filiform needles with reducing method and retain the needles for 15—20 minutes manipulating them two to three times.

2. Damp—heat Retention in the Liver and Gallbladder

Principle: Clear heat, resolve dampness, soothe the liver and promote the function of the gallbladder by needling points mainly from The Liver Channel of Foot—*Jueyin* and The Gallbladder Channel of Foot—*Shaoyang*.

Prescription: Qimen (LR14)   Riyue (GB24)

                  Zhigou (SJ 6)   Yanglingquan (GB34)

                  Qiuxu (GB40)   Xingjian (LR 2)

Explanation: Qimen (LR14) and Riyue(GB24), points where the *Qi* of the liver and gallbladder flows together, can be used with reducing method to regulate *Qi,* and blood in the liver and gallbladder. Zhigou (SJ 6) and Yanglingquan (GB34), points in set for hypochondriac pain, have the function to regulate *Qi* of the *Shaoyang* channels. These two points in combination with Qiuxu (GB40) and Xingjian (LR 2), respective the *Yuan*—source point of the gallbladder channel and the *Ying*—spring point of the liver channel, have the function to clear up the damp—heat from the liver and gallbladder. These six points in combination are able to clear up heat, resolve dampness, soothe the liver, promote the function of the gallbladder, and stop pain.

Point Modification: Add Guanchong (SJ 1) for severe fever; Zhongwan(RN12) and Neiguan(PC 6) for nausea and vomiting; and Ximen(PC 4) for restlessness.

Method: Apply filiform needles with reducing method and retain the needles for 15—20 minutes, manipulating them two to three times.

3. Blood Stasis Type

Principle: Activate the circulation of *Qi* and blood, resolve blood stasis and stop pain by needling points mainly from The Liver Channel of Foot—*Jueyin* and The Bladder Channel of Foot—*Taiyang*.

Prescription: Geshu (BL17)　Ganshu (BL18)
　　　　　　　Taichong (LR 3)　Sanyinjiao (SP 6)
　　　　　　　Qimen (LR14)　Zhigou (SJ 6)

Explanation: Geshu (BL17), the Influential Point of blood, in combination with Ganshu (BL18) and Sanyinjiao (SP 6), may resolve the blood stasis by activating blood circulation. Qimen (LR14) and Taichong (LR 3) soothe the liver, regulate the circulation of *Qi* and blood and remove the blood stasis. Zhigou (SJ 6) promotes the *Qi* circulation of the *Sunjiao* in a way to activate *Qi* and blood circulation. The hypochondriac pain may disappear spontaneously when the circulation of blood returns to its normal status.

Point Modification: Add local Ahshi points provided that the pain in the hypochondrium is ascribed to traumatic factors.

Method: Apply filiform needles with reducing method and retain the needles for 15—20 minutes, manipulating them two to four times.

4. Liver *Yin* Deficiency Type

Principle: Nourish *Yin* and blood, regulate *Qi* circulation and relieve pain by needling points selected mainly from The Bladder Channel of Foot—*Taiyang* and The Stomach Channel of Foot—*Yangming*.

Prescription: Ganshu (BL18)   Shenshu (BL23)
 Qimen (LR14)   Taichong (LR 3)
 Zusanli (ST36)   Sanyinjiao (SP 6)

Explanation: Ganshu (BL18) and Shenshu (BL23) in combination with Qimen (LR14), the Front—*Mu* point of the liver, and Taichong (LR 3), the *Yuan*—source point of the liver channel, replenish the essence, nourish blood, soothe the liver and relieve pain. Zusanli (ST36) and Sanyinjiao (SP 6) strengthen the spleen and stomach, the source for providing the acquired energy, to reinforce the manufacturing of *Qi* and blood. The joint use of these points replenish both *Yin* and blood, nourish the channles and collaterals, and stop pain.

Point Modification: Add Gaohuangshu(BL43) for tidal fever; Baihui(DU20) and Fengchi(GB20) for dizziness and vertigo.

Method: Apply filiform needles with reinforcing method and retain the needles for 20—30 minutes, manipulating them once or twice.

Alternative Treatment

1. Auricular Acupuncture

Prescription: Liver Gallbladder Ear—shenmen Chest
 Subcortex

Method: Apply filiform needles with moderate stimulation and retain the needles for 20 minutes. Embedding of subcutaneous needles or ear seeds is also applicable.

2. Plum—blossom Needling

Prescription: The tenderness in the hypochondriac region, and three Back—*Shu* points at the same level, respectively superior, inferior and horizontal to the tender point.

Method: Tap gently till local redness with moisture appears, which is then followed by cupping. Such a method is contraindicated in hypochondriac pain due to traumatic injuries.

1.20 Dizziness Syndrome

Dizziness is the general term for blurred vision and vertigo. The former refers to visionary sparkling or the blurring of vision with darkness appearing in front of the eyes. The latter refers to a subjective feeling that the body or surrounding objects are turning around with difficulty to keep balance. They are always mentioned together since both may appear at the same time. Mild dizziness may be stopped by instant closing of the eyes. In the severe case, the patient feels as if he is on a fast—moving train or sailing boat that makes him unable to stand firmly. It may be accompanied by nausea, vomiting, sweating or fainting in more severe condition.

Dizziness may be seen in many cases in modern medicine such as auditory vertigo, cerebral arteriosclerosis, hypertention, hypotention, vertebrobasilar ischemia, anemia, neurasthenia and those cerebral conditions with dizziness as the main symptom. For the above mentioned conditions, the differentiation and treatment in this section can be referred to.

Cause and Mechanism

Dizziness is mostly due to melancholy and excessive anger

that consumes the liver *Yin* and results in hyperactivity of liver *Yang* disturbing the head; or injured *Qi* of the heart and spleen by weakness after prolonged illness or overthinking that leads to hypofunction of the spleen in the manufacturing of *Qi* and blood, and poor nourishment of the brain; or emptiness of the marrow sea and over consumption of the kidney essence caused by over sexual indulgence. A diet of greasy and sweet food may on the other hand cause impairment of the digestive function of the spleen and stomach leading to the assembled dampness to form phlegmatic obstruction in the middle—*Jiao*. Such a phlegmatic obstruction impairs the normal ascending of clear *Yang* and descending of turbid *Yin*, thus giving rise to the onset of dizziness and vertigo.

Differentiation

1. Hyperactivity of Liver *Yang*

The chief manifestations include dizziness, tinnitus, distending pain in the head aggravated by overstrain or shortness of temper, flushed face, congested eyes, irritability, dream—disturbed sleep, bitter taste in the mouth, red tongue proper with thin yellow coating, and wiry rapid pulse.

2. Deficiency of *Qi* and Blood

The chief manifestations include dizziness, blurred vision aggravated by exertion or overstrain, pale complexion, poor spirit, palpitation and insomnia, pallor lips and nails, shortness of breath, reluctant speech, weak limbs, poor appetite, pale tongue proper, and thin weak pulse.

3. Deficiency of Kidney Essence

The chief manifestations include dizziness, poor memory, weakness of the lumbus and knees, seminal emission, tinnitus, and poor sleep. Patients with kidney *Yang* deficiency may also have cold limbs, pale tongue proper with thin deep pulse. Patients with kidney *Yin* deficiency may also have feverish palms, soles and chest, night sweating, red tongue proper with thin wiry pulse.

4. Phlegm—damp Obstruction in the Middle—*Jiao*

The chief manifestations include dizziness, lassitude, heaviness of head, nausea, vomiting, fullness in the chest and epigastrium, sticky mouth with no thirst, poor appetite, dream—disturbed sleep, numbness of the limbs, white greasy tongue coating, and soft slippery pulse.

Treatment

1. Hyperactivity of Liver *Yang*

Principle: Nourish *Yin* and reduce hyperactivity of liver *Yang*, calm the liver, quench the liver wind by needling points mainly from The Liver Channel of Foot—*Jueyin* and The Kidney Channel of Foot—*Shaoyin*.

Prescription: Fengchi (GB20) Taichong (LR 3)
Xiaxi (GB43) Ganshu (BL18)
Shenshu (BL23) Taixi (KI 3)

Explanation: Fengchi (GB20) in combination with Taichong(LR 3) and Xiaxi(GB43), respectively the *Yuan*—source point of the liver channel and the *Ying*—spring point of the gallbladder channel, may soothe the liver, quench the liver wind, and clear away the pathogenic heat from the liver and gallbladder. This is a method for treating the symptomatic *Biao*. Ganshu (BL18) nourishes liver *Yin*. Shenshu (BL23) and Taixi (KI 3) reinforce kidney *Yin*. This is the method to deal with the root cause *Ben*. The joint use of these points nourish *Yin* and reduce *Yang*, soothe the liver, quench the wind, and relieve the dizziness.

Method: Apply filiform needles with both reinforcing and reducing methods. Reducing method is applied at Fengchi (GB 20), Taichong (LR 3) and Xiaxi (GB43); and reinforcing method at Shenshu (BL23), Taixi (KI 3) and Ganshu (BL18). Retain the needles for 20—30 minutes, manipulating them three to four times.

2. Deficiency of *Qi* and Blood

Principle: Invigorate *Qi,* nourish blood, strengthen the spleen and stomach by needling points mainly from The Bladder Channel of Foot—*Taiyang* and The Stomach Channel of Foot—*Yangming*.

Prescription: Zusanli (ST36) Sanyinjiao (SP 6)
               Pishu (BL20) Shenshu (BL23)
               Guanyuan (RN 4) Baihui (DU20)

Explanation: Zusanli (ST36), Sanyinjiao (SP 6) and Pishu (BL20) are selected to strengthen the spleen and stomach in providing the acquired energy for transforming essence and manufactring blood to replenish the acquired source of *Qi* and blood. Shenshu (BL23) and Guanyuan (RN 4) may invigorate the *Yuan*—source *Qi,* and Baihui (DU20) to help ascend both *Qi* and blood. The joint use of these points can ease the dizziness by means of replenishing *Qi* and blood.

Point Modification: Add Neiguan (PC 6) and Shenmen (HT 7) for palpitation and insomnia.

Method: Apply filiform needles with reinforcing method and retain the needles for 15—30 minutes, manipulating them two to three times. Moxibustion may also be applied to Pishu (BL20), Zusanli (ST36) and Guanyuan (RN 4) for 10 minutes. Baihui

(DU20) is mainly applied with moxibustion for 30 minutes.

3. Defieicny of Kidney Essence

Principle: Reinforce kidney and tonify the *Yuan*–source *Qi* by needling points mainly from The Kidney Channel of Foot–*Shaoyin* and The *Ren* Channel.

Prescription: Guanyuan (RN 4)   Shenshu (BL23)
Taixi (KI 3)   Zusanli (ST36)

Explanation: Guanyuan (RN 4) is used to strengthen *Yuan*–source *Qi*. Shenshu (BL23) and Taixi (KI 3) are used to reinforce the kidney *Yin*. Zusanli (ST36) is used to regulate the function of the spleen and stomach in manufacturing essence and blood. Dizziness can be spontaneously eased if the kidney essence is replenished and the sea of marrow is nourished.

Point Modification: Add moxibustion to Mingmen (RN 4), Baihui (DU20) for deficiency of kidney *Yang*.

Method: Apply filiform needles with reinforcing method and retain the needles for 15–30 minutes, manipulating them one to three times. Moxibustion is also applicable to Guanyuan (RN 4) and Shenshu (UB23) in addition to acupuncture.

4. Phlegm–damp Obstruction in the Middle–*Jiao*

Principle: Strengthen spleen, pacify the stomach, eliminate phlegm and resolve the dampness by needling points mainly from The Stomach Channel of Foot–*Yangming* and Back–*Shu* as well as Front–*Mu* points.

Prescription: Zhongwan (RN12)   Pishu (BL20)
Zusanli (ST36)   Fenglong (ST40)
Baihui (DU20)   Neiguan (PC 6)

Explanation: Zhongwan (RN12), the Front–*Mu* point of the stomach, in combination with Pishu (BL20), Zusanli (ST36) and

Fenglong (ST40) are able to strengthen spleen, pacify the stomach and resolve phlegm and dampness. Baihui (DU20) ascends the clear *Yang* and regulates the *Qi* of the channel in the local area. Neiguan (PC 6) is used to relieve fullness sensation in the chest, regulate qi, pacify the stomach and stop vomiting. The joint use of these points may adjust the *Qi* of the spleen and stomach, resolve dampness, separate the clean from the turbid, and relieve the dizziness.

Method: Apply filiform needles with even method, or with reducing method and retain the needles for 15–20 minutes, manipulating them two to three times.

Alternative Treatment

1. Auricular Acupuncture

Prescription: Kidney Ear–shenmen Subcortex
Inner ear

Method: Apply filiform needles with moderate stimulation and retain the needles for 15–30 minutes. Besides, either embedding of ear seeds or subcutaneous needles is applicable.

2. Scalp Acupuncture

Prescription: Bilateral dizzy–auditory areas

Method: Apply moderate stimulation at the dizzy–auditory areas and retain the needles for 30–40 minutes. Three to five minutes of needling rotation is repeated for two to three times in each treatment. Electric stimulation with dense–sparse wave for 40–60 minutes is also applicable.

1.21 Windstroke

Windstroke refers to a disease characterized by sudden fainting with loss of consciousness, hemiplegia, slurred speech, and deviation of eyes and mouth. Because of its abrupt onset and drastic changes bearing the wandering and changing nature of wind, it acquires the term windstroke by convention.

For many diseases such as cerebral hemorrhage, cerebral thrombosis, cerebral emblism, subarachaoid hemorrhage, cerebral angiospasm as well as their sequelae, the differentiation and treatment in this section can be referred to.

Cause and Mechanism

Windstroke is often caused by constitutional deficiency of *Qi* and blood and imbalance of *Yin* and *Yang* among the three organs of heart, liver and kidney. Emotional upset or depression, alcoholic indulgence, improper diet, over sexual indulgence or invasion of exogenous pathogenic factors can lead to a sudden rise of liver *Yang* that forces excessive flow of *Qi* and blood to ascend and the turbid dampness to disturb the clear organ. Therefore, the obstruction of channels and collaterals develops into windstroke attack. Upward distrubance of *Yang* and wind obstructing the clear organ is known as the obstructive windstroke. The windstroke will be manifested by collapse if such symptoms and signs appear as critical condition of the patient, exhaustion of *Yuan*—source energy and separation of *Yin* from *Yang*. However, there may also appear the windstroke that only involves *Qi* obstruction of the channels and collaterals with deviation of eyes and mouth and hemiplegia.

Differentiation

1. Windstroke Attacking the *Zangfu*

The condition is critical with sudden onset. It is manifested by sudden falling down, confused mental state, hemiplegia, running saliva from the mouth corner and rigid tongue. According to the difference in etiology and mechanism, it is further divided into obstructive type windstroke and collapsing type windstroke.

(1) Obstructive Type Windstroke

The chief manifestations include sudden falling down with loss of consciousness, locked jaws, clenched teeth, tight fists, rough sound due to phlegm in the throat, dysuria, constipation, thick yellow or grey dark tongue coating, and wiry slippery but forceful pulse.

(2) Collapsing Type Windstroke

The chief manifestations include sudden falling down with loss of consciousness, closed eyes, opening mouth, weak nasal breathing, incontinence of urine and stools, flaccid tongue and weak thready pulse. In the severe case, there may also appear cold limbs, flushed face, fainting pulse or rootless superficial pulse.

2. Windstroke Attacking The Channels and Collaterals

The condition is less severe than the last type of windstroke with a slow onset. The chief manifestations include hemiplegia, numbness of skin and limbs, deviation of mouth and eyes, rigid tongue with poor speech, yellow greasy tongue coating, and wiry or slippery slow pulse. It may also be accompanied by headache, dizziness and vertigo, mental depression and shortness of temper.

Treatment

1. Windstroke Attacking The *Zangfu*

(1) Obstructive Type Windstroke

Principle: Bring back resuscitation, quench the wind, eliminate fire and clear up phlegm by needling points mainly from The *Du* Channel, The Liver Channel of Foot- *Jueyin* plus some of the *Jing*—well points.

Prescription: Renzhong (DU26)   Laogong (PC 8)

Taichong (LR 3)　Yongquan (KI 1)

Fenglong (ST40)　12 *Jing*—well points

Explanation: Renzhong (DU26), the point for firstaid, is able to bring back resuscitation and clear up obstruction. Pricking the 12 *Jing*—well points helps to eliminate heat and bring back resuscitation. Laogong(PC 8), the *Ying*—spring point of the pericardium channel, is applied with reducing method to eliminate heat from the heart. Taichong(LR 3), the *Yuan*—source point of the liver channel, may soothe the circulation of liver *Qi,* sedate liver *Yang* and reomve obstruction of stasis in the channels and collaterals. Yongquan (KI 1), the *Jing*—well point of the kidney channel, guides the heat to flow downward. Fenglong (ST 40), the *Luo*—connecting point of the stomach channel, promote the *Qi* mechanism of the spleen and stomach and resolve dampness and phlegm. The joint use of the above points may quench liver wind, sedate fire, clear up phlegm and bring back resusciation.

Point Modification: Add Jiache (ST 6) and Dicang (ST 4) for locked jaws.

Method: Apply filiform needles with reducing method and retain the needles for 2—40 minutes, manipulating them three to five times. The *Jing*—well points are pricked with a three—edged needle to cause bleeding.

(2) Collapsing Type Windstroke

Principle: Reinforce *Yuan*—source *Qi* and restore *Yang Qi* from collapse by needling points mainly from The *Ren* Channel.

Prescription: Shenque (RN 8)　Qihai (RN 6)

Guanyuan (RN 4)

Explanation: The *Ren* Channel is the sea of the *Yin* channels. According to the principle of interdependence of *Yin* and *Yang* and the doctrine that "sole *Yang* will not grow if the sole *Yin* is not promoted," it is imperative to save *Yang* by reinforcing *Yin* if the original *Yang* is exhausted. Guanyuan (RN 4) intersects The *Ren* Channel with the three *Yin* channels of the foot as well as the place where *Qi* of the *SanJiao* infuses. It connects with the real *Yang* of the vital gate and a point from the *Yin* channel that contains part of the *Yang*. Qihai (RN 6), also named Dantian, is the point where *Qi* of the channel develops. Umbilicus is considered the root of life according to the theory of traditional Chinese medicine. Shenque(RN 8) is located in the center of the umbilicus, linking with the real life energy. Therefore, moxibustion is applied at these three points in order to restore the collapsed *Yang* energy. The regaining of *Yang* energy ensures the body consolidation and defence so that the patient can be saved from the collapse of *Yang Qi*.

Point Modification: Add Neiguan(PC 6) and Taiyuan(LU 9) for windstroke patients with fainting pulses; and Zusanli (ST 36) for cold limbs.

Method: Apply ignited moxa cones at these points till the stop of sweating, increase of body temperature and repulsation disregarding the number of moxa cones that will be used in the treatment.

2. Windstroke Attacking the Channels and Collaterals

Principle: Regulate the circulation of *Qi* and blood, quench the wind and reomove obstruction from channels and collaterals by needling the points mainly from The *Du* Channels plus points from the *Yang* channels on the affected side of the body.

Prescription: Baihui (DU20) Fengfu (DU16)

Renying (ST 9)

For hemiplegia involving the upper limb, add Jianyu (LI15), Quchi (LI11), Waiguan (SJ 5) and Hegu (LI 4); for hemiplegia involving the lower limb, add Huantiao (GB 30), yanglingquan(GB34), Fengshi (GB31) and Zusanli (ST36); for deviation of the eyes and mouth, add Jiache (ST 6), Dicang (ST 4), Xiaguan (ST 7), Hegu (LI 4) and Taichong (LR 3); and add Yamen (DU15) and Lianquan (RN23) for poor speech conducting.

Explanation: The *Du* Channel is the sea of the *Yang* channels. Baihui (DU20) and Fengfu (DU16) eliminate wind and remove obstruction from the channels and collaterals. Renying (ST 9), a point from the stomach channel that is more abundant with *Qi* and blood, is used to regulate the *Qi* and blood of the general body, and remove channel obstruction both in the upper and lower portion of the body. *Yang* dominates the body movement. Impaired body movement is related to the dysfunction of *Yang*. This is the reason why points from the three *Yang* channels of the hand and foot are used to promote and *Qi* and blood circulation in the channels and collaterals. The active antipathogenic *Qi* will help the recovery of body movement. Both distal and local points are used to regulate the circulation of *Qi* and eliminate wind for deviation of eyes and mouth. Yamen(DU15) and Lianquan (RN23) are used to strengthen the root of the tongue.

Method: Apply filiform needles with even method and retain the needles for 20–30 minutes, manipulating them one to three times. Points only from the affected side are selected for the first few treatments soon after the attack. Points from both sides are used for the subsequent treatments or for windstroke involving a longer history.

Alternative Treatment: Scalp Acupuncture

Prescription: Motor area   Speech area

Method: Apply filiform needles with continous rotating for three to five minutes out of every ten minutes and retain the needles for 30—40 minutes. Electric stimulation may also be applied for 60 minutes. Advise the patients to perfome exercices when the neeldes are rotated. This will help achieve better therapeutic effect.

1.22   Deviation of the Eye and Mouth

Deviation of eye and mouth, also called facial paralysis, is manifested by deviated eye and mouth and unilateral looseness of facial muscle. It may happen in patients at any age, but more common in the young and the middle aged. The disease is the same as the peripheral facial paralysis (Bell's paralysis) in modern medicine.

Cause and Mechanism

When the channels and collaterals are hypofunction, the pathogenic wind—cold may seize the chance to attack the *Yangming* and *Shaoyang* channels as well as the tendenomuscular structure, leading to the *Qi* obstruction of the channels, poor nourishment of the tendenomuscular structure and looseness of the facial muscles to develop the disease.

Differentiation

The onset of the disease is abrupt, mostly afftecting only one side of the face. Subsequently, the patient fcels a stiff and numb sensation on the affected side of the face. This is accompanied by incomplete closure of the eye, lacrimation, drop of the mouth corner, slivation and inability to frown, to raise the eyebrow, to blow out the cheek, to close the eye, to show the teeth or to whistle. Some patients may also complain pain in the posterioinferior auricular region and migraine. In severe cases, there may appear hypogeusthesia or ageusia on the anterior 2 / 3 of the tongue.

Treatment

Principle: Eliminate wind, remove obstruction from the channels and collaterals and regulate *Qi* and blood circulation by needling points mainly from The Large Intestine Channel of Hand—*Yangming* and The Stomach Channel of Foot—*Yangming*.

Prescription: Fengchi (GB20)   Yifeng (SJ17)

Yangbai (GB14)   Sibai (ST 2)

Taiyang (EX—HN5)   Dicang (ST 4)

Jiache (ST 6)   Yingxiang (LI20)

Hegu (LI 4)   Neiting (ST44)

Explanation: Fengchi (GB20) and Yifeng (SJ17), points of the *Shaoyang* channels, are able to eliminate wind and stop pain. Taiyang (EX—HN5), Yangbai (GB 14), Sibai (ST 2), Dicang (ST 4), Jiache (ST 6), Yingxiang (LI20) are local points to eliminate wind from the channels and collaterals and regulate the circulation of *Qi* and blood. Hegu (LI 4) and Neiting (ST44), points of the *Yangming* channels, have the effect of promoting the *Qi* circulation of the *Yangming* channels and eliminating wind from facial and head areas. The joint use of the above points may eliminate wind from the channels and collaterals, regulate *Qi* and blood and wram up the local muscle and tendenostructure in order to help the recovery of facial paralysis.

Point Modification: Add Zanzhu (BL 2) and Tongziliao (GB 1) for incomplete closure of the eye; add Chengjiang (RN24) or Jiachengjiang (Extra) for deviation of mentolabial sulcus; add Juliao (ST 3) for difficulty for showing the teeth; and add Wangu (GB12) and Waiguan (SJ 5) for pain in the posterioinferior auricular region.

Method: Apply filiform needles with even method and retain the needles for 15–20 minutes. Or, apply reducing method in the early period of the treatment and reinforcing method for later period of treatment. Needles are manipulated for one to three times during each treatment. Fengchi (GB20) and Yifeng (SJ17) for 15–20 minutes after acupuncture treatment. Penetrating method may also be applied from Yangbai (GB14) to Yuyao(Extra) from Dicang (ST 4) to Jiache (ST 6), and from Taiyang (EX–HN5) to Xiaguan (ST 7).

Alternative Treatment

1. Plum–blossom Needling Therapy

Prescription: Yangbai (GB14)   Taiyang (EX–HN5)
Sibai (ST 2)   Dicang (ST 4)   Jiache (ST 6)

Method: Tap these points with gentle stimulation till local redness appears once every other day. This kind of treatment is suitable for rehabilitation or sequela of facial paralysis.

2. Cupping

Prescription: Jiache (ST 6)   Xiaguan (ST 7)
Taiyang (EX–HN5)

Method: Apply cupping with small sizes of cups after acupuncture treatment once every two to three days. Each point is cupped for five to ten minutes. Cupping can also be applied after tapping with the plum–blossom needle.

3. Scar–causing Plastering

Prescription: Yifeng (SJ17)   Taiyang (EX–HN5)

Method: Stick the herbal plasters in the above mentioned areas. The patient will soon feel a feverish sensation or even burning sensation in the local area. Remove the plasters in two to three hours. At this time, there will be purplish colour in the local area. Some patients may have blisters of different sizes. Prick the blisters with a three—edged needle to let out the fluid in the blisters. No special handling is necessary.

1.23 Chest *Bi*—Syndrome

Chest *Bi*—syndrome refers to suffocating sensation, fullness and pain in the chest. There is only fullness as if the chest is being oppressed in the mild case, but angina pectoris, shortness of breath and asthmatic breathing in the severe cases. Since chest cavity is the anotomical residence of the heart and lungs, chest *Bi*—syndrome is closely related to the dysfunction of these two organs.

Chest *Bi*—syndrome is commonly seen in coronary arteriosclerotic cardiopathy in modern medicine. If the chest pain occurs as a major symptom in case of chroinc bronchitis, pulmonary emphysema, etc., the differentiation and treatment in this section can be referred to.

Cause and Mechanism

Chest *Bi*—syndrome is mostly caused by constitutional deficiency of either heart *Qi* or heart *Yang*, leading to the invasion of pathogenic cold. Cold retention in the interior and stagnation of *Qi* due to cold retention cause obstruction of the channels and collaterals.Impairment of the spleen and stomach due to improper diet such as over indulgence of sweet, greasy, raw or cold food can cause accumulation of phlegm–damp obstructing the chest *Yang*. Nevertheless, prolonged stagnation of *Qi* due to emotional disturbance cause poor blood circulation. And Stasis of blood in the vessels results in chest *Bi*–syndrome.

Differentiation

1. Deficient Cold Type

The chief manifestations include chest pain aggravated by cold and radiating towards the back, palpitation, fullness sensation in the chest, shortness of breath, aversion to cold, white greasy tongue coating, and deep thin pulse.

2. Turbid Phlegm Retention Type

The chief manifestations include stuffy sensation in the chest, chest pain radiating towards the back and shoulder, palpitation, shortness of breath, dyspnea, cough, profuse white sticky sputum, fullness in the epigastrium and abdomen, poor appetite, listlessness, white greasy tongue coating, and soft slow pulse.

3. Blood Stasis Type

The chief manifestations include paroxysmal pricking pain or colic pain in the chest radiating towards the shoulder and back, fullness of the chest, shortness of breath, palpitation, purplish lips, dark tongue proper, and thin uneven or intermittent pulse.

Treatment

1. Deficient Cold Type

Principle: Activate *Yang*, eliminate cold and promote the circulation of *Qi* and blood by needling points mainly from The Bladder Channel, The *Sun Jiao* Channel of Hand–*Shaoyang* and The Pericardium Channel of Hand–*Jueyin*.

Prescription: Xinshu (BL15) Juque (RN14)

Jueyinshu (BL14)   Danzhong (RN17)

Neiguan (PC 6)   Tongli (HT 5)

Explanation: Xinshu (BL15) and Juque (RN14), the combination of Front–*Mu* and Back–*Shu* points, may tonify the *Qi* of the heart and warm up heart *Yang*. Jueyinshu (BL14) and Danzhong (RN17), another combination of Front–*Mu* and Back–*Shu* points, may promote *Qi* circulation in the chest and eliminate cold. Neiguan (PC 6), the *Luo*–connecting point of the pericardium channel, is combined with Tongli (HT 5), the *Luo*–connecting point of the heart channel, to assist the above in eliminating cold, removing obstruction from the channels and collaterals, promoting the circulation of *Qi* and blood and stopping pain.

Point Modification: Add moxibustion at Feishu (BL18) and Fengmen (BL12) for aversion to cold; and moxibustion at Qihai (RN 6) and Guanyuan (RN 4) for cold limbs.

Method: Apply filiform needles with reinforcing or even method and retain the needles for 20–30 minutes, manipulating them two to three times. Moxibustion may also be applied at Xinshu (BL15) and Jueyinshu (BL14) in addition to acupuncture treatment for 10–15 minutes.

2. Turbid Phlegm Retention Type

Principle: Promote *Yang Qi* and resolve the pathogenic turbid dampness by needling points mainly from The *Ren* Channel, The Pericardium Channel of Hand–*Jueyin* and The Stomach Channel of Foot–*Yangming*.

Prescription: Juque (RN14)   Danzhong (RN17)

Ximen (PC 4)   Jianli (RN11)

Fenglong (ST40)   Sanyinjiao (SP 6)

Explanation: Juque (RN14) and Danzhong (RN17) are used in combination with the *Xi*−cleft point of the pericardium channel Ximen (PC 4) to activate heart *Yang*, promote *Qi* in the chest and stop pain. Jianli (RN11) warm up the middle−*Jiao*, strengthen the stomach and resolve dampness. Fenglong (ST40), the *Luo*−connecting point of the stomach channel, is combined with Sanyinjiao (SP 6) to strengthen spleen, pacify the stomach and resolve the turbid plegm. The joint use of the above points may promote *Yang Qi*, resolve dampness and phlegm, activate blood and stop pain.

Point Modification: Add Pishu (BL20), Xinshu (BL15) for spinal pain; and moxibustion at Qihai (RN 6) and Neiguan (PC 6) for shortness of breath.

Method: Apply filiform needles with reducing and retain the needles for 15−30 minutes, manipulating them two to three times.

3. Blood Stasis Type

Principle: Activate blood, resolve stasis and stop pain by needling points mainly from The Bladder Channel of Foot−*Taiyang*, The *Ren* Channel and The Heart Channel of Hand−*Shaoyin*.

Prescription: Zhiyang(DU 9) Yinxi(HT 6) Xinshu(BL15)
Juque (RN14) Geshu (BL17)
Danzhong (RN17)

Explanation: Zhiyang (DU 9) promotes the circulation of heart and eases heart pain. Yinxi (HT 6), the *Xi*−cleft point of the heart channel, is combined with Juque (RN14) and Xinshu (BL15) to regulate both *Qi* and blood, resolve stasis and stop pain. Geshu (BL17) and Danzhong (RN17) are used to promote *Qi* circulation and activate blood. The joint use of the above points may promote the circulation of both *Qi* and blood, and resolve the blood stasis so that the pain will ease.

Point Modification: Add Shaochong (HT 9) and Zhongchong (PC 9) by pricking with a three—edged needle to cause bleeding for purplish lips and tongue.

Method: Apply filiform needles with reducing method and retain the needles for 15–30 minutes, manipulating them two to three times.

Alternative Treatment: Auricular Acupuncture

Prescription: Heart Small intestine Ear—shenmen
Sympathetic Subcortex Lung chest

Method: Apply filiform needles at three to four points with moderate stimulation and retain the needles for 20 minutes. Embedding of ear seeds or subcutaneous needles is also applicable.

1.24 Palpitation

Palpitation is cardiac condition charaterized by unduely rapid heart beat with nervousness and anxiety. It generally occurs in paroxymal attacks. Such attacks or their aggravated conditions are often the consequence of emotional disturbance or overstrain.

Cause and Mechanism

Palpitation is mostly due to constitutional deficieny of heart *Qi* or insufficiency of heart blood related to prolonged illness. Sudden frightenings or fear cause the disturbed heart and mind because "the heart loses its reliance and the mind has no place to house." Impairment of the spleen due to improper diet can cause phlegm—fluid retention in the interior. Overthinking or overstrain can cause stagnation of *Qi* turning into fire and phlegm—fluid disturbance in the interior. Pathogenic wind, cold, dampness and heat affecting the heart in chronic *Bi*—syndrome causes *Qi* stagnation and blood stasis obstructing the blood vessels of the heart.

Differentiation

1. Heart—mind Disturbance Type

The chief manifestations include palpitation, easy frightening or fear, restlessness, dream—distrubed sleep that often wakens the patient, poor appetie, thin white tongue coating, and rapid thready pulse.

2. *Qi* and Blood Deficiency Type

The chief manifestations include palpiation, restlessness, shortness of breath, lassitude, pallor complexion, dizziness, vertigo, pale tongue proper, and weak thready or choppy pulse.

3. Plegm—fire Disturbance Type

The chief manifestations include intermittent palpitation, restlessness, fullness sensation in the chest,dizziness, insomnia with dream—disturbed sleep, easy frightenings, forgetfulness, bitter taste in the mouth, cough, with sticky sputum, yellow urine, slightly dry stools, yellow greasy tongue coating, and rapid slippery pulse.

4. Blood Stasis Type

Worsening palpitation for years asthmatic breathing up on exertion, occasional cardiac pain, sallow emaciated complexion, and thready, choppy pulse. In severe cases, there may appear cold limbs, asthmatic breathing that makes it difficult for the patient to lie down, cold sweating, and puffiness.

Treatment

1. Heart—mind Disturbance Type

Principle: Calm the heart and mind and sedate frightenings by needling points mainly from The Heart Channel of Hand–Shaoyin, and The Pericardium Channel of Hand–*Jueyin*.

Prescription: Shenmen (HT 7)   Xinshu (BL15)
　　　　　　 Neiguan (PC 6)   Jianshi (PC 5)
　　　　　　 Juque (RN14)

Explanation: Shenmen (HT 7), the *Yuan*–source point of the heart, is combined with Jianshi (PC 5) and Neiguan (PC 6) to calm the heart and mind, sedate the patient from frightening and tranquilize the palpitation. Xinshu (BL14) and Juque (RN14), the combination of Back–*Shu* and Front–*Mu* points, regulate and reinforce the heart *Qi*. The joint use of the above points may stop frightening, calm the mind and heart and ease the palpitation.

Point Modification: Add Daling (PC 7) for easy frightenings.

Method: Apply filiform needles with reinforcing method and retain the needles for 15–30 minutes, manipulating them one to two times.

2. *Qi* and Blood Defieicny Type

Principle: Strengthen *Qi*, nourish blood and sedate palpitation by needling points mainly from The Bladder Channel, The *Ren* Channel and The Heart Channel of Hand–*Shaoyin*.

Prescription: Xinshu (BL15)   Juque (RN14)
　　　　　　 Geshu (BL 17)   Pishu (BL20)
　　　　　　 Zusanli (ST36)   Qihai (RN 6)
　　　　　　 Shenmen (HT 7)   Neiguan (PC 6)

Explanation: Xinshu (BL15) and Juque (RN14) tonify heart and promote heart *Yang*. Geshu (BL17), the Influential Point of blood, may tonify blood and nourish the heart and mind. Pishu (BL20), Zusanli (ST36) strenghten the spleen and stomach in order to promote the source for providing the acquired energy.

Qihai (RN 6)reinforces *Qi*. Shemen (HT 7) and Neiguan (PC 6) calm the heart and mind. The joint use of the above points may reinforce *Qi* and nourish blood, calm the mind and ease palpitation.

Point Modification: Add Baihui (DU20) and Fengchi (GB20) for dizziness and vertigo.

Method: Apply filiform needles with reinforcing method and retain the needles for 15–30 minutes, manipulating them two to three times. The Back–*Shu* points, Zusanli (ST 36) and Qihai (RN 6) may be applied with both acupuncture and moxibustion.

3. Phlegm–fire Disturbance Type

Principle: Eliminate fire, resolve phlegm and calm the heart and mind by needling points mainly from the three *Yin* channels of the hand and The Stomach Channel of Foot–*Yangming*.

Prescription: Lingdao (HT 4)　Ximen (PC 4)

Feishu (BL13)　Chize (LU 5)

Fenglong (ST40)　Yanglingquan (GB34)

Explanation: Lingdao (HT 4) and Ximen (PC 4) calm the heart and mind and ease palpitation. Chize (LU 5) and Feishu (BL13) sedate lung fire. Fenglong (ST 40) and Yanglingquan (GB 34) eliminate fire from the liver and stomach, descend the adverse flow of *Qi* and resolve dampness. The joint use of the above points may eliminate heat, resolve dampness, calm the heart and mind so as to ease palpitation.

Point Modification: Add Lidui(ST45) for insomnia, dreamdisturbed sleep and forgetfulness; Jianshi(PC 5) for restlessness; and Dachangshu(BL25) for constipation.

Method. Apply filiform needles with reducing method and retain the needles for 15–20 minutes, manipulating them two to

three times.

4. Blood Stasis Type

Principle: Activate blood, resolve blood stasis, strengthen the heart and ease palpitation by needling points mainly from The Heart Channel of Hand—*Shaoyin,* The Pericardium Channel of Hand—*Jueyin* and The Bladder Channel of Foot—*Taiyang*.

Prescription: Neiguan (PC 6) Quze (PC 3)

Shaohai(HT 3) Geshu(BL17)

Qihai(RN 6)

Explanation: Pericardium is the palace of heart. Therefore, Neiguan (PC 6) is combined with Quze (PC 3) and Shaohai (HT 3) to strengthen the heart and ease palpitation and pain. These three points are aimed to deal with the symptomatic *Biao*. Qihai (RN 6) reinforces *Yang Qi*. Geshu (RN17) activates blood and resolve blood stasis, aiming at dealing with the root cause *Ben*.

Method: Apply filiform needles with even method and retain the needles for 15—30 minutes, manipulating them one to two times.

Alternative Treatment: Auricular Acupuncture

Prescription: Heart Sympathetic Ear—Shenmen

Subcortex Small intestine

Method: Apply filiform needles with mild stimulation and retain the needles for 15—20 minutes. Embedding of ear seeds is also apllicable.

1.25 Insomnia

Insomnia is a condition that makes the patient unable to acquire normal hours of sleep. It is usually accompanied by dizziness, headache, palpitation and poor memory. However, insomnia does present different clinical manifestations. In the mild cases, there may be difficulty to fall into sleep, dream—disturbed sleep that often wakes up the patient with frightening or makes him unable to fall into sleep again. In severe cases, there can often be no sleep for the whole night.

Cause and Mechanism

Insomnia can be due to various causative factors. Impairment of the heart and spleen by overthinking or overstrain causes insufficiency of *Qi* and blood which fail to nourish the heart and calm the mind. Impairment of the kidney due to sexual indulgence cancause kidney *Yin* deficiency and hyperactive fire that leads to dysharmony between the heart *Yang* and kidney *Yin*. Impairment of the spleen and stomach due to improper diet leads to excessive accumulation of dampness and phlegm. And stagnant phlegm produces fire which flares up to disturb the heart and mind. Stagnation of liver *Qi* turning into fire due to emotional disturbance can cause flaring up of liver fire to disturb the heart and mind, resulting in insomnia.

Differentiation

1. Deficiency of Heart and Spleen

The chief manifestations include difficulty to fall into sleep if waked up during sleep, dream—disturbed sleep that can often wake up the patient, palpitation, poor memory, general lassitude, pallor complexion, poor appetite, epigastric distention, loose stools, pale tongue proper, thin white tongue coating, and feeble thready pulse.

2. Dysharmongy Between the Heart and Kidney

The chief manifestations include restlessness, poor sleep, dizziness, tinnitus, dry mouth with lack of fluid, feverish sensation in the palms and soles, poor memory, palpitation, seminal emission, lumbar sourness, red tongue proper with less coating, and thin rapid pulse.

3. Derangement of Stomach

The chief manifestations include poor sleep disturbed by dreams, feverish sensation in the chest, distention or distending pain in the epigastrium and abdomen, occasional nausea or vomiting, belching, acid regurgitation, difficult defecation, yellow greasy tongue coating, and slippery or wiry pulse.

4. Flaring up of Liver Fire

The chief manifestations include dizziness, head distention, restlessness, shortness of temper, difficulty to fall into sleep, probable congested eyes, bitter taste in the mouth and hypochondriac pain, thin yellow tongue coating, and wiry rapid pulse.

Treatment

1. Deficiency of Heart and Spleen

Principle: Reinforce heart and spleen, nourish blood and calm the mind by needling points mainly from The Heart Channel of Hand—*Shaoyin,* The Spleen Channel of Foot—*Taiyin* and The Bladder Channel of Foot—*Yangming*.

Prescription: Pishu(BL20) Xinshu(BL15) Yinbai(SP 1)
               Shenmen(HT 7) Sanyinjiao(SP 6)

Explanation: Pishu (BL20) and Xinshu(BL15) reinforce heart and spleen. Yinbai(SP 1), the *Jing*—well point of the spleen channel, can treat patient for dream—disturbed sleep with frightenings, Sanyinjiao(SP 6) and Shenmen(HT 7) reinforce *Qi,* nourish blood and calm the mind. The joint use of the above points can reinforce heart and spleen, strengthen *Qi,* produce blood and calm the heart and mind so that sleep will become normal again.

Point Modification: Add Zhishi (BL52) and Baihui (BL20) for poor memory.

Method: Apply filiform needles with reinforcing method and retain the needles for 15—30 minutes. Moxibustion is also applicable.

2. Dysharmony Between Heart and Kidney

Principle: Regain the harmony between heart and kidney by needling points mainly from The Urinary Bladder Channel of Foot—*Taiyang*, The Kidney Channel of Foot—*Shaoyin* and The Heart Channel of Hand—*Shaoyin*.

Prescription: Xinshu(BL15) Shenshu(BL23) Taixi(KI 3)
Daling(PC 7) Shenmen(HT 7) Zhaohai(KI 6)

Explanation: Xinshu(BL15) and Daling(PC 7) are combined with Shenmen(HT 7) to sedate heart fire, relieve frightened feelings and calm the mind. Shenshu(BL23) is combined with Taixi(KI 3), the *Yuan*—source point of the kidney channel, to promote kidney water. Zhaohai(KI 6) reinforces kidney *Yin*, eliminate heart from heart and calm the heart and mind. The joint use of the above points may help descend heart to meet the ascending kidney water so that heart and kidney will be harmonious state and heart and mind will be calmed.

Point Modification: Add Fengchi(GB20) for dizziness; Tinggong(SI 19) for tinnitus; and Zhishi(BL52) for seminal emission.

Method: Apply filiform needles with both reinforcing and reducing method and retain the needles for 15—30 minutes, manipulating them two to three times.

3. Deragnement of Stomach *Qi*

Principle: Strengthen the spleen and stomach, eliminate

dampness and resolve phlegm by needling points mainly from The *Ren* Channel, The Stomach Channel of Foot—*Yangming* and The Spleen Channel of Foo—*Taiyin*.

Prescription: Zhongwan(RN12) Fenglong(ST40)
Zusanli (ST36) Lidui (ST45) Yinbai (SP 1)
Shenmen (HT 7)

Explanation: Zhongwan(RN 12), the Front—*Mu* point of the stomach, is combined with the *Luo*—connecting point of the stomach channel, and Zusanli (ST36), the *He*—sea point of the stomach channel, to pacify the stomach, appeace the middle—*Jiao* and resolve phlegm. Lidui (ST 45) and Yinbai(SP 1), respectively the ending point of the stomach channel and the starting point of the spleen channel, are indicated in insomnia with dream—disturbed sleep. Shenmen(HT 7) calms the heart and mind. The joint use of the above points may pacify the stomach and relieve insomnia.

Point Modification: Add Neiguan(PC 6) for feverish sensation in the chest and nausea.

Method: Apply filiform needles with reducing method and retain the needles for 15—30 minutes, manipulating them two to three times.

4. Flaring up of Liver Fire

Principle: Eliminate liver fire, moisten *Yin* and sedate hyperactive *Yang* by needling points mainly from The Gallbladder Channel of Foot—*Shaoyang,* The Liver Channel of Foot—*Jueyin* and The Heart Channel of Hand—*Shaoyin*.

Prescription: Ganshu(BL18) Danshu(BL19)
Xingjian (LR 2) Foot—Qiaoyin (GB44)
Shenmen (HT 7)

Explanation: Ganshu(BL18) and Xingjian(LR 2) sedate liver fire, benifit *Qi* and nourish *Yin*. Danshu(BL19) and Foot—Qiaoyin(GB44) sedate fire from the gallbladder and relieve restlessness. Shenmen(HT .7) calms the heart and mind. The joint use of the above points may sedate fire from the liver and gallbladder, benifit *Yin*, sedate *Yang* and relieve insomnia.

Point Modification: Add Taiyang(EX—HN5) for congested eyes.

Method: Apply filiform needles with reducing method and retain the needles for 15—20 minutes, mani pulating them two to three times. Taiyang (EX—HN5) can be pricked with a three—edged needle to cause bleeding.

Alternative Treatment

1. Auricular Acupun cture

Prescription: Subcortex Sympathetic Ear—Shenmen Heart Spleen Kidney Endocrine

Method: Apply filiform needles at three to five points with mild stimulation and retain the needles for 30 minutes. Embedding of ear seeds or subcutaneous needles is also applicable.

2. Plum—blossom Needling Therapy

Prescription: Sishencong (EX—HN 1) Anmian Huatuojiaji

Method: Tap with mild stimulation untill local redness appears. Tap the Huatuojiaji points from top down to the bottom repeatedly for two to three times. Treatment is given once every other day.

1.26 Somnolence

Somnolence, Known as sleepiness or drwosiness, is characterized by low spirit with drowsiness that bothers the patient all day long, being easily waked up during the state of drowsiness and falling asleep soon after the awakened state.

In modern medicine, for such conditions as paroxysmal sleeping, neurosis and psychosis with similar symptoms to somnolence, the differentiation and treatment in this section can be referred to.

Differentiation

1. Excessive Dampness Accumulating in the Spleen

The chief manifestations include drowsiness as if the head is wrapped up, general heavy sensation, lassitude, fullness sensation in the chest, anorexia, nausea or puffiness, white greasy tongue coating and soft slow pulse.

2. Deficiency of Spleen *Qi*

The chief manifestations include sleepiness after meal, general lassitude that is relieved after quarters of sleeping, sallow complexion, poor appetite, loose stools, thin white tongue coating, and deficient weak pulse.

3. Deficiency and Decline of *Yang Qi*

The chief manifestations include full drowsiness in the day, reluctant speech, poor spirit, cold limbs, poor memory, pale tongue proper, yellow coating, and feeble thready pulse.

4. Blood Stasis Obstruction

The chief manifestations include dizziness, headache, drowsiness from time to time, general lassitude, poor memory, dark purplish tongue proper with purplish spots, and deep unsmooth pulse. Some patients may have traumatic history of the head.

Treatment

1. Excessive Dampness Accumulating in the Spleen

Principle: Strengthen the spleen, resolve dampness and invigorate the spirit by needling points mainly from The Spleen Channel of Foot—*Taiyin,* The Stomach Channel of Foot—*yangming* and The *Du* Channel.

Prescription: Zhongwan(RN12)   Fenglong(ST40)
Yinlingquan(SP 9) Baihui(DU20)
Taiyang(EX—HN5)

Explanation: Zhongwan (RN 12) is combined with Fenglong (ST 40), the *Luo*—connecting point of the stomach channel, and Yinlingquan (SP 9), the *He*—sea point of the spleen channel, to strengthen the spleen, pacify the stomach and resolve dampness.

Baihui (DU20) and Taiyang (EX—HN5) clear the mind state. The joint use of the above points may strengthen the spleen, resolve dampness, and clear the mind and brain.

Point Modification: Add Zusanli (ST36) and Neiguan (PC 6) for poor appetie and nausea.

Method: Apply filiforn needles with reinforcing or even method and retain the needles for 15—20 minutes, manipulating them two to three times.

2. Deficiency of Spleen *Qi*

Principle: Strengthen spleen *Qi* and clear the mind by needling points mainly from The Spleen Channel of Foot—*Taiyin* and The Stomach Channel of Foot—*Yangming,* plus some Back—*Shu* and Front—*Mu* points.

Prescription: Pishu(BL20)   Zhangmen(LR13)
Yinbai(SP 1)   Zusanli (ST36)
Jiexi (ST41)   Baihui (DU20)

Explanation: Pishu(BL20) and Zhangmen(LR13), the combination of Back—*Shu* and Front—*Mu* points, reinforce spleen *Qi.* Yinbai (SP 1), the *Jing*—well point of the spleen channel, reinforces spleen *Qi* and resolves dampness from the spleen. Jiexi (ST 41), the *Jing*—river point of the stomach channel, pertains to fire according to the five element theory. It is the mother of earth. It is used in combination with Zusanli(ST 36), the *He*—sea point of the stomach channel, to strengthen functions of the spleen and stomach as well as the transformation and transportation. Baihui(DU 20) clears the brain and invigorates the spirit. The joint use of the above points may strengthen the *Qi* of the spleen so that spleeen will regain its normal transformation and transportation, and the clear *Yang* will be ascended to invigorate the spirit.

Method: Apply filiform needles with reinforcing method and retain the needles for 20—30 minutes, manipulating them one to two times. Moxibustion can also be applied at Pishu (BL20), Zhangmen (LR 13) and Zusanli (ST 36).

3. Deficiency and Decline of *Yang Qi*

Principle: Reinforce and warm up the *Yang Qi* by needling points mainly from The Bladder Channel, The Spleen Channel of Foot—*Taiyin* and The Kidney Channel of Foot—*Shaoyin*.

Prescription: Gaohuangshu(BL43)   Shenshu(BL23)

Qihai (RN   6)   Sanyinjiao (SP   6)

Dazhong (KI   4)   Shenmai (BL62)

Explanation: Gaohuangshu (BL43) reinforces the deficient *Qi*. Shenshu (BL23) and Qihai (RN   6) warm up and strengthen kidney *Yang*. Sanyinjiao (SP   6) reinforces spleen *Qi* and regulates the *Qi* of the three *Yin* channels of the foot. Dazhong (KI   4), the *Luo*—connecting point of the kidney channel, reinforces and regulates the kidney *Qi*. Shenmai (BL 62), generated by The *Yangqiao* Channel, indicates in drowsiness. The joint use of the above points may reinforce the kidney and spleen, strengthen *Yang* and clear the mind.

Point Modification: Add Shenmen(HT 7) for poor memory.

Method: Apply filiform needles with reinforcing method and retain the needles for 15−30 minutes, manipulating them once or twice. Moxibustion can also be used at Gaohuangshu(BL43), Qihai (RN 6) and Shenshu(BL 23) for 10−15 minutes.

4. Blood Stasis Obstruction

Principle: Activate blood circulation, remove obstruction from the channels and collaterals, clear the mind and invigorate the spirit by needling points mainly from The Bladder Channel of Foot−*Taiyang*, The Stomach Channel of Foot−*Yangming* and The Liver Channel of Foot−*Jueyin*.

Prescription: Geshu(BL17) Ganshu(BL18)

Hegu(LI14) Taichong(LR 3)

Taiyang(EX−HN5) Baihui(DU20)

Explanation: Geshu (BL17) and Ganshu (BL18) soothe the liver *Qi*, activate blood and resolve blood stasis. Hegu (LI 4), having the ascending and dispersing, is good for activating the circulation of *Qi* and blood and remove obstruction from the channels and collaterals. Taichong (LR 3) soothes the liver and help to resolve blood stasis. It is used in combination with T jung (EX−HN5) and Baihui(DU20) to clear the mind and invigorate the spirit.

Method: Apply filiform needles with reducing method and retain the needles for 15−20 mintes, manipulating them two to three times.

1.27　Poor Memory

Poor memory refers to a condition characterized by hypomensia and forgetfulness. Refer to the differentiation and treatment for poor memory seen in patients suffering from neurasthenia, cerebral arteriosclerosis in modern medicine.

Cause and Mechanism

Although poor memory invloves a perplexing etiology, it is mostly caused by impairment of the heart and spleen as well as deficiency of heart and spleen due to overthinking. Kidney *Yin* deficiency due to excessive sexual indulgence may create a dysharmony between the heart and kidney, resulting in poor memory. Besides, poor nourishment of the brain due to kidney deficiency in the aged and deficiency of heart *Qi,* or obstruction of the heart by phlegm–fluid retention and blood stasis may also cause poor memory.

Differentiation

1.　Deficiency of Heart and Spleen

The chief manifestations include forgetfulness, listlessness, weakness of the four limbs, palpitation, poor sleep and appetite, shortness of breath, low voice, pallor complexion, pale tongue proper with teeth marks on the edge, thin white or white greasy tongue coating, and weak thready pulse.

2.　Dysharmony Between Heart and Kidney

The chief manifestations include forgetfulness, lumbar soreness, knee joint weakness or seminal emission, dizziness, tinnitus, or feverish sensation in the palms and soles, restlessness, poor sleep, red tongue proper, and thin rapid pulse.

3.　Aging–related Poor Spirit

The chief manifestations include forgetfulness, poor appetite, lassitude, trance, shortness of breath, lumbar soreness and knee joint weakness, frequent urination, palpitation, poor sleep, thin white tongue coating, and weak thready pulse.

4. Phlegm—fluid and Stasis Obstruction

The chief manifestations include forgetfulness, low speech, dull response, ecchymosis over the tongue, white greasy tongue coating, and slippery or thin rapid pulse.

Treatment

1. Deficiency of Heart and Spleen

Principle: Nourish heart and strengthen spleen by selecting mainly the Back—*Shu* points and points from The *Ren* Channel.

Prescription: Xinshu(BL15)   Pishu(BL20)

Geshu(BL17)   Qihai (RN 6)

Explanation: Xinshu(BL15) and Pishu(BL20) reinforce heart and spleen. The patient will be spiritful and sharp in response if the heart *Qi* is invigorating. The food essence can be normally absorbed and transported if the spleen does normal transporting and transforming. Geshu(BL17) tonifies blood while Qihai(RN 6) reinforces *Qi*. Only when there is aboundant *Qi* and blood to nourish the heart and spleen, can the founctions of the two organs become normal.

Method: Apply filiform needles with reinforcing method and retain the needles for 20—30 minutes, manipulating them one to two times. Moxibustion is also applicable for 10 minutes at each point.

2. Dysharmony Between Heart and Kidney

Principle: Regain the harmony between the heart and kidney by using mainly the Back—*Shu* points and points from the *Shaoyin* channels of both the hand and the foot.

Prescription: Xinshu(BL15) Taixi(KI 3) Shenshu(BL23)
Laogong(PC 8) Shenmen(HT 7)

Explanation: Xinshu(BL15) and Shenshu(BL23) reinforce the heart and kidney so the heart fire and kidney water can mutually assist each other. Taixi(KI 3) tonifies kidney water. Laogong(PC 8) eliminates heart fire. Shenmen(HT 7) tranquilizes the mind. The harmonized state between the heart and kidney ensures a clear mind and sharp response, provided that the kidney water is not deficient nor the heart fire is hyperactive.

Method: Apply filiform needles with both reinforcing and reducing methods. Xinshu(BL15), Shenshu(BL23) and Taixi(KI 3) are done with reinforcing method and Laogong(PC 8) and Shenmen(HT 7) with reducing method. Needles are retained for 15—20 minutes, manipulating them one to two times.

3. Aging—related Poor Spirit

Principle: Reinforce kidney, nourish heart, strengthen spleen and promote intellegence by using mainly the Back—*Shu* points and points of The Kidney Channel of Foot—*Shaoyin*.

Prescription: Shenshu(BL23) Taixi(KI 3) Xinshu(BL15)
Pishu(BL20) Sishencong(EX—HN1)

Explanation: Shenshu(UB23) is used in combination with the *Yuan*—source point of the kidney channel Taixi(KI 3) to reinforce kidney *Qi* and kidney essence, and produce marrow to fill in the brain to promote the intellegence. Xinshu(BL15) and Pishu(BL20) nourish heart and spleen. Sishencong (EX—HN1), clearing the mind and promoting the intellegence, is an emperical point for poor memory. The joint use of the above points may invigorate the kidney *Qi*, refill the kidney essence, strengthen the *Qi* of the heart and spleen. The poor memory and other symptoms and signs can be helped when the sea of the marrow is nourished.

Method: Apply filiform needles with reinforcing method and retain the needles for 20—30 minutes, manipulating them one to two times. Shenshu(BL23), Xinshu(BL15), Pishu(BL20) and Taixi(KI 3) may be applied with both acupuncture and moxibustion, or only with moxibustion for 10—15 minutes at each point.

4. Phlegm—fluid and Stasis Obstruction

Principle: Strengthen heart *Qi* and resolve phlegm by using mainly the points from the *Yangming* and *Jueyin* channels.

Prescription: Fenglong(ST40) Zusanli(ST36)
　　　　　　　　Shenmen(HT 7) Daling(PC 7)
　　　　　　　　Sanyinjiao(SP 6) Xingjian(LR 2)

Explanation: Fenglong (ST 40) resolves phlegm. Zusanli (ST 36) regulates the function of the spleen and stomach in order to assist Fenglong(ST40) to eliminate the turbid phlegm. Daling (PC 7) and Shenmen(HT 7) resolve phlegm, clear the mind and calm the heart. Sanyinjiao (SP 6), regulating blood, is used in combination with Xingjian(LR 2) to soothe the circulation of *Qi* of the liver and spleen and resolve the stagnant *Qi*. The joint use of the above points may resolve the phlegm and dissolve the stasis, promote the circulation of *Qi* and blood and ensure the heart to house the mind.

Method: Apply filiform needles with reducing method and retain the needles for 15—20 minutes, manipulating them two to three times.

Alternative Treatment: Auricular Acupuncture

Prescription: Heart Spleen Kidney Ear—Shenmen
　　　　　　　Sympathetic Brainstem

Method: Apply filiform needles at three to four points with mild stimulation and retain the needles for 15–20 minutes. Embedding of ear seeds is also applicable.

1.28 Maniac Depression and Insanity

Both maniac depression and mental insanity are considered as abnormal conditions of the mental state. The former is characterized by a quiet physical state such as emotional dejection, apathy, dull or incoherent speech. The later is characterized by a hyperactive physical and mental state such as restlessness, abnormally hyperactive mentality, excessive motor activity or violent behavior. Maniac depression belongs to *Yin* in nature while mental in sanity belongs to *Yang* in nature. Pathologically, there is certain relationship between them. Conditions of both may intertransform. There fore, both are always mentioned together.

The TCM definition of the above syndrome may include schizophrenia, reactive psychosis and mental disorders caused by cerebral organic conditions in modern medicine.

Cause and Mechanism

Maniac depression is mostly due to overthinking, grief or emotional depression that causes the liver unable to maintain the free flow of *Qi* and poor transporting of spleen *Qi*. Therefore, fluid stagnates into phlegm and disturbs upward to result in the mind disorder.

Mental insanity is mostly related to depressive liver *Qi* due to failure in achieving ambitions. In this case, the stagnation of liver *Qi* turns into fire to dry up the body fluid which then stagnates into phlegm—fire to disturb upward and to obstruct the heart. Therefore, mental insanity occurs due to the mental confusion.

Differentiation

1. Maniac Depression

This condition is characterized by a gradual onset. At the beginning, the patient may experience some emotional dejection, mental dullness. The subsequent manifestations include incoherent speech, abnormal mood changing such as excessive joy or anger, somnolence, no sense to mind clean or dirty, no desire for food, illusions, thin greasy tongue coating, and thready thin, or thready slippery pulse.

2. Mental Insanity

The sudden onset of mental insanity is often characterized by irritability, less sleep and no desire for food. The subsequent manifestations include excessive mental activity, increased physical energy with violent behavior and rage shouting, running around in nude, destroying surrounding objects and harming familiar or unfamiliar persons for no reason at all. Yellow greasy tongue coating, and rapid thready slippery pulse.

Treatment

1. Maniac Depression

Principle: Soothe the stagnant liver Qi, resolve the phlegm and regain the founction of the heart to house the mind by using mainly the points from The Heart Channel of Hand—*Shaoyin*, The Liver Channel of Foot—*Jueyin* plus some of the Back—*Shu* points.

Prescription: Shenmen(HT 7) Daling(PC 7)

　　　　　　　Xinshu(BL15) Ganshu(BL18)

　　　　　　　Pishu(BL20) Taichong(LR 3)

　　　　　　　Fenglong(ST40) Tanzhong(RN17)

Explanation: Daling (PC 7) is the *Yuan*—source point of

The Pericardium Channel of Hand—*Jueyin* and one of the thirteen shost points for treating mental disorders. Shenmen (HT 7), the *Yuan*—source point of The Heart Channel of Hand—*Shaoyin*, is good for dullness due to poor function of the heart in housing the mind. The above two points in combination may calm the heart and mind. Xinshu(BL15), Pishu(BL20) and Ganshu(BL18) clear the heart, promote spleen *Qi* transforming and soothe the stagnant liver *Qi*. Taichong(LR 3), the *Yuan*—source point of the liver channel, may soothe the liver *Qi* and relieve the stagnation of liver *Qi*. Tanzhong(RN 17), the Influential Point of *Qi*, is used in combination with Fenglong (ST40) to regulate *Qi* circulation and resolve phlegm. The joint use of the above points may soothe the liver *Qi*, resolve phlegm, and calm the heart and mind.

Point Modification: Add Zhongwan(RN12) and Zusanli (ST 36) for no desire for food; Jianshi(PC 5) for abnormal joy or anger; Jingming(BL 1) for photism, and Tinggong(SI19) for auditory hallucination.

Method: Apply filiform needles with even method and retain the needles for 15—30 minutes, manipulating them two to three times.

2. Mental Insanity

Principle: Clear the heart, dispel the phlegm and resuscitate the mind by using the points mainly from The *Du* Channel and The Pericardium Channel of Hand—*Jueyin*.

Prescription: Dazhui(DU14)　Fengfu(DU16)
　　　　　　　Shuigou(DU26)　Fenglong(ST40)
　　　　　　　Jianshi(PC 5)　Laogong(PC 8)

Explanation: Dazhui (DU14), the merging point of all *Yang*, is used in combination with Shuigou(DU26) to eliminate the *Yang* heat and resuscitate the mind. Fengfu(DU16) promote brain marrow and calms the mind. Jianshi (PC 5) is used in combination with Fenglong(ST40) to clear the heart and resolve the phlegm. Laogong(PC 8), the *Ying*—spring point of the pericardium channel, may clear the pericardium, eliminate the fire from the heart, and calm the mind. The joint use of the above points may eliminate the phlegm—fire, calm the mind and ease the mental insanity.

Method: Apply filiform needles with reducing method and retain the needles for 15—30 minutes, manipulating them two to four times. Reducing method may also be carried out without retention of needles. Dazhui(DU14) may be pricked with three—edged needle to cause bleeding.

Alternative Treatment: Auricular Acupuncture

Prescription: Heart   Subcortex   Kidney   Occipital

forehead   Ear—Shenmen   Sympathetic

Method: Apply filiform needles at three to four points for 15—20 minutes with mild stimulation to maniac depression, and strong stimulation for mental insanity without needling retention. Embedding of ear seeds or subcutaneous needles is also applicable.

1.29   Epilepsy

Epilepsy, a mental disorder in paroxysmal attacks, is characterized by a sudden falling down in a fit, mouthful foams, eyes staring upward, convulsions and screamings as if shoutings of domesticated pigs and sheep. However, the patient appears normal when he regains consciousness.

The condition described here is similar to that in modern medicine. The differentiation and treatment in this section can be referred to disregarding whether it is a case of primary or secondary epilepsy.

Cause and Mechanism

In most cases epilepsy is caused by stagnant *Qi* circulation of the heart and liver due to fear, depression or anger, or by dampness formed in case of spleen deficiency due to improper diet. Stagnation of *Qi* that turns into fire in a long run evaporates the dampness to form phlegm. Consequently the fire carrying phlegm to preserve into the channels and rushes up to disturb the mind, resulting in an epilepsy attack, a temporary incoordination between the *Yin* and *Yang*.

Differentiation

1. During the Seizure

Patient first experiences dizziness, headache and suffocating sensation in the chest. This is then followed by a sudden falling down with loss of consciousness, pallor complexion, clenched jaws, upward staring of the eyes, limb convulsions, mouthful foams, screamings as pigs and sheep, and even incontinence of urine and feces. Not long after that, the patient regains consciousness and becomes asymptomatic. Apart from the fatigue and weakness, the patient appears normal. The tongue coating is white greasy and the pulse is thready slippery.

2. After the Seizure

The chief manifestations include listlessness, lustreless complexion, dizziness, palpitation, loss of appetite, profuse sputum, lumbar soreness and knee weakness, pale tongue proper with white greasy coating, and thin slippery pulse.

Treatment

1. During the Seizure

Principle: Dissolve the phlegm to resuscitate the patient, soothe the liver and quench the wind by puncturing points mainly from The *Du* Channel, The *Ren* Channel and The Liver Channel of Foot—*Jueyin*.

Prescription: Shuigou(DU26) Jiuwei(RN15)
                    Dazhui(DU14) Jianshi(PC 5)
                    Taichong(LR 3) Fenglong(ST40)

Explanation: Shuigou(DU26) is an important point to resuscitate patients. Jiuwei(RN15) is the *Luo*—connecting point of The *Ren* Channel. Dazhui(DU15) merges all *Yang* of the body. These two poitns in combination may harmonize the disorderly *Yin* and *Yang*. Jianshi (PC 5) regulates *Qi* circulation of The Pericardium Channel of Hand—*Jueyin*. Taichong(LR 3) soothes the liver and quenches wind. It is also applied here to clear the mind and calm the heart. Fenglong(ST40) pacifies the stomach and helps descned the turbid *Qi,* particularly in eliminating heat and resolving phlegm. The joint use of the above points may dissolve phlegm, resuscitate the patient, soothe the liver and quench the wind, and tranquilize the mind.

Point Modification: Add Yongquan(KI 1) and Qihai(RN 6) for loss of consciousness during the seizure.

Method: Apply filiform needles with reducing method and retain the needles for 15—20 minutes, manipulating them two to three times. Generally, Shuigou(DU26) is punctured first. This is followed by puncturing Taichong(LR 3)and Yongquan(KI 1) with lifting, thrusting and rotating until the patient resuscitates.

2. After the Seizure

Principle: Nourish the heart, calm the mind, strengthen the spleen and reinforce the kidney by puncturing points mainly from

The Heart Channel of Hand—*Shaoyin* and The Spleen Channel of Foot—*Taiyin.*

Prescription: Xinshu(BL15) Yintang(EX—HN)
Shenmen(HT 7) Sanyinjiao(SP 6)
Taixi(KI 3) Yaoqi(EX—B9)

Explanation: Xinshu(BL15), Yintang(EX—HN3) and Shenmen(HT 7) are used in combination to nourish the heart and tranquilize the mind. Sanyinjiao(SP 6) and Taixi(KI 3) strengthen spleen and reinforce kidney. Yaoqi (EX—B9) is the empirical point for the treatment of epilepsy.

Point Modification: Add Shenmai(BL62) if attacks mostly take place in the daytime; Zhaohai(KI 6) if attacks mostly take place at night; and Fenglong (ST40) for profuse sputum.

Method: Apply filiform needles with reinforcing or even method and retain the needles for 20—30 minutes, manipulating them one to two times.

Comment: Attention is paid to treat the patient for primary epilepsy even for the treatment of the secondary attacks. Comprehensive treatment is necessary if the patient is accompanied by high fever and loss of consciousness during the attacks.

1.30   Melancholy

Melancholy is a general term for diseases caused by emotional depression and *Qi* stagnation. Its main symptoms are depression, restlessness, fullness sensation in the chest, ditending pain in the hypochondrium, irritability or feeling of a lump in the throat.

The diseases such as hysteria, neurosis and menopause syndrome in modern medicine can be treated according to the differentiation and treatment in this ection, section.

Cause and Mechanism

Melancholy is mostly due to emotional depression and violent rage resulting in the failure of the liver to maintain the free flow of *Qi* and stagnation of liver which makes upward attacks on the heart and mind. Forming and accumulation of phlegm due to impairment of spleen from over thinking or poor function of spleen in transforming and transporting will turn into fire in a long run to disturb the heart and mind. leading to disturbance of the heart and mind. Excessive anxiety or fear may also lead to melancholy because the impaired *Qi* mechanism helps to consume nutrient blood in a hidden way.

Differentiation

1. Liver *Qi* Stagnation Type

The chief manifestations include emotional depression, restlessness, fullness in the chest and distending pain in the hypochondrium, abdominal distention and eructation, anorexia or abdominal pain, nausea and vomiting, thin greasy tongue coating, and wiry pulse.

2. *Qi* Stagnation Turning into Fire

The chief manifestations include irritable temper, fullness in the chest and hypochondriac region, dryness and bitter taste in the mouth, headache, congested eyes, tinnitus or aid regurgitation, constipation, red tongue proper and rapid wiry pulse.

3. Phlegmatic *Qi* Stagnation Type

The chief manifestations include depression, chest fullness, discomfort sensation of the throat with a lump feeling but not difficulty in swallowing, thin greasy tongue coating, and wiry slippery pulse.

4. Blood Deficiency Type

The chief manifestations include frequent sorrow without any obvious causes, abnormal joy or rage, unreasonable suspicion or fear, palpitation and irritability, unsound sleep, thin white tongue coating, and wiry pulse. Sometimes, there may be sudden fullness sensation in the chest, hiccups, sudden loss of voice, and convulsions. In severe cases, there may be sudden syncope.

Treatment

1. Liver *Qi* Stagnation Type

Principle: Soothe the liver *Qi* and regulate the *Qi* circulation of the middle—*Jiao* by using points mainly from The *Ren* Channel and The Liver Channel of Foot—*Jueyin*.

Prescription: Danzhong(RN17)   Ganshu(BL18)

Taichong(LR 3)   Zhongwan(RN12)

Zusanli(ST36) Gongsun(SP 4)

Explanation: Danzhong(RN17), the Influential Point of *Qi,* may regulate the mechanism of *Qi* circulation. Ganshu(BL 18) and Taichong(LR 3) soothe the liver *Qi* and release the *Qi* stagnation. Zusanli(ST36) and Zhongwan(RN12) pacify the stomach to keep the adverse *Qi* downwards. Gongsun(SP 4), the *Luo*—connecting point of the spleen channel, strengthens the spleen and pacifies the stomach. The joint use of these points helps the liver to maintain free flow of *Qi,* pacify the *Qi* mechanism of the spleen and stomach and relieve all of the symptoms and signs.

Method: Apply filiform needles with even method and retain the needles for 15—20 minutes, manipulating them two to three times.

2. Qi Stagnation Turning into Fire

Principle: Eliminate liver fire, soothe the liver *Qi,* regulate *Qi* circulation and pacify the middle−*Jiao* by using points mainly from The *SanJiao* Channel of Hand−*Shaoyang,* The Gallbladder Channel of Foot−*Shaoyang,* The Liver Channel of Foot−*Jueyin* and The Stomach Channel of Foot−*Yangming.*

Prescription: Xingjian(LR 2) Xiaxi(GB43)

Zhigou(SJ 6)

Yanglingquan(GB34) Shangwan(RN13)

Zusanli(ST36)

Explanation: Xingjian(LR 2) and Xiaxi(GB43), respectively the *Ying*−spring points of the liver channel and the gallbladder channel, may sedate the fire from the liver and gallbladder. Zhigou(SJ 6) and Yanglingquan(GB34) may regulate the *Qi* circulation of the *Shaoyang* channels and soothe the liver *Qi.* Shangwan(RN13) and Zusanli(ST36) pacify the stomach and regulate *Qi* circulation. The joint use of the above points sedates liver fire, regulates *Qi* circulation, pacifies the middle−*Jiao* and calms the mind.

Method: Apply filiform needles with reducing method and retain the needles for 15−20 minutes, manipulating them two to three times.

3. Phlegmatic *Qi* Stagnation Type

Principle: Soothe the liver, promote *Qi* circulation and resolve phlegm by using points mainly from The Liver Channel of Foot−*Jueyin* and The *Ren* Channel.

Prescription: Tiantu(RN22) Danzhong(RN17)

Neiguan(PC 6) Fenglong(ST40)

Taichong(LR 4)

Explanation: Tiantu (RN 22) helps to descned Qi, clear the throat and promote the diaphragm. Neiguan (PC 6) has the function to relieve chest fullness and regulate Qi circulation. Taichong (LR 3) soothes the liver Qi. Danzhong(RN17) and Fenglong (ST 40) activate Qi and resolve phlegm. The joint use of the above points may soothe the liver Qi, relieve Qi stagnation, resolve phlegm, relieve fullness in the chest and clear the throat.

Method: Apply filiform needles with even method and Retain the needles for 15—20 minutes, manipulating them two to three times.

4. Blood Deficiency Type

Principle: Regulate the liver, nourish blood and calm the heart and mind. by using points mainly from The Heart Channel of Hand—*Shaoyin* and The Liver Channel of Foot—*Jueyin*.

Prescription: Taichong(LR 3)　Shenmen(HT 7)
　　　　　　　Xinshu(BL15)　Neiguan(PC 6)
　　　　　　　Sanyinjiao(SP 6)　Juque(RN14)

Explanation: Taichong (LR 3), the *Yuan*—source point of the liver channel, may regulate the liver and nourish blood, soothe liver Qi and relieve the stagnation of Qi. Xinshu(BL15) in combination with Juque(RN14), the Front—*Mu* point of the heart, and Shenmen(H7), the *Yuan*—source point of the heart channel, may calm the heart and mind. Sanyinjiao(SP 6) may tonify the *Yin* and nourish blood. Neiguan (PC 6) relieves the fullness in the chest as well as the Qi stagnation. The joint use of the above points may refill the deficient *Yin* blood, calm the heart and mind and relieve the melancholy.

Point Modification: Add Tongli(HT 5) and Lianquan(RN 23) for horseness of voice; Tiantu(RN 22) for hiccup; Hegu(LI 4),

Yanglingquan(GB34); and Shuigou(DU26) and Yongquan(KI 1) for syncope.

Method: Apply filiform needles with even method and retain the needles for 15—20 minutes, manipulating them one to two times.

Alternative Treatment: Auricular Acupuncture

Prescription: Heart Subcortex Occipital Liver Brainstem Endocrine Ear—Shenmen

Method: Apply filiform needles at three to four points with mild stimulation at each treatment and retain the needles for 15—20 minutes. Embedding of ear seeds or subcutaneous ear needles is also applicable.

1.31 Headache

Headache is a subjective symptom that may appear in many acute and chronic diseases. The headache stated here refers to that as a main symptom in many exogenous or miscellaneous internal diseases. It does not include the headache as an accompanying symptom in the progression of certain diseases.

Headache can be seen in many infectious diseases with fever in modern medicine such as hypertension, intracranial diseases, psychoneurosis and migraine.

Cause and Mechanism

Exogenous type of headache is often caused by the invasion of wind, cold, dampness or heat in the channels and collaterals in the head, leading to the obstruction of the lucid *Yang* in the head. Endogenous type of headache is mostly caused by emotional stimulation that further causes the stagnation of liver *Qi*. The *Qi* stagnation then turns into fire to disturb the head, the clear organ. Kidney *Yin* deficiency can lead to the failure of kidney water to irrigate the wood so that there will be hyperactivity of liver to cause headache. Improper diet such over intake of greasy oily food can impair the function of the spleen in transforming and transporting and production of turbid dampness in the interior of the body. The dampness formed in the interior will halt the lucid *Yang* to develop headache. Blood deficieny due to prolonged illness or excessive loss of blood may also cause headache because of inadequate up going blood to nourish the head.

Lingering headache over a long period of time can affect the collaterals, leading to stasis of blood in the collaterals. Traumatic injuries affecting the brain and its marrow may also lead to poor circulation of *Qi* and blood, leading to stasis type of headache.

Differentiation

1. Exogenous Type of Headache

This type of heache is characterized by a sudden onset of pain in paroxysmal attacks. The pain is severe in nature and may radiate to the back. It can sometimes be a kind of pricking pain in a fixed location. The tongue coating is thin and white and the pulse is wiry and tense.

2. Endogenous Type of Headache

This type of headache is characterized by a slow onset of dull, hallow pain with dizzy sensation. It may bother the patient off and on, but definitely worse with overstrain.

(1)Liver *Yang* Type of Headache

The chief manifestations include pain, dizziness, irritability, shortness of tempor, poor sleep, redness of the face, congested eyes, bitter taste in the mouth, red tongue proper, thin yellow tongue coating, and wiry forceful pulse.

(2)Turbid Phlegm Type of Headache

The chief manifestations include pain in the forehead as if the head is wrapped up, fullness sensation in the chest, nausea, vomiting of saliva in severe case, loose stools, white greasy tongue coating, and wiry slippery pulse.

(3)Blood Deficiency Type of Headache

The Chief manifestations include headache, dizziness, lingering pain worsened by overstrain and alleviated by rest, lassitude, shortness of breath, palpitation, poor memory, poor appetite, pallor complexion, pale tongue proper, thin white coating, and thready feeble pulse.

(4)Blood Stasis Type of Headache

The chief manifestations include a fixed stabbing pain that lasts for a long time, blurring of vision, poor memory, purplish spots on the tongue, and thready hesitant pulse.

Treatment

1. Exogenous Type of Headache

Principle: Eliminate wind, remove obstruction from the channels, activate blood and stop pain by using mainly the local points plus points from the affected channels.

Prescription: Fengchi(GB20)　Touwei(ST　8)

　　　　　　　　Baihui(DU20)　Hegu(LI　4)

Explanation: Fengchi (GB20) is used to eliminate wind and stop pain, viz, to relieve the *Shaoyang* headache and dispel the wind from the neck and nape areas. Touwei(ST 8) further eliminates wind from the channels and stop pain, particularly the wind from the *Yangming* channel. Baihui(DU20) where The Liver Channel of Foot—*Jueyin* merges in the vertex is used to quench the wind in the vertex. Head is the merging of all yang while face is the home place of *Yangming* channels. Therefore, Hegu(LI 4) is used to eliminate wind from the facial area. The joint use of the above points may eliminate wind and relieve pain.

Point Modification: Add Shangxing(DU23), Yangbai(GB14) and Yintang(Extra) for frontal headache; Tianzhu(BL10), Kunlun(BL60) and Houxi(ST 3) for occipital headache; Taiyang(EX—HN3) , Shuaigu(GB 8) and Waiguan(SJ 5) for temporal headache; Tongtian(BL 7), Naokong (GB 19) and Taichong(LR 3) for pain in the vertex.

Method: Apply filiform needles with reducing method and retain the needles for 15—20 minutes, manipulating them two to three times. If the pain is severe during the attack, continue to manipulate the needles until the pain lessens.

2. Endogenous Type of Headache

(1)Liver *Yang* Type of Headache

Principle: Soothe liver, sedate its *Yang* and quench the wind by using points mainly from the Gallbladder Channel of Foot—*Shaoyang,* and The Liver Channel of Foot—*Jueyin.*

Prescription: Fengchi(GB20) Xuanlu(GB 5)
　　　　　　　 Taiyang(EX—HN5) Xingjian(LR 2)
　　　　　　　 Xiaxi(GB43) Taixi(KI 3)

Explanation: Fengchi (GB20) and Xuanlu (GB 5), points from The Gallbladder Channel of Foot—*Shaoyang,* have the effect of eliminating heat, quenching the wind and stoping pain. They just quench the wind that is disturbing the head. Taiyang (EX—HN5) promotes the circulation of *Qi* in the local area. Xingjian(LR 2) and Xiaxi(GB 43), respectively the *Ying*—spring points of the liver and gallbladder channels, eliminate the pathogenic heat from these two channels. Taixi(KI 3) tonifies kidney water in order to build up *Yin* to restrict hyperactive *Yang*. The joint use of the above points may soothe the liver, quench the wind and stop pain.

Point Modification: Add Guanchong(SJ 1) for pricking for congestion in the eyes; Ganshu(BL18) and Jianshi (PC 5) for restlessness and shortness of tempor.

Method: Apply filiform needles with reducing method except Taixi(KI 3) that is punctured with reinforcing method, and retain the needles for 10—20 minutes, manipulating them two to three times. Taiyang (EX—HN5) may also be applied with three—edged needle to cause bleeding.

(2)Turbid Phlegm Type of Headache

Principle: Resolve phlegm and sedate the turbidity, remove obstruction from the channels and collaterals and stop pain by using points mainly from The *Ren* Channel and The Stomach Channel of Foot—*Yangming*.

Prescription: Zhongwan(RN12)   Fenglong(ST40)
              Baihui(DU20)   Yintang(EX—HN 3)
              Xuanzhong(GB39)

Explanation: Zhongwan(RN 12) is used in combination with Fenglong(ST40) to strengthen the spleen and stomach and re-solve dampness. This is to treat the root cause of the disease. Xuanzhong(GB39) eliminates the turbid dampness from the *SanJiao*. Baihui(DU20) and Yintang(EX—HN3) helps to disperse the lucid *Yang* in the head, remove obstruction from the channels and collaterals and stop pain. The joint use of the above points may resolve the phlegm, remove obstruction and stop pain.

Point Modification: Add Neiguan(PC 6) for vomiting of saliva; Tianshu(ST25) for loose stools.

Method: Apply filiform needles with reducing method and retain the needles for 15—20 minutes, manipulating them two to three times.

(3)Blood Deficiency Type of Headache

Principle: Reinforce *Qi,* nourish blood, promote channel circulation and stop pain by using mainly the Back—*Shu* points.

Prescription: Ganshu(BL18)　Pishu(BL20)
　　　　　　　 Shenshu(BL23)　Geshu(BL17)
　　　　　　　 Qihai(RN　6)　Baihui(DU20)
　　　　　　　 Zusanli(ST36)　Sanyinjiao(SP　6)

Explanation: The Liver stores the blood. The spleen governs the blood. Brain is the sea of marrow, and the marrow is manufactured by the kidney. Therefore, the Back—*Shu* points of the liver, spleen and kidney, plus Geshu(BL 17) and Sanyinjiao(SP 6) are used to nourish both *Qi* and blood. Zusanli (ST36) is used to strengthen the source for providing the acquired energy. Qihai (RN　6) regulates *Qi* of the general body. Baihui(DU20) lifts the lucid *Yang* in order to guide *Qi* and blood to go upward to nourish the brain. The joint use of the above points may replenish *Qi* and blood, nourish the sea of marrow and stop headache.

Method: Apply filiform needles with reinforcing method and retain the needles for 20—30 minutes, manipulating them one to two times.

(4)Blood Stasis Type of Headache

Principle: Activate blood, resolve blood stasis, promote *Qi* circulation and stop pain by using points mainly from The Large Intestine Channel of Hand—*Yangming* and The Spleen Channel of Foot—*Taiyin,* plus some Ahshi points.

Prescription: Ahshi point　Hegu(LI 4)　Sanyinjiao(SP 6)
　　　　　　　Geshu(BL17)

Explanation: Ahshi point is used to eliminate the local blood stasis and promote the circulation of *Qi* in the local area. Hegu (LI 4) is good for treating head and facial disorders because of its ascending and dispersing property. Sanyinjiao(SP 6) is used in combination with Geshu(BL17) to activate blood and resolve blood stasis. The joint use of the above points may resolve blood stasis and stop pain.

Point Modification: Add Zanzhu(BL 2) for pain in the superciliary ridge; Taiyang (EX—HN5) for migraine; Yuzhen(BL 9) for occipital headache; and Sishencong (EX—HN1) for pain in the vertex.

Method: Apply filiform needles with even method or both reinforcing and reducing methods. Hegu(LI 4) is applied with reducing method and the rest of the points with even method. Retain the needles for 15—20 minutes, manipulating them two to three times. Ahshi point is applied with three—edged needle to cause bleeding.

Alternative Treatment:

1. Auricular Acupuncture

Prescription: Subcortex　Vertex　Occipital　Taiyang
　　　　　　　Ear—Shenmen　Liver　Spleen　Kidney

Method: Apply filiform needles at three to four points each time with moderate stimulation and retain the needles for 15—20 minutes. Strong stimulation is suggested for severe headache. Pricking the veins on the ear dorsum is also applicable for the severe headache. Embedding of ear seeds or subcutaneous ear seeds is also applicable.

2. Plum—blossom Needle Therapy

Prescription: Taiyang(EX—HN5) Yintang(EX—HN3) Ahshi
point

Method: Use the plum—blossom needles to tap in the local area until the skin turns red. This method is used for headache due to invasion of exogenous pathogenic wind and that due to hyperactivity of liver *Yang*.

1.32 Facial Pain

Facial pain refers to some severe aching that may be paroxysmal, temporal or burning in the facial region. It mostly affects one side of the face in the lateral aspect of the forehead, superior maxillary bone or inferior maxillary bone, but rarely affects both sides. At the beginning, the attack of aching only lasts for a short time with very long intervals. The longer history it has, the more frequent attacks there will be. Facial pain is often complained by patients in their middle ages, but more common in middle aged women. It is similar to trigeminal neuralgia in modern medicine.

Cause and Mechanism

Facial pain is mostly caused by invasion of exogenous pathogenic wind—cold into the *Yangming* channels in the facial region. The contracting cold stagnates the channels and collaterals and obstructs the normal circulation of *Qi* and blood. Invasion of exogenous pathogenic wind—heat on the other hand can also affect the normal circulation of *Qi* and blood in the facial, region, giving rise to painful attacks. Ascending of excess fire from the liver and stomach or flaring up of deficient fire due to the *Yin* deficiency of kidney accounts for another major reason for facial pain.

Differentiation

The abrupt onset of pain appears paroxysmal and radiative with electric shock sensation. The pain that is relieved in a few seconds or a few minutes can be described as if the affected part of the face is being cut, stabbed or burnt. There may be many attacks daily with irregular intervals. The location of the aching usually involves the cheek and inferior maxillary region, but rarely affects the forehead. The pain can simply be induced by exposure to wind, washing the face, speaking and eating.

1. Wind—cold Type

The chief manifestations include painful cheek, facial muscular spasm and twitching, aggravation of pain or new attack due to exposure to cold and alleviation by warmth. The accompanying symptoms and signs include headache, aversion to cold, nasal discharge, thin white tongue coating, and wiry tense pulse.

2. Wind—heat Type

The chief manifestations include burning pain in the cheek, feverish sensation on one side of the face, congestion of the eyes, running tears, restlessness, dry mouth and throat, thin yellow tongue coating, and wiry rapid pulse.

3. Excess Heat from the Liver and Stomach

The chief manifestations include burning pain in the cheek, restlessness with shortness of tempor, bitter taste in the mouth, congestion of the eye, dizziness and vertigo, fullness sensation in the chest, distention in the hypochondriac region, constipation, dry red tongue proper, thick yellow coating, and wiry rapid or full rapid pulse.

4. Hyperactivity of Fire due to *Yin* Deficiency

The chief manifestations include pain in the cheek in repeated attacks, redness in the cheek, rough facial skin, dizziness, blurring of vision, feverish sensation in the palms and soles, emaciation, red tongue proper with less coating, and thin rapid pulse.

Treatment

Principle: Remove obstruction from the channels and collaterals and stop pain by using points mainly from the *Yangming*, *Shaoyang* and *Taiyang* channels.

Prescription: (Based on the location of the pain)

Forehead pain: Zanzhu(BL 2) Yangbai(GB14) Touwei(ST 8)
　　　　　　　Shuaigu(GB 8) Zhongzhu(SJ 3)

Superior maxillary pain:
　　　　　　　Sibai(ST 2) Quanliao(SI18)
　　　　　　　Taiyang(EX−HN5) Yingxiang(LI20)
　　　　　　　Hegu(LI 4)

Inferior maxillary Pain:
　　　　　　　Chengjiang(RN24) Jiache(ST 6) Xiaguan(ST 7)
　　　　　　　Yifeng(SJ17) Xiangu(ST43)

Point Modification:
　　　(1)Add Fengchi (GB20), Fengfu (DU16) and Lieque (LU 7) for wind−cold invasion;
　　　(2)Add Dazhui(DU14)and Quchi(LI11)for wind−heat invasion;
　　　(3)Add Xingjian(LR 2) and Neiting(ST44) for ascending heat from the liver and stomach;
　　　(4)Add Fengchi(GB20)and Taixi(KI 3)for hyperactivity of fire due to *Yin* deficiency.

Explanation: The above grouping of points is primarily based on the use of local points plus some distal ones in an attempt to promote *Qi* and blood circulation in the facial region and promote *Qi* and blood in order to remove the obstruction from the channels and collaterals and stop pain. Fengfu(DU16) and Fengchi(GB20) are used to eliminate wind. Lieque(LU 7) is used to dispel cold and wind. Dazhui(DU14) and Quchi(LI11) are used to dispel wind−heat. Xingjian(LR2) and Neiting(ST44), the *Ying*−spring points of their respective channels, are used to disperse heat, Taixi(KI 3) is used to reinforce kidney water to put off the deficient fire while Fengchi(GB20) is applied to sedate the hyperactive *Yang*.

Method: Apply filiform needles with reducing method except Taixi(KI 3) which is used with reinforcing method for hyperactivity of fire due to *Yin* deficiency. Retain the needles for 15−30 minutes, manipulating them two to four times. Electirc stimulation can also be applied at two points each time with densedisperse wave for 30 minutes.

Alternative Treatment:

Auricular Acupuncture

Prescription: Cheek Superior maxillary Inferior maxillary
          Forehead Ear−Shenmen Sympathetic Subcortex

Method: Apply filiform needles at three to four needles with strong stimulation and retain the needles for 20−30 minutes. Embedding of subcutaneous ear needles is also applicable.

1.33 *Bi* Syndrome

Bi is a Chinese concept. *Bi* syndrome means obstruction. Conditions characterized by the following chief manifestations, such as aching, numbness and heavy sensation involving the limbs, joints and muscles as well as swollen joints and limited movement due to poor circulation as well as obstruction of *Qi* and blood caused by exogenous pathogenic invasion into the channels and collaterals, are called in general the *Bi* syndrome.

Bi syndrome, commonly seen in the clinic, also bears the characteristics of progressive pain or pain in repeated attacks.

The concept of *Bi* syndrome in traditional Chinese medicine covers rheumatic fever, rheumatic arthritis, rheumtoid gout and rheumatic myofibrositis in modern medicine.

Cause and Mechanism

Factors such as poor defensive energy with empty skin pores, exposure to wind with sweating after physical exertion, catching cold in the water or dwelling in damp place for a long time may cause invasion of exogenous pathogenic wind, cold and dampness into the body when the body is defieient. The invasion if perverses into the channels and collaterals will cause poor circulation of *Qi* and blood to develop *Bi* syndrome.

The clinical symptoms and signs complained about by patients vary greatly due to the difference in body constitution and invasion of different pathogenic factors. Wandering *Bi* syndrome is basically due to a prevailing wind invasion. Painful *Bi* syndrome is basically due to a prevailing cold invasion. Fixed *Bi* syndrome is basically due to a prevailing dampness invasion. Febrile *Bi* syndrome is complained by patients of *Yang* type of body constitution with retention of heat in the interior. In this case, patient also experience an invasion of exogenous pathogenic wind, cold and dampness which then also turns into heat in the body. When newly formed heat encounters interior heat, they jointly flow into the channels and collaterals to develop a febrile *Bi* syndrome. And stubborn *Bi* syndrome takes place in patient with long history of general *Bi* syndrome because they have had a long time of poor circulation of *Qi* and blood and obstruction of channels and collaterals due to blood stasis. Both of them have virtually affected the bones.

Differentiation

1. Wandering *Bi* Syndrome

The chief manifestations include wandering pain and soreness in the body limbs, joints and muscles, particularly in the wrist joints, elbow, knee and ankle areas, limited movements of the joints, or fever with aversion to cold, thin greasy tongue coating, and superficial wiry pulse.

2. Painful *Bi* Syndrome

The chief manifestations include severe pain in the limbs and joints as if being stabbed or pricked in worse cases, fixed pain that is alleviated by warmth but aggravated by cold, better in the daytime, but worse at night, limited movements of the joints, no local redness nor feverish sensation, cold sensation in the affected parts, thin white tongue coating, and wiry tense pulse.

3. Fix *Bi* Syndrome

The chief manifestations include pain and heavy sensation in relatively fixed areas of body limbs or joints, numbness of the muscles, aggravation of the condition in rainy days, white greasy tongue coating, and soft slow pulse.

4. Febrile *Bi* Syndrome

The chief manifestations include painful limb or joints, local burning sensation with redness, pain worsened by touching, limited movement involving one or several joints, or fever, thirst, restlessness, desire for cold drinks, aversion to heat, yellow tongue coating, and slippery rapid pulse.

5. Stubborn *Bi* Syndrome

Stubborn *Bi* syndrome has a long history of repeated attacks that have already deformed the affected joints. Some of the joint areas may have black spots. The chief manifestations include a severe pain in the local areas, limited movement, soreness and numbness, redness and swelling of the joints, or fevre, thirst, short scanty urine, or cold sensation in the joints, worsened condition in the cold seasons, alleviation of pain by warmth, purplish dark tongue with spurplish spots, and thready hesitant pulse.

Treatment

Principle: Strengthen the anti—pathogenic *Qi,* reomve wind and cold from the channels and collaterals and resolve dampness by using mainly the local points according to the local of pain. Both Ahshi points and distal are also combined in the prescriptions.

Prescription: (Based on locations of pain)

Shoulder: Jianyu(LI15)   Jianliao(SJ14)   Naoshu(SI10)
           Hegu(LI 4)

Elbow: Quchi(LI11)   Tianjing(SJ10)   Chize(LU 5)
           Waiguan(SJ 5)

Wrist: Yangxi(LI 5) Yangchi(SJ 4) Waiguan(SJ 5)
           Wangu(SI 4)

Hip: Huantiao(GB30)   Juliao(GB29)
           Xuanzhong(GB39)

Femur: Zhibian(BL54)   Chengfu(BL36)
           Yinmen(BL37)   Kunlun(BL60)

Knee: Liangqiu(ST34) Xuehai(SP10) Xiyan(EX—LE5)
           Yanglingquan(GB34) Yinlingquan(SP 9)

Ankle: Jiexi(ST41) Shangqiu(SP 5) Kunlun(BL60)
           Taixi(KI 3) Qiuxu(GB40)

Back and Lumbar region:

        Shenzhu(DU12) Yaoyangguan(DU 3)

        Dazhui(DU14) Huatuojiaji(Extra)

Point Modification:

    (1)Add Fengchi(GB20), Xuehai(SP10)and

        Geshu(BL17) for wandering *Bi* syndrome.

    (2)Add Guanyuan(RN 4) and Shenshu(BL23) for

        painful *Bi* syndrome.

    (3)Add Pishu(BL20), Zusanli(ST36) and

        Yanglingquan(GB34) for fixed *Bi* syndrome.

    (4)Add Dazhui (DU14), Quchi (LI11) and

        Weizhong (BL40) for febrile *Bi* syndrome.

    (5)Add Pishu(UB20), Ganshu(BL18),

        Shenshu(BL23), Geshu (BL17) and Dashu (BL11)

        for stubborn *Bi* syndrome.

Explanation: Local points and distal plints are used in combination in order to promote *Qi* and blood circulation, eliminate wind and cold, resolve dampness, strengthen the anti–pathogenic *Qi* and harmonize the nutrient and defensive *Qi* so that *Bi* syndrome can be relieved because the body does not provide shelter any more for pathogenic factors. Fengchi(GB 20), Xuehai (SP 10) and Geshu (BL17) are added to eliminate wind and activate blood circulation in the channels and collaterals. Guanyuan (RN 4) and Shenshu (BL23) are used to strengthen kidney *Yang* and dispel cold. Zusanli (ST36), Pishu (BL20) and Yinlingquan (SP 9) are used to strengthen the spleen and stomach and resolve dampness. Dazhui (DU14), Quchi (LI11)and Weizhong (BL40) are used to climinate wind, dispel heat and activate blood circulation in the channels. Pishu (BL20), Ganshu (BL18),

Shenshu (BL23), Geshu (BL17) and Dashu (BL11) are used to strengthen the anti-pathogenic *Qi,* eliminate the pathogenic factors, activate blood, resolve dampness, remove obstruction from the channels and collaterals and stop pain.

Method: Apply filiform needles with reducing or even method and retain the needles for 20—30 minutes manipulating them two to three times. Acupuncture and moxibustion are used at the same time in case of painful, fixed and stubborn *Bi* syndromes.

Alternative Treatment

1. Plum—blossom Needle Therapy

Prescription: Back—*Shu* points, Huatuojiaji plus local points where the joints have swellings.

Method: Tap the above mentioned areas with moderate stimulation until local redness appears slightly. This is then followed by cupping. Treatment is given once every other day.

2. Moxibustion Therapy

Prescription: Shenque (RN 8)

Method: Cut ginger slices in 2 mm thickness and prick many holes with needles on the ginger slice to be put over Shenque. Ignite five to seven pieces of moxa cones at the point in order. This method is applicable for painful, fixed and stubborn *Bi* syndromes.

1.34 *Wei* Syndrome

Wei syndrome refers to some paralytic conditions, especially that of the lower limbs, related to softness and weakness of the hand or feet accompanied by muscular atrophy, or loss of motor function.

Wei syndrome is often complained about by patient suffering from polyneuritis, acute and chronic myelitis, progressive myatrophy, myathenia gravis, periodic paralysis, muscular trophoneurosis, hysterical paralysis and paralysis due to traumatic injuries in terms of modern medicine.

Cause and Mechanism

Wei syndrome is mostly caused by invasion of pathogenic heat that attacks the lung. The heat in the lung consumes *Yin* fluid and body fluid may not be normally dispersed by the lung to the superficial portion of the body. The muscles and tendons in the general body will suffer from malnutrition. Improper diet characterized by intake of spicy, pungent, sweat or oily food usually causes accumulation of heat in the spleen and stomach to dry the body fluid. Malnutrition of the muscles and tendons gradually forms *Wei* syndrome. Dwelling in a damp place over a long period of time or being caught in rain or water makes the patient suffer from dampness invasion. Lingering dampness in the body will turn into heat to steam the *Yangming* channels so that there will be looseness and softness of the tendons and muscles. Both weak body constitution due to prolonged illness or over indulgence in sex can cause deficiency of liver blood and kidney essence. Malnutrition of the tendons and muscles will also develop into *Wei* syndrome. Besides, impairment of channels and collaterals with poor circulation of *Qi* and blood and malnutrition of tendons will also lead to softness and looseness of muscles to result in *Wei* syndrome.

Differentiation

1. Excessive Heat in the Lung and Stomach

The chief manifestations include sudden weakness of the body limbs that accompanied by fever, cough, restlessness, thirst, short scanty urine, loose stools, red tongue proper, yellow coating, and thready rapid or rapid slippery pulse.

2. Retention of Damp—heat

The chief manifestations include heavy sensation of the body, soreness, weakness of the body, or slight swelling with feverish sensation. The accompanying symptoms and signs include fever, profuse sweating, fullness sensation in the chest and epigastric region, turbid urine, yellow greasy tongue coating, and soft rapid pulse.

3. *Yin* Deficiency of the Liver and Kidney

The chief manifestations include gradual weakness of the feet, soreness and weakness of the back and lumbar region, dizziness, blurring of vision, seminal emission, prospermia, pallor complexion, or palpitation, spontaneous sweating, irregular menstruation, red tongue proper with less coating, and thready weak pulse.

4. *Wei* Syndorme due to Traumatic Injuries

Most of these patients have traumatic history. They complain numbness of the limbs, weakness of the limbs, or incontinence of urine, thin white tongue coating, and slow or hesitant pulse.

Treatment

Principle: Promote the circulation of *Qi* and blood and nourish tendons and bones by using points mainly from The Large Intestine Channel of Hand—*Yangming,* The Stomach Channel of Foot—*Yangming,* The *SanJiao* Channel of Hand—*Shaoyang,* The Gallbladder Channel of Foot—*Shaoyang,* The Lung Channel of Hand—*Taiyin* and The Spleen Channel of Foot—*Taiyin*. Besides, eliminate heat and moisten the lung if there is accumulation of heat in the lung and stomach. Nourish the liver and blood and refill the kidney essence in case of *Yin* deficiency of the liver and kidney. Strengthen *Qi* and blood and remove obstruction from the channels and collaterals in case traumatic injuries.

Prescription:

Upper Limb: Jianyu(LI15) Quchi(LI11) Waiguan(SJ 5)
           Hegu(LI 4)

Lower Limb: Biguan(ST31) Liangqiu(ST34)
           Zusanli(ST36) Yanglingquan (GB34)
           Huantiao(GB30) Xuanzhong(GB39)
           Jiexi(ST41)

Point Modification:

    (1)Add Chize(LU 5), Feishu(BL13) and Neiting (ST44) for heat accumulation in the lung and stomach.

    (2)Add Pishu(BL20) and Yinlingquan(SP 9) for retention of damp—heat in the body.

    (3)Add Ganshu(BL18), Shenshu(BL23) and Taixi (KI 3) for *Yin* deficiency of the liver and kidney.

    (4)Add the coresponding Huatuojiaji for *Wei* syndrome due to traumatic injuries.

Explanation: *Yangming* is the sea of food essenc and part of the source for providing the acquired energy. *Huangdi Neijing* says, " Select points only from the *Yangming* channels in the treatment of *Wei* syndrome". It is for this reason why points from The Large Intestine Channel and The Stomach Channel are used alternately to eliminate heat and promote the circulation *Qi*. Yanglingquan(GB34), the Influcntial Point of the tendons, is used in combination with Xuanzhong(GB39), the Influential

Point of marrow, to nourish both tendons and bones. Chize(LU 5), Feishu(BL13) and Neiting (ST44) are used to eliminate heat from the stomach and lung. Pishu(BL20) and Yinlingquan (SP 9) are used to eliminate pathogenic heat and dampness. Ganshu (BL18), Shenshu(BL23) and Taixi(KI 3) are selected to tonify the *Yin* of the liver and kidney. The corespond-ing Huatuojiaji points are used to promote the circulation of both *Qi* and blood in the local area and remove obstruction from the channels and collaterals.

Point Modification: Add Dazhui(DU14) for fever; Hegu (LI 4) and Fuliu(KI 7) for profuse sweating; Zhongji(RN 3) and Sanyinjiao (SP 6) for incontinence of urine; and Dachangshu (BL 25) and Ciliao(BL 32) for incontinence of stools.

Method: Apply filiform needles with reducing method heat accumulation in the stomach and lung and damp—heat retention in the body, and reinforcing method for *Yin* deficiency of the liver and kidney. Even method is applied for *Wei* syndrome due to traumatic injuries. Retain the needles for 15—30 minutes, manipu-lating them two to three times.

Alternative Treatment: Plum—blossom Needle Therapy

Prescription: Feishu(BL13) Ganshu(BL18) Pishu(BL20)
Weishu(BL21) Shenshu(BL23) or the lines of the
Yangming channels of the foot and hand.

Method: Use the plum—blossom needle to tap gently until local redness appears. Treatment is given once every other day.

1.35   Lumbar Pain

Lumbar pain, also broadly known as lumbospinal pain, may involve either the spine, or one side or both sides of the lumbar region. It is a commonly encountered condition in the clinic.

Lumbar pain often refers to soft tissue injury, muscular rheumatism and lumbar disc degeneration in modern medicine. This section mainly covers the lumbar pain due to cold—damp invasion, lumbar pain due to kidney *Yin* deficiency and that due to traumatic injuries. Knowledge of lumbar pain due to other factors can referred to in the chapters concerned.

Cause and Mechanism

Lumbar pain is often the consequence of impaired circulation of *Qi* and blood in the lumbar region due to invasion of pathogenic cold—damp into the local channels. The malnutrition of local channels due to such factors as kidney deficiency after prolonged illness, over sexual indulgence with excessive consumption of kidney essence, or impairment of the channels caused by twisting while carrying heavy load, incidental falling down or being hit, etc. may also lead to the stagnation of *Qi* and blood and develop into lumbar pain.

Traditional Chinese medicine holds that lumbar region is the residence of kidney. The *Du* Channel distributes along the spinal column. The two kidneys are located on both sides of the lumbar region. The Urinary Bladder Channel of Foot—*Taiyang* bifurcates on either side of the spinal column to connect with the kidney in the lower back. Therefore, pain in the lumbar region is closely related to both the kidney and the urinary bladder.

Differentiation

1. Lumbar Pain due to Cold—damp Invasion

The patient has a history of cold—damp invasion. The pain is characterized by a rapid onset of aching and soreness, lumbar rigidity that makes the patient feel difficult to bend forward or extend backward. The pain sometimes even involve the sacrum, hip and the popliteal area. The pain aggravates and alleviates from time to time with local aversion to cold and worsened condition in rainy days. The tongue coating is white greasy and the pulse is deep and weak or deep slow.

2. Lumbar Pain due to Kidney Deficiency

The chief manifestations include a slow onset of hidden pain, in the lumbar region that lasts for a long time, weakness of lumbus and knees, lassitude, cold limbs worsened by exertion or fatigue, pale tongue proper with white coating, and deep thready pulse.

3. Lumbar Pain due to Traumatic Factors

In addition to the traumatic history, the chief manifestations include a fixed local pain and rigidity that worsens by pressing or turning of body position, slightly red or dark purplish tongue, and wiry choppy pulse.

Treatment

1. Lumbar Pain due to Cold—damp Invasion

Principle: Warm up the channels and collaterals, eliminate cold and resolve dampness by selecting points mainly from The Urinary Bladder Channel of Foot—*Taiyang*.

Prescription: Shenshu(BL23) Yaoyangguan(DU 3)

Guanyuanshu(BL26) Ciliao (BL32)

Weizhong(BL40)

Explanation: Lumbus is the home of the kidney. The Back—*Shu* points are used to reinforce the kidney *Qi*. Yaoyangguan(DU 3), located in the lower back, may activate the *Yang Qi* of The *Du* Channel. Yaoyangguan(DU 3) in combination with Guanyuanshu (BL26) and Ciliao(BL32) regulates *Qi* of the affected channel, removes obstruction and stops pain. Weizhong(BL40) is an important point for the treatment of lumbar pain. The joint use of the above points can strengthen the lumbus, clear away pathogenic cold and dampness and ease the pain.

Method: Apply filiform neddles with even method and retain the needles for 15—20minutes, manipulating them two to three times. Moxibustion is also applicable for 15 minutes in the treatment.

2. Lumbar Pain due to Kidney Deficiency

Principle: Tonify kidney *Qi* and strengthen the lumbar region by using points mainly from The *Du* Channel, The Bladder Channel of Foot—*Taiyang* and The Kidney Channel of Foot—*Shaoyin*.

Prescription: Shenshu(BL23)　Mingmen(DU　4)

　　　　　　　Zhishi(BL52)　Taixi(KI　3)

　　　　　　　Weizhong(BL40)

Explanation: Shenshu (BL23) is used to warm up and tonify the kidney *Qi*. Mingmen (DU　4), Zhishi (BL52) and Taixi (KI　3) are used to nourish kidney *Yang* and strengthen kidney essence. Weizhong (BL 40) removes obstruction from the affected channel and strengthens the lumbus. The combination of these points can build up kidney *Yang*, promote the circulation of *Qi* and stop pain.

Method: Apply filiform needles with reinforcing method, and retain the needles for 20—30 miuntes, manipulating them one to two times. Shenshu (BL23), Mingmen (DU　4) and Zhishi (BL 52) may also be applied with moxibustion for 15—20 minutes, or with direct warming needles.

3. Lumbar Pain due to Traumatic Factors

Principle: Activate blood circulation, remove obstruction from the channels and collaterals, resolve blood stasis and stop pain by using points mainly from The Bladder Channel of

Foot—*Taiyang* plus some local Ahshi points.

Prescription: Ahshi points   Geshu(BL17)   Ciliao(BL32)

Weizhong(BL40)   Houxi(SI   3)

Explanation: Ahshi points are used to promote *Qi* and blood circulation in the local area. Geshu(BL17) and Ciliao(BL32) are used to activate blood circulation, resolve stasis and stop pain. Weizhong(BL40) is used to as a distal point to remove obstruction from the channels and collaterals. Houxi(SI   3), one of the Eight Confluent Points, has the effect of communicating with The *Du* Channel. It is used here to sedate pain in the lumbar region. The joint use of the above points have the effect of activating *Qi* and blood circulation, resolving stasis of blood and stopping pain.

Point Modification: Add Shuigou(DU26) if the pain is severe.

Method: Apply filiform needles with reducing method and retain the needles for 15—20 minutes, manipulating them three to four times. Weizhong(BL 40) may also be pricked with three—edged needle to cause bleeding. For acute pain in the lumbar region, the paitent is expected to do lumbar exercices when needles at Shuigou (DU26) or Houxi (SI   3) are frequently manipulated. Pricking is applied on Ahshi points, which is then followed by cupping in order to suck out the stagnant blood as much as possible.

Alternative Treatment: Auricular Acupuncture

Prescription: Lumbar vertebra   Sacral vertebra   Kidney

Ear—Shenmen   Subcortex

Method: Apply filiform needles with strong stimulation for 20 minutes. Implanting of ear seeds is also applicable. The patient is expected to do some lumbar exercices when the ear points are stimulated, for instance, lifting hand, bending forward or turning to either side.

1.36   Frozen Shoulder

Frozen should is a condition that bothers most of its victims at the age around fifty. It therefore is also known as fifty shoulder. It is characterized by a heavy aching on one or two shoulders and limited movement.

The condition of frozen shoulder is described as peripheral shoulder arthritis in modern medicine.

Cause and Mechanism

Frozen shoulder is mostly caused by weakness of the nutrient and defensive systems, asthenia of muscles and joints as well as wind−cold invasion. However, twisting and contusion due to careless exertion or stagnation of *Qi* and blood due to habitual onesided sleep pressing the channels and collaterals may also cause frozen shoulder.

Differentiation

Pain initially starts on one or two shoulders. It alleviates in the daytime and worsens at night, and may also involve the upper arm, nape and back. The condition also aggravates with cold but alleviates with warmth. At the advanced stage, there may be difficulty in raising the arm, limited arm abduction and backward stretching. Prolonged frozen shoulder may result in muscular atrophy.

Treatment

Principle: Expel wind−cold, promote *Qi* and blood circulation and remove the obstruction from the channels and collaterals by using points mainly from the three *Yang* channels of the hand.

Prescription: Jianyu(LI15)   Jianzhen(SI 9)
                  Binao(LI14)   Quchi(LI11)

Waiguan(SJ 5) Hegu(LI 4)
Houxi(SI 3)

Explanation: Jianyu(LI 15), Jianzhen(SI 9) and Binao(LI 14) are local points to promote *Qi* and blood circulation, remove obstruction from the channels and collaterals and stop pain. Quchi (LI11), Waiguan(SJ 5)and Hegu(LI 4) are distal points to promote *Qi* circulation in the *Yangming* channels and eliminate wind—cold. Houxi(SI 3)is a significant point to search out wind—cold in the shoulder area because The Small Intestine Channel of Hand—*Taiyang* also distributes in the shoulder area. In addition, this point can also activate blood circulation and stop pain. The joint use of the above points can relieve the pathogenic factors, promote *Qi* and blood circulation and stop pain.

Point Modification: Add Tianzhu(BL10), Bingfeng(SI12) and Quyuan(SI13) if the pain radiates to the neck and back.

Method: Apply filiform needles with even method and retain the needles for 20—30 minutes, manipulating them two to three times. Mostly, acupuncture and moxibustion are combined in the treatment. Moxibustion is applied at Jianyu (LI15)for 20 minutes or direct warming needle.

Alternative Treatment: Auricular Acupuncture

Prescription: Shoulder Shoulder joint Clavicle Sympathetic Subcortex

Method: Apply filiform needles at three to four points with moderate stimulation and retain the needles for 20 minutes. Advise the patient to do some exercises when the needles are frequently manipulated. Embedding of ear seeds is also applicable.

1.37　Diabetic Syndrome

Diabetic syndrome is a condition characterized by polydipsia, polyphagia, polyuria, emaciation and sweet urine. It is called diabetes in modern medicine.

Cause and Mechanism

Diabetic syndrome is mostly due to hyperactive heart fire and over consumption of lung *Yin*. Retention of heat in the spleen and stomach due to improper food intake over—consumes the body fluid. Also, sexual indulgence may impair the kidney, causing the deficiency of kidney essence. These factors respectively cause the diabetic syndromes of the upper, middle and lower—*Xiao*.

Differentiation

1. Upper—*Xiao* Diabetes

The chief manifestations include thirst with desire to drink, and dry mouth and tongue. The accompanying symptoms and signs include profuse urine, polydipsia, redness in the tip of the tongue, thin yellow tongue coating, and full rapid pulse.

2. Middle—*Xiao* Diabetes

The chief manifestations include great increase of appetite, easy hunger, discomfort sensation in the stomach, restlessness with feverish sensation, profuse sweating, emaciation, or dry stools. It is accompanied by profuse drinking of water, polyuria, dry yellow tongue coating, and rapid slippery pulse.

3. Lower—*Xiao* Diabetes

The chief manifestations include frequent urination, in heavy quantity and turbid quality, dry mouth and tongue, desire for profuse drinking, dizziness, blurring of vision, red cheeks, restlessness due to *Yin* deficiency, easy hunger but not good appetite, soreness and weakness of the lumbus and knees, red tongue proper, and rapid thready pulse. There will be dark complexion, aversion to cold, profuse urinary discharge, pale tongue proper with white coating, and deep thready weak pulse if the chronic *Yin* deficiency has affected *Yang* of the body. And there will be impotence and amenorrhea respectively as well.

Treatment

Principle: Eliminate the heat retained in the *Sanjiao* by using points in consideration of the three different types of diabetic syndromes. For upper *Xiao* diabetes, select points mainly from The Lung Channel of Hand—*Taiyin* and The Heart Channel of Hand—*Shaoyin*. For middle—*Xiao* diabetes, select points mainly from The Stomach Channel of Foot—*Yangming* and The Spleen Channel of Foot—*Taiyin*. And for lower *Xiao* diabetes, select points mainly from The Kidney Channel of Foot—*Shaoyin* and The Liver Channel of Foot—*Jueyin*, plus some Back—*Shu* points as well as some extra points.

Prescription:(Based on different diabetic conditions)

Upper—*Xiao* Diabetes: Shaofu(HT 8)   Xinshu(BL15)
                        Taiyuan(LU 9)   Feishu(BL13)
                        Yishu(Extra)

Middle—*Xiao* Diabetes: Neiting(ST44)   Sanyinjiao(SP 6)
                         Pishu(BL20)   Weishu(BL21)
                         Yishu(Extra)

Lower—*Xiao* Diabetes: Taixi(KI 3)   Taichong(LR 3)
                        Ganshu(BL18)   Shenshu(BL23)
                        Yishu(Extra)

Explanation: For upper—*Xiao* diabetes, Shaofu(HT 8), the

Ying—spring point of the heart channel, is used in combination with Xinshu (BL15) to clear away heart fire. Taiyuan(LU 9), the *Shu*—stream and *Yuan*—source points of the lung channel, is combined with Feishu(UB13)to reinforce *Yin* of the lung. For middle—*Xiao* diabetes, the principle of treatment is to regulate the function of the spleen and stomach, eliminate gastric heat and nourish the *Yin* of the stomach. Therefore, Sanyinjiao (SP 6), Pishu (BL20) are used to reinforce the function of spleen to ascend fluid. Neiting(ST44), the *Ying*—spring point of the stomach channel, is used to eliminate gastric heat. The principle of treatment for lower—*Xiao* diabetes is to reinforce the liver and kidney. Therefore, Taixi(KI 3), the *Yuan*—source point of the kidney, is combined with Shenshu (BL23) to strengthen the function of kidney to receive *Qi*, Taichong (LR 3) and Ganshu (BL18) soothe the liver and sedate the fire. The extra point Yishu (Extra) is the empirical point for the treatment of the three type of diabetes.

Point Modification: Add Lianquan(RN23) and Chengjiang (RN24) for dry mouth; Zhongwan(RN12) and Neiguan(PC 6) for gastric discomfort sensation with acid regurgitation and polyorexia; Gaungming (GB37) for blurred vision; Shangxing(DU23) for dizziness; Mingmen(DU 4) for *Yang* deficiency.

Method: Apply filiform needles with both reinforcing and reducing methods. Specifically, Shaofu(HT 8), Xinshu(BL15), Neiting (ST44), Taichong (LR 3) and Ganshu (BL18) with reducing method; Taiyuan(LU 9), Feishu(BL18), Pishu(BL20), Taixi(KI 3), Shenshu(BL23) and Yishu (Extra)with reinforcing method. Retain the needles for 20—30minutes, manipalating them two to three times.

Alternative Treatment

1. Auricular Acupuncture

Prescription:Pancreas　Endocrine　Kidney　Spleen
　　　　　　　　Stomach　Lung　*Sanjiao*　Ear—Shenmen
　　　　　　　　Heart　Liver Root of auricular vagus nerve

Method: Apply filiform needles at three to five points with mild stimulation and retain the needles for 20 minutes. Embedding of ear seeds is also applicable.

2. Plum—blossom Needle Therapy

Prescription: Huatuojiaji from T7 to T10 or the Back—*Shu* points at the corresponding levels.

Method: Use a plum—blossom needle to tap on the areas suggested with gentle stimulation until local redness appears.

Remarks: Diabetic patients have deficiency of anti—pathogenic *Qi*. Strict disinfection is required for them because they may easily develop in fection. For severe case of diabetic syndrome, comprehensive treatment with herbs is necessary. Patients are advised to adjust the diet when they receive acupuncture treatment.

1.38　Beriberi

Beriberi refers to flaccid feet, swollen feet and lower portion of the legs, or weakness and numbness of the feet even though there may not be any swelling involved. Since the condition starts from the feet, hence the name feet flaccidity or beriberi. It includes feet conditions due to VB₁ deficiency in modern medicine. The differentiation and treatment here can be referred to for other feet conditions that bear the similar manifestations such as feet malnutrition and polyneuritis.

Cause and Mechanism

Beriberi is mostly due to invasion of damp—water from rain or dew, or dwelling from damp place that causes dampness invading into the muscles and tendons. Improper diet damaging the spleen and stomach can also lead to beriberi. This is because the poor function of spleen and stomach in transforming and digesting gives rise to heat accumulation in the lower—*Jiao*. The heat continues to flow down to the feet to develop pain and swelling. Nevertheless, constitutional *Yin* deficiency of the liver and kidney makes it easy for the dampness turn into heat and further into dryness to cause blood deficiency. Consequently malnutrition of tendons and muscles will develop beriberi.

Differentiation

At the beginning of beriberi, patients only feel flaccidity of the feet. But gradually, swelling of foot dorsum, numbness and pain of the feet, and difficult walking will appear. According to the difference in clinical manifestations, beriberi can be divided into damp type beriberi, dry type beriberi and beriberi affecting the heart.

1. Damp Type Beriberi

The chief manifestations include swelling of foot dorsum, pain and numbness of toes which gradually affects the legs, soreness and heaviness of the feet and knee joints, weakness of the feet with difficulty in walking. There will be cold sensation in the feet that responds to warmth if cold—damp is more prevailing. There will be feverish sensation in dorsum of the feet that responds to cooling if the damp—heat is more prevailing. Other manifestations of the damp—heat type may include fever with aversion to cold, short scanty urine, white greasy or slightly yellow tongue coating, rapid soft pulse.

2. Dry Beriberi

The chief manifestations include weakness of both feet, numbness and pain of legs and knees with occasional tendon spasm, limited movement, gradual atrophy of foot muscles or even severe atrophy of foot muscles, constipation, yellow urinary discharge, slightly red tongue proper, thin white tongue coating or slightly coated tongue, and rapid thready pulse.

3. Beriberi Affecting the Heart

The chief manifestations include swelling, pain or numbness with atrophy and weakness for walking, sudden onset of shortness of breath, palpitation, nausea, vomiting, suffocating sensation in the chest, restlessness and even loss of consciousness in the severe case, disorderly speech, purplish lips, rapid thready pulse of a feeble nature.

Treatment

1. Damp Type Beriberi

Principle: Promote *Qi* and blood circulation in the channels and collaterals, clear up heat and resolve dampness by using points mainly from The Urinary Bladder Channel of Foot—*Taiyang*, The Stomach Channel of Foot—*Yangming* and The Gallbladder Channel of Foot—*Shaoyang*.

Prescription: Zusanli(ST36)   Sanyinjiao(SP 6)
                    Yanglingquan(GB34)   Bafeng(EX—LE10)

Explanation: Pathogenic dampness is a kind of *Yin* pathogenic factor that has the characteristic to descend. Beriberi of this type is caused by retention of dampness in the lower limbs. Therefore, Zusanli (ST36), Sanyinjiao (SP 6) are used to invigorate the *Qi* mechanism in order to resolve the damp—water from The Stomach Channel of Foot—*Yangming* and The Spleen Channel of Foot—*Taiyin*. Pathogenic wind can also help to produce dampness. The Gallbladder Channel of Foot—*Shaoyang* is a wind—wood channel according to the five element theory. Therefore, Yanglingquan (GB34) and Bafeng(Ex—LE 10) are used to eliminate wind, resolve dampness and clear up heat. Once the damp—heat is removed. there will be smooth circulation of *Qi* and blood in the channels and collaterals so that swelling and pain can disappear.

Point Modification: Add Hegu(LI　4), Dazhui(DU14) and Waiguan (SJ　5) for fever with aversion to cold; Yinlingquan (SP 9) and Kunlun (BL60) for short scanty urine.

Method: Apply filiform needles with reducing method and retain the needles for 20--30 minutes, manipulating them two to three times. Moxibustion can be applied for 10—15 minutes if cold—damp is prevailing. Pricking with a three—edge needle at Bafeng (Extra) can be applied for beriberi due to severe damp—heat.

2. Dry Type of Beriberi

Principle: Nourish *Yin* and blood by using points mainly from The Stomach Channel of Foot—*Yangming* and The Spleen Channel of Foot—*Taiyin*.

Prescription: Jiexi(ST41)　Yinshi(ST33)　Fuliu(KI　7)
　　　　　　　Zhaohai(KI　6)　Xuehai(SP10)
　　　　　　　Xuanzhong(GB 39)

Explanation: Jiexi (ST41), Yinshi (ST33) and Xuehai(SP 10) are used to strengthen the spleen and stomach in order to nourish qi and blood. Zhaohai(KI　6), Xuanzhong(GB39)　and

Fuliu(KI 7) are used to reinforce kidney *Yin* in order to refill the kidney essence. Sufficient *Qi*, blood and essence will ensure nourishment to the tendons and bones so beriberi with difficult walking and muscular atrophy can be alleviated.

Point Modification: Add Chengshan(BL57) for muscular spasm; Weizhong (BL 40) for lumbar pain; Xiyan (Ex—LE5) and Fengshi(GB 31) for swollen knees.

Method: Apply filiform needles with reinforcing method and retain the needles, manipulating them one to two times.

3. Beriberi Affecting the Heart

Principle: Promote the function of lung in descending and dispersing and clear away damp—heat from the heart by using points mainly from The Lung Channel of Hand—*Taiyin*, The Pericardium Channel of Hand—*Jueyin*, The Heart Channel of Hand—*Shaoyin* and The Kidney Channel of Foot—*Shaoyin*.

Prescription: Chize(LU 5) Danzhong(RN17)
              Laogong(PC 8) Shenmen(HT 7)
              Zusanli(ST36) Yongquan(KI 1)

Explanation: Chize (LU 5), the *He*—sea point of the lung channel, is combined with Danzhong(RN17), the Influential Point of *Qi*, to promote the function of lung in descending and dispersing. Laogong(PC 8), Shenmen (HT 7) calm the heart and mind. Zusanli(ST36) pacifies stomach and descneds the dampness. Yongquan(KI 1), the *Jing*—well point of the kidney channel, is used to guide the pathogenic damp—heat to the foot to be dispelled. The joint use of these points may promote lung in descending and dispersing, clear up pathogenic damp—heat from the heart and calm the heart and mind.

Point Modification: Add Renzhong(DU26) for loss of consciousness; Qihai (RN 6) and Guanyuan(RN 4) for collapse of *Yang Qi*.

Method: Apply filiform needles with even mothod and retain the needles for 15—20 minutes.

Alternative Treatment: Auricular Acupuncture

Prescription: Toe Ankle Knee Spleen Stomach
              Lung Kidney Ear—Shenmen

Method: Apply filiform needles at three to four points with moderate stimulation for 20 minutes. Embedding of ear seeds is also applicable.

1.39   Drum Belly

Drum belly is a term applied in traidtional Chinese medicine only, referring to abnormal abdominal distention like the drum, hence the name. It is characterized by distended abdomen and yellowish skin. There will be visible green vessels on the abdomen, with normal limbs or slightly swollen limbs. According to the different clinical manifestations, drum belly is generally divided into *Qi* distention, water distention and blood distention.

The condition described here can be seen in the advanced stage of various chronic diseases in terms of modern medicine such as hepatocirrhosis, tubercular peritonitis, abdominal tumor, etc. The differentiation and treatment in this section can be referred to for similar symptoms and signs appearing in the above conditions.

Cause and Mechanism

Drum belly is mostly caused by the dysfunction of liver, spleen and kidney. Improper food intake and over alcoholic indulgence, emotional impairment or accumulation of jaundice that is inadequately treated will lead to stagnation of *Qi*, stasis of blood and water retention in the abdomen to form the drum belly.

Drum belly can also be sometimes caused by the effect of pathogenic water or parasites which were not dispelled in time.

Differentiation

1. *Qi* Distention

The chief manifestations include abdominal and epigastric fullness and distention, unchanged abdominal skin colour, depression upon hand pressing but soon rebounding when the hand is removed, aggravation of distention during emotional upset, alleviation by belching, sighing or passing wind, percussing sound on abdomen, fullness sensation in the epigastric and hypochondriac regions, short yellow urine, dry stools or constipation, thin white tongue coating, and wiry thready pulse.

2. Water Distention

The chief manifestations include abdominal distention like the belly of a frog, lustrous abdominal colour, depression that is slow to rebound, or occasional edema in the lower limbs, distention in epigastric and abdominal areas, pallor complexion, aversion to cold, lassitude, difficult urination, loose stools, white greasy tongue coating, and deep slow pulse.

3. Blood distention

The chief manifestations include distention in the abdomen and epigastrium with hard abdominal wall, visible vessels surrounding the umbilicus, mass in the hypochondriac region with pricky pain, scaled skin, dimmish complexion or dark pallor complexion with red threads, bloody moles appearing in neck, chest and arms, tidal fever, dry mouth with no desire for drinks, or occasional black stools, purplish dark tongue proper with possible stagnant spots, hesitant or wiry thready pulse.

Treatment

1. *Qi* Distention

Principle: Soothe the liver *Qi,* pacify the stomach and relieve distention by using points mainly from The Liver Channel of Foot—*Jueyin,* The Stomach Channel of Foot—*Yangming* and The *Ren* Channel.

Prescription:　Danzhong(RN17)　Zhongwan(RN12)

　　　　　　　　　Qihai(RN　6)　Zusanli(ST36)

　　　　　　　　　Tianshu(ST25)　Taichong(LR 3)

Explanation: Danzhong(RN17) is used to regulate *Qi* circulation of the upper—*Jiao;* Zhongwan (RN12), the middle—*Jiao* and Qihai (RN 6), the lower—*Jiao* Taichong(LR 3) soothes the liver and relieve *Qi* stagnation. Zusanli(ST36) and Tianshu(ST 25) promote the function of the stomach and intestines in order to pacify the stomach and relieve distention. The joint use of these points may soothe the liver *Qi,* promote *Qi* circulation, and relieve the distention.

Point Modification: Add Fujie(SP14) for constipation; Zhigou(SJ 6) and Yanglingquan (SP34) for hypochondriac pain; and Yinlingquan(SP 9) for yellow urine.

Method: Apply filiform needles with reducing method and retain the needles for 20—30 minutes, manipulating them two to three times.

2. Water Distention

Principle: Strengthen the spleen and tonify the kidney, promote *Qi* circulation and enhence water discharge by using mainly the Back—*Shu* points, and points from The Spleen Channel of

Foot—*Taiyin*, The Kidney Channel of Foot—*Shaoyin* and The *Ren* Channel.

Prescription:　Pishu(BL20)　Shenshu(BL23)
　　　　　　　　Shuifen (RN　9)　Fuliu (KI　7)
　　　　　　　　Gongsun(SP　4)

Explanation: Shuifen (RN 9) is an important point for relieving abdominal water. Part of the spleen's function is to transport and transform water and dampness. The kidney dominates water discharge. Therefore, Pishu(BL 20) and Gongsun (SP 4) are used to strengthen spleen *Qi* in transporting and transforming water and dampness. Shenshu(BL 23) and Fuliu(KI 7) are used to reinforce kidney *Qi* and open the water passage. The joint use of the above points can strengthen the *Qi* of the spleen and kidney, resolve the water and dampness, and promote the function of the water passage so that water distention can be relieved.

Point Modification: Add Tianshu (ST25) and Shangjuxu (ST37) for loose stools; and Mingmen(DU 4) and Qihai (RN 6) for aversion to cold.

Method: Apply filiform needles with both reinforcing and reducing method. Pishu(BL20) and Shenshu(BL23) are applied with reinforcing method. The rest of the points are applied with even method. Retain the needles for 20—30 minutes, manipulating them two to three times. Moxibustion can be applied at Shuifen (RN 9) for 15—20 minutes.

3. Blood Distention

Principle: Activate blood, resolve stasis, promote *Qi* circulation and water discharge by using points mainly from The Liver Channel of Foot—*Jueyin* and The Spleen Channel of Foot—*Taiyin*.

Prescription: Qimen (LR14)   Zhangmen(LR13)

Shimen(RN 5)   Sanyinjiao(SP 6)

Explanation: Blood distention is mostly developed from masses in the hypochondriac region. The masses are often involve with liver and spleen diseases. Therefore, Qimen(LR 14) and Zhangmen (LR 13), respectively the Front−*Mu* points of the liver and spleen, are used to regulate the *Qi* and blood circulation of the two organs. Sanyinjiao(SP 6), the intersecting point of the three *Yin* channels of the foot, is used in combination with Shimen(RN 5), the Front−*Mu* point of the triple heater, to activate blood, resolve stasis, and promote *Qi* circulation and water discharge.

Point Modification: Add Liangmen (ST21) for distention; Yanggang(BL48) for jaundice; and Taixi (KI 3) and Gaohuangshu(BL 43) for tidal fever.

Method: Apply filiform needles with reducing method and retain the needles for 20−30minutes, manipulating them three to four times.

Alternative Treatment: Auricular Acupuncture

Prescription: Liver   Kidney   Pancrease   Large intestine

Small intestine   Sanjiao   Auricular concha

Method: Apply filiform needles with moderate stimulation at 4−5 points each time and retain the needles for 15−20 minutes. Embedding of ear seeds is also applicable.

1.40   Edema

Edema refers to retention of fluid in the body, resulting in the puffiness of the head, face, eyelids, limbs, abdomen and even the general body. It can be divided into *Yang* type edema and *Yin* type edema in terms of etiology and pathogenisis.

The condition elaborated here includes the edema caused by acute and chronic nephritis, congestive heart failure, endocrinal disorder and dystrophy in modern medicine.

Cause and Mechanism

Yang edema is mostly due to wading through water or being caught in rain, exposure to cold after bath, invasion of pathogenic heat into the interior due to furuncle effect. These factors may cause the dysfunction of the lung in dispersing and descending, and that of the spleen in transforming and transporting, leading to the eventual retention of pathogenic damp-water flooding over the body superficies.

Yin edema is often due to improper diet, deficiency of spleen *Qi,* impairment of kidney *Qi* caused by overstrain, or over sexual indulgence. The deficient spleen results in poor transforming and transporting, and internal retention of damp-water. The deficiency of kidney leads to poor water metabolism and failure of kidney to control over urination, resulting in flooding of the damp-water to the exterior of the body.

Lingering *Yang* edema may turn into the *Yin* type due to gradual consumption of anti-pathogenic *Qi*. *Yin* edema on the other hand may manifest some symptoms and signs of the *Yang* type due to recurrent exogenous pathogenic invasion and sudden worse swelling.

Differentiation

1. *Yang* Type Edema

This type of edema, mostly acute in nature, is characterized by incipient puffiness of the face, eyelids, limbs affecting the general body, lustrous skin, swelling of the scrotum, and dysuria.

Depressions appearing upon hand pressing may rebound quickly. The accompanying symptoms and signs include fullness sensation in the chest, cough, uneven breathing, soreness and aching of the limbs, white slippery tongue coating with moisture, superficial slippery or superficial rapid pulse.

2. *Yin* Type Edema

This type of edema is characterized by a slow onset, light swelling of the face in the incipient stage which then spreads to the abdomen and the whole body, especially the areas below the waist. Depressions appearing upon hand pressing rebound slowly. The accompanying symptoms and signs include short urine, epigastric distention, loose stools, lassitude and aversion to cold, weak limbs, pale tongue proper with white coating, deep thready or deep slow pulse.

Treatment

1. *Yang* Type Edema

Principle: Eliminate wind, clear up heat, disperse lung and promote water metabolism by using points mainly from The Urinary Bladder Channel of Foot—*Yangming*, The Spleen Channel of Foot—*Taiyin* and The Large Intestine Channel of Hand—*Yangming*.

Prescription: Feishu (BL13)   Sanjiaoshu (BL22)
           Pianli (LI 6)   Yinlingquan(SP 9)
           Waiguan(SJ 5)   Hegu(LI 4)

Explanation: The dispersing mechanism is applied to edema in the upper part of the body. Feishu(BL13) and Pianli (LI 6) are used to disperse the lung and eliminate cold. Waiguan(SJ 5) and Hegu(LI 4) are used to dispel wind, clear up heat and cause sweating so that the damp—water in the superficial portion of the body will follow the sweat to be removed. Sanjiaoshu(BL 22) has the function of regulating the water passage. Yinlingquan(SP 9) strengthens the spleen and promotes water metabolism so that the internal water retention is sent down to the urinary bladder to be discharged, thus separating the clean from the turbid, and subduing the edema.

Method: Apply filiform needles with reducing method and retain the needles for 15—20 minutes, manipulating them two to three times.

2. *Yin* Type Edema

Principle: Tonify the spleen and warm up the kidney'to strengthen the *Yang Qi* in steaming water by using points main from The *Ren* Channel, The Stomach Channel of Foot—*Yangming* and The Kidney Channel of Foot—*Shaoyin,* plus some Back—*Shu* points.

Prescription: Pishu(BL 20)   Shenshu(BL 23)

Shuifen(RN 9)   Qihai(RN 6)

Taixi(KI 3)   Zusanli (ST 36)

Explanation: For the edema involving the upper portion of the body, the mechanism is to separate the clean from the turbid. Pishu (BL20) and Zusanli (ST36) are used to strengthen the spleen and eliminate the dampness. Shenshu(BL 23) and Taixi(KI 3) warm up the kidney *Yang*. Qihai (RN 6) assists the *Yang* in steaming water. Shuifen (RN 9) separates the clean from the turbid. Normal *Qi* circulation leads to the normal function of the water passage, thus swelling subdues with the normal water metabolism.

Point Modification: Add Zhongwan(RN12) for epigastric distention; and Tianshu(ST 25) for loose stools.

Method: Apply filiform needles with reinforcing or even method and retain the needles for 15−30 minutes, manipulating them two to three times. Moxibustion is also applicable for 20−30 minutes, particularly with heavy moxibustion on Qihai(RN 6).

Alternative Treatment: Auricular Acupuncture

Prescription: Liver   Spleen   Kidney   Lung

                        Urinarybladder   Subcortex   Lung

Method: Apply filiform needles with moderate stimulation at three to four points each time and retain the needles for 20 minutes. Embedding of ear seeds is also applicable.

1.41 *Lin* Syndrome

Lin syndrome refers to a condition characterized by frequent, incontinent urinary discharge with pain, spasm of the lower abdomen, and umbilical pain. According to the different etiology and pathogenisis in the clinic, it is divided into five types altogether. They include heat *Lin,* stone *Lin,* blood *Lin, Qi Lin* and turbid *Lin* syndromes.

Lin syndrome is mainly seen in some urinary system diseases with abnormal stimulation or infections of the uretha, such as pyelonephritis, cystitis, renal tuberculosis, stones in the urinary tract, acute and chronic prostatitis, carcinoma of the urinary bladder, and chylous urine. The differentiation and treatment in this section can be referred to for their treatments.

Cause and Mechanism

Frequent urination and feverish pain due to poor *Qi* transforming and downward flowing of damp−heat resulted from either exogenous pathogenic damp−heat invasion or poor function of spleen in resolving dampness to form heat *Lin* syndrome.

Stone *Lin* syndrome is due to stones formed in a long time of damp—heat accumulation. It is characterized by sandy stones obstructing the uretha and irritative pain during urinary discharge. Accumulation of damp—heat affecting the blood system or hyperactivity of deficient fire affecting the collaterals results in blood *Lin* syndrome. This is indicated by bloody urination. *Qi Lin* syndrome is often complained by the aged patients with severe deficiency of kidney *Qi*. The poor function of the urinary bladder in transforming *Qi* leads to difficult urination characterized by lingering dripping of urine. Turbid *Lin* syndrome is related to chronic deficiency of spleen and kidney. Deficient spleen causes difficulty in transporting the food essence while deficiency of kidney leads to the inability of kidney itself to control the urinary bladder so that there will be milky urine because the turbid is not separated from the clean.

Differentiation

1. Heat *Lin* Syndrome

The chief manifestations include rapid onset of urinary dripping, frequent urination, dark yellow urine with feverish and painful sensation, hasty urinary discharge, pain involving the umbilicus, or fever with aversion to cold, bitter taste in mouth, red tongue proper with yellow greasy tongue coating, and rapid soft pulse.

2. Stone *Lin* Syndrome

The chief manifestations include difficult urination with occasional sandy substance in the urine or dysuria with pain involving the lower abdomen that makes the patient feel difficult to tolerate, or on and off urinary discharge with stabbing lumbar pain that involves both the lower abdomen and external genitalia, occasional bloody urine, thin white or yellow tongue coating, wiry or rapid pulse.

3. Blood *Lin* Syndrome

The chief manifestations include short reddish urine in hast or that with dark purplish clots, severe burning pain, difficulty in discharging the urine, distending pain in the uretha in severe cases which invloves the umbilicus, red tongue tip, thin yellow tongue coating, rapid forceful pulse.

4. *Qi Lin* Syndrome

The chief manifestations include distending pain in the lower abdomen and pubic region, weakness in discharging the urine, dripping of urine of clear quality and high frequency, reluctant speech, poor spirit, lumbar soreness, pale tongue with thin white coating, and weak thready pulse.

5. Turbid *Lin* Syndrome

The chief manifestations include turbid milky urine that soon sediments with catkin substance at the bottom, but faty oily substance at the surface of the urine container with coalgulation or bloody, diffiutlt urinary discharge with feverish pain, or soreness in the lumbar region and knees, dizziness, lassitude, red tongue proper, slightly white greasy coating, soft rapid or rapid thready pulse.

Treatment

Principle: Regulate the *Qi* mechanism of the urinary bladder, eliminate heat and promote urinary discharge by using points mainly from the three *Yin* channels of the foot plus some of the Back−*Shu* points.

Prescription: Pangguangshu(BI 28)   Zhongji(RN   3)

Yinlingquan (SP   9)   Xingjian(LR   2)

Taixi(KI 3)

(1)Hegu (LI 4) and Waiguan (SJ 5) for heat *Lin* syndrome;

(2)Weiyang (BL39) and Rangu (KI 2) for stone *Lin* syndrome;

(3)Xuehai (SP10) and Sanyinjiao (SP 6) for blood *Lin* syndrome;

(4)Qihai (RN 6) and Shuidao (ST28) for *Qi Lin* syndrome;

(5)Qihai (RN 6), Shenshu(BL 23) and Baihui (DU 20) for turbid *Lin* syndrome.

Explanation: Pangguangshu (BL28) is combined with Zhongji (RN 3), the Front—*Mu* point of the urinary bladder, to regulate the *Qi* mechanism of the urinary bladder. Yinlingquan (SP 9), the *He*—sea point of the spleen channel, is tused to promote urinary discharge, and restore the normal *Qi* mechanism of the urinary bladder. Pain can be stopped if normal urinary discharge is regained. Xingjian(LR 2) is used to sedate the fire from the liver channel and stop pain because the liver channel curves around the reproductive organ. Taixi(KI 3), the *Yuan*—source point of the kidney channel, is used to tonify the kidney water and clear the source. The joint use of the above points can regulate the *Qi* mechanism of the urinary bladder and promote urinary discharge.

Method: Apply filiform needles with reducing or even method and retain the needles for 15—30 minutes, manipulating them two to three times.

Alternative Treatment: Auricular Acupuncture

Prescription: Urinary bladder Kidney Sympathetic

Occipital bone   Adrenal gland   Endocrine

Method: Apply filiform needles at three to four points with strong stimulation and retain the needles for 20—30 minutes. Embedding of ear seeds is also applicable.

1.42   Seminal Emission

Seminal emission refers to the involuntary seminal discharge that takes place often apart from during sexual intercourse. Specifically, nocturnal emission happens during dreams in sleep while spermatorrhea happens when the patient has no dreams or completely clear during sleep. However, occasional seminal emission in adult males, married or unmarried, is not considered as a disease condition.

For seminal emission caused by prostatitis, neurasthenia, seminal vesiculitis and other diseases in modern medicine, the differentiation and treatment in this section can be referred to.

Cause and Mechanism

Nocturnal emission in dreams is mainly due to overstrain or stress, or excessive sexual indulgence that leads to flaring up of heart fire and over consumption of kidney *Yin*. In this case, the heart fire does not descend to control the kidney water while the kidney water can not ascend to cool the heart fire, thus appearing the dysharmony between the heart and kidney. The hyperactive heart fire disturbs the sperms, causing nocturnal emission in dreams. Also, functional impairment of the spleen and stomach due to over eating of sweat, greasy, fatty or pungent food can cause damp—heat accumulation in the middle—*Jiao*. The downward flowing of such a damp—heat can induce dreams and disturb the sperms, resulting in nocturnal emission.

Spermatorrhea is often due to damage of the kidney after prolonged illness, over indulgence in sex or habitual masturbation. Exhausted kidney essence due to stubborn nocturnal emission causes the deficiency of kidney Qi which fails to consolidate sperms. The kidney can not store sperms because the spermal gate is not firm.

Differentiation

1. Nocturnal Emission

This kind of seminal emission takes place at night when the sleep is not profound. There can be several emissions a night or one emissions every several nights with dreaming of penis erecting or with premature ejaculation. The accompanying symptoms and signs include dizziness, vertigo, restlessness, poor sleep, lumbar soreness, tinnitus, lassitude, poor spirit, yellow urine, red tongue proper, and thready rapid pulse.

2. Spermatorrhea

This kind of emission may happen without any dreams at any time during the day or the night. There may be emission on sexual thoughts in severe cases. The accompanying symptoms and signs include emaciation, pallor complexion, soreness and cold sensation in the lumbar region, pale tongue proper with white coating, and deep thready pulse.

Treatment

1. Nocturnal Emission

Principle: Sedate heart fire, nourish Yin and consolidate sperms by using points mainly from The Heart Channel of Hand—*Shaoyin,* The Kidney Channel of Foot—*Shaoyin,* plus some Back—*Shu* points.

Prescription: Xinshu (BL15)   Shenmen (HT 7)

Shenshu (BL23)   Taixi(KI 3)
Guanyuan (RN 4)   Zhishi(BL52)

Explanation: Xinshu (BL 15) is combined with Shenmen (HT 7), the *Yuan*—source point of the heart channel, to sedate heart fire and guide the heart fire to go downward to control the kidney water. Shenshu (BL23) is combined with Taixi (KI 3), the *Yuan*—source point of kidney channel to reinforce the kidney water in order restrict the heart fire. Guanyuan (RN 4), the point crossing the three *Yin* channels of the foot and The *Ren* Channel, is the root of *Yuan*—source *Qi* of the body. Zhishi(BL 52), also known as spermal room, is added in combination with the above points to nourish *Yin,* regain the harmony between the heart and kidney, promote the function of kidney in storing essence and consolidate sperms.

Point Modification: Add Zusanli (ST36) for lassitude and poor spirit; Baihui(DU 20) for dizziness; and Yinlingquan (SP 9) and Sanyinjiao (SP 6) for short scnaty or dripping of urine due to down—flowing of damp—heat.

Method: Apply filiform needles with both reinforcing and reducing methods and retain the needles for 20—30 minutes, manipulating them two to three times.Xinshu (BL15), Shenmen (HT 7) are used with reducing method and the rest of the points with reinforcing method.

2. Spermatorrhea

Principle: Tonify the kidney *Qi* and regain consolidation over the spermal gate by using points mainly from The Kidney Channel of Foot—*Shaoyin* and The *Ren* Channel.

Prescription: Shenshu(BL23)   Sanyinjiao(SP 6)
Guanyuan (RN 4)   Qihai (RN 6)

Taixi(KI 3) Dahe (KI12)
Zusanli (ST36)

Explanation: Sanyinjiao (SP 6) is an important point at the crossing of the three *Yin* channels of the foot. It is used here to strengthen the liver, spleen and kidney and clear up the deficient fire. Shenshu (BL23), Qihai (RN 6), Guanyuan(RN 4) and Taixi(KI 3) warm up the primary *Yang,* reinforce *Qi* and consolidate the sperms. Dahe (KI 12) firms the spermal gate. Zusanli (ST 36) strengthens the spleen and stomach in order to promote the source for providing the acquired energy. The joint use of the above points can reinforce *Qi*, strengthen deficiency and firm the spermal gate.

Method: Apply filiform needles with reinforcing method and retain the needles for 20—30 minutes, manipulating them two to three times. Moxibustion can be combined with acupuncture treatment.

Alternative Treatment: Auricular Acupuncture

Prescription: Sperm Palace   Endocrine   Ear—Shenmen
Heart   Kidney

Method: Apply filiform needles with mild stimulation and retain the needles for 20 minutes. Embedding of ear seeds or subcutaneous ear needles is also applicable

1.43 Impotence

Impotence refers to weakness of penis erecting during sexual intercourse, characterized by poor erecting or erection that lasts only for seconds. For impotence as a main symptom due to sexual neurasthenia or some other chornic diseases, the differentiation and treatment in this section can be referred to.

Cause and Mechanism

Impotence is often the consequence of deficiency of the essential *Qi* and decline of life gate fire due to over sexual indulgence or juvenile masturbation. Over consumption of *Qi* of the heart, spleen and kidney due to fear, fright or worry can also cause impotence. Internal damp—heat retention affecting the liver and kidney with looseness of penis accounts for another factor to cause impotence.

Differentiation

1. Life Gate Fire Decline

The main manifestations include poor erecting of penis or erection that lasts only for seconds, pallor complexion, cold limbs, dizziness, blurring of vision, poor spirit, soreness in the lumbar region and knee joints, frequent urination, pale tongue proper with white coating, and deep thready pulse. There will also be palpitation and insomnia if the impairment of heart and spleen is involved.

2. Downward Flowing Damp—heat

The chief manifestations include inability of the penis to erect and wet scrotum with foul smell. It can be accompanied by bitter taste in the mouth, thirst, short scanty urine, soreness in the lower limbs, greasy tongue coating, and rapid soft pulse.

Treatment

1. Life Gate Fire Decline

Principle: Reinforce kidney *Yang* and warm up the lower—*Jiao* by using points mainly from The *Ren* Channel and The Kidney Channel of Foot—*Shaoyin*.

Prescription: Shenshu (BL23)   Mingmen (DU 4)

Guanyuan (RN 4)   Sanyinjiao(SP 6)

Taixi(KI 3)

Explanation: Shenshu(BL23), Mingmen(DU 4) and Taixi(KI 3), the *Yuan*-source point of the kidney channel, can reinforce kidney *Yang*, strengthen kidney essence, warm up the lower-*Jiao* and consolidate the primary *Qi*. Sanyinjiao (SP 6) strengthens basically the spleen and the liver and kidney as well. It is an important point for treating diseases of the reproductive system. Guanyuan (RN 4) may refill *Qi* and essence and invigorate *Yang Qi*. The joint use of the above points can activate the primary *Qi,* refill both blood and essence so that strengthened kidney *Qi* saves the patient from impotence.

Point Modification: Add Xinshu (BL 15), Daling (PC 7) for deficiency of both heart and spleen; Baihui(DU20) and Zusanli(ST 36) for dizziness and blurring of vision.

Method: Apply filiform needles with reinforcing method and retain the needles for 20−30 minute, manipulating them two to three times. Direct the needle towards the pubic region in order to let the needling sensation radiate to the penis when Guanyuan (RN 4) is needled. Moxibustion can also be applied at Guanyuan (RN 4), Shenshu (BL 23) and Mingmen (DU 4) for 15−20 minutes.

2. Downward Flowing of Damp−heat

Principle: Eliminate damp−heat by using points mainly from The *Ren* Channel and The Spleen Channel of Foot−*Taiyin*.

Prescription: Zhongji(RN 3)   Sanyinjiao (SP 6)
　　　　　　　　Yinlingquan (SP 9)   Xingjian (LR 2)
　　　　　　　　Zusanli (ST 36)

Explanation: Zhongji(RN 3), Sanyinjiao (SP 6) and Yinlingquan (SP 9), the *He−sea* point of the spleen channel, have the function of promoting urinary dishcarge and eliminating damp—heat. The collateral of the liver channel connects with the reproductive organ. Therefore, Xingjian(LR 2) is used to eliminate damp—heat from the liver channel. Zusanli (ST 36) strengthens the spleen in transforming and resolving damp—heat because heat will have no condition to exist in the body if dampness is resolved. The joint use of the above points may eliminate damp—heat from the lower—*Jiao* in order to treat the patient for seminal emission.

Method: Apply filiform needles with reducing method and retain the needles for 15—20 minutes, manipulating them two to three times.

Alternative Treatment: Auricular Acupuncture

Prescription: Sperm Palace   External genitalia   Kidney
                    Testis   Endocrine

Method: Apply filiform needles with moderate stimulation and retain the needles for 20 minutes. Embedding of ear seeds is also applicable.

1.44   Enuresis and Incontinence of Urine

Enuresis refers to involuntary discharge of urine during sleep at night. The victim is not aware of it until he or she is waked up. It is often seen in children over the age of three and a very small number of adults. Incontinence of urine refers involuntary urinary discharge when the patient is conscious of it. It is mostly seen in the aged patients, women patients or patients who survived some morbid conditions. The urine drips spontaneously without control.

The conditions described here include enuresis complained

of by children and adults as well as that caused by neural dysfunction and pathological changes of the urinary system in terms of modern medicine.

Cause and Mechanism

Enuresis and incontinence of urine are consequences of poor function of lower—*Jiao* and dysfunction of the urinary bladder in controlling urination due to weak constitution and kidney *Qi* deficiency. Insufficiency of kidney *Qi* in the aged or impairment of the kidney due to over sexual indulgence may also cause incontinence of urine because of cold retention in the lower—*Jiao* and poor opening function of the urinary bladder. Internal injuries due to seven emotional disturbances such as fear, fright and over thinking affecting the spleen and lung can cause deficiency of the two. And the superior deficiency cannot control the inferior so that the urinary bladder will lose its control over urinary discharge. Accumulation of damp—heat that flows down to the urinary bladder too leads to enuresis or incontinence of urine. Also, blood stasis due to various reasons obstructing in the urinary bladder will cause the dysfunction of urinary bladder in transforming *Qi*. Therefore, enuresis or incontinence of urine appears because the urinary bladder does not control urination.

Differentiation

1. Kidney *Yang* Deficiency Type

Enuresis takes place during sleep. The patient is not aware of it until he wakes up. There can be frequent urination with dripping of urine or incontinence of urine in severe cases. The accompanying symptoms and signs include emaciation, lassitude, cold limbs, pallor complexion, soreness and weakness of the lumbar region and knees, pale tongue proper, and deep slow pulse weak in nature.

2. *Qi* Deficiency of the Lung and Spleen

The patient has frequent and hasty urine with occasional enuresis and incontinence of urine. The accompanying symptoms and signs include pallor complexion, shortness of breath, lassitude, weakness of the four limbs, poor appetite, loose stools, pale tongue proper, and slow or deep thready pulse.

3. Downward Flowing of Damp—heat

The chief manifestations include frequent urination with burning sensation in the uretha, occasional enuresis or incontinence of urine, short scanty urine with odour or dripping urine, lumbar sorenss, lower grade fever, thin greasy tongue coating, and rapid thready pulse.

4. Blood Stasis in the Lower—*Jiao*

The chief manifestations include dripping of urine, abdominal distention with dull pain, masses felt by palpating, occasional enuresis, dark purplish tongue proper, and hesitant or rapid thready pulse.

Treatment

1. Kidney *Yang* Deficiency Type

Principle: Warm up the kidney *Yang* by using points mainly from The Urinary Bladder Channel of Foot—*Taiyang* and The *Ren* Channel.

Prescription: Shenshu (BL23)　　Pangguangshu (BL28)
　　　　　　　　Guanyuan (RN　4)　Zhongji (RN　3)
　　　　　　　　Taixi(KI　3)　Sanyinjiao(SP　6)

Explanation: Shenshu (BL 23) is combined with Taixi (KI 3), the *Yuan*—source point of the kidney channel, to reinforce both kidney *Qi* and kidney *Yang*. Sanyinjiao (SP 6) tonifies the spleen, kidney and liver and strnegthens the *Yuan*—source energy. Guanyuan(RN 4), the root of the *Yuan*—source *Qi,* can strengthen the *Yuan*—source *Qi* and promote the *Qi* transforming. Zhongji(RN 3), the Front—*Mu* point of the urinary bladder, may activate the *Qi* mechanism of the urinary bladder. The joint use of the above points may reinforce kidney and strengthen kidney *Yang*. Sufficient *Qi* of the kidney will ensure the function of the urinary bladder in controlling urination, so that enuresis and incontinence of urine can be relieved.

Point Modification: Add Baihui(DU 20) and Shenmen (HT 7) for profound sleep; Qihai (RN 6) and Mingmen (DU 4) for incontinence of urine in the aged with *Qi* deficiency.

Method: Apply filiform needles with reinforcing method and retain the needles for 20—30 minutes, manipulating them two to three times. Moxibustion are mostly applied to Shenshu (BL 23), Pangguangshu (BL 28) and Guanyuan (RN 4) at the same time for 15—20 minutes.

2. *Qi* Deficiency of the Spleen and Lung

Principle: Reinforce lung and strengthen the spleen by using points mainly from The *Ren* Channel, The Lung Channel of Hand—*Taiyin,* The Spleen Channel of Foot—*Taiyin* and The Stomach Channel of Foot—*Yangming.*

Prescription: Feishu (BL13)   Taiyuan (LU 9)

　　　　　　　Pishu (BL20)   Zusanli (ST36)

　　　　　　　Qihai (RN 6)   Sanyinjiao (SP 6)

Explanation: Feishu(BL13) is combined with Taiyuan (LU 9), the *Yuan*—source point of the lung channel, to reinforce the lung *Qi* and regulate the water passage. Pishu (BL20), Zusanli (ST36)and Sanyinjiao(SP 6) are used to strengthen the spleen and stomach, and reinforce the liver and kidney. in order to promote the transforming and dispersing of body fluid. Qihai (RN 6) warms up kidney *Yang,* strengthens the *Yuan*—source *Qi* and reinforces the lower—*Jiao* function. The joint use of the above points can help ascend the spleen *Qi,* descend the lung *Qi* and regain the control of urinary bladder over urination to let the patient have normal urinary discharge.

Point Modification: Add Baihui(DU20) and Ciliao (BL32) for frequent urination.

Method: Apply filiform needles with reinforcing method and retain the needles for 20—30 minutes. Feishu (BL13), Pishu(BL 20), Zusanli (ST36) and Qihai (RN 6) can be applied with both acupuncture and moxibustion.

3. Downward Flowing of Damp—heat

Principle: Eliminate damp—heat from the lower—*Jiao* by using points mainly from The Urinary Baldder Channel of Foot—*Taiyang,* The Spleen Channel of Foot—*Taiyin* and The Kidney Channel of Foot—*Shaoyin.*

Prescription: Pangguangshu (BL28)　Zhongji(RN　3)
　　　　　　　　Yinlingquan(SP　9)　Foot—Tonggu(BL66)
　　　　　　　　Weiyang(BL39)　Sanyinjiao(SP　6)

Explanation: Pangguangshu (BL28) and Zhongji(RN 3), known as the combination of Back—*Shu* and Front—*Mu* points, are used to eliminate damp—heat from the lower—*Jiao* and promote the function of urinary bladder in discharging urine. Yinlingquan (SP 9) is used in combination with Sanyinjiao (SP 6) to strengthen the spleen and resolve damp—heat in the lower—*Jiao* Weiyang (BL39) and Foot Tonggu(BL66), respectively the Lower *He*—sea point of the *Sanj iao* channel and the *Ying*—spring point of the urinary bladder channel, are used to eliminate heat retention in the urinary bladder. The joint use of the above points can eliminate the damp—heat from the lower—*Jiao* Dispelling of damp—heat from the urinary bladder helps the urinary bladder to control urinary discharge so that urination will become normal again.

Method: Apply filiform needles with reducing method and retain the needles for 15—20 minutes, manipulating them two to three times.

4. Blood Stasis in the Lower—*Jiao*

Principle: Activate blood circulation and resolve stasis of blood by using points mainly from The *Ren* Channel and The Spleen Channel of Foot—*Taiyin*.

Prescription: Zhongji(RN 3)　Ciliao(BL32)　Sanyinjiao
　　　　　　　(SP 6)　Qihai(RN 6)　Geshu(BL17)

Explanation: Zhongji(RN 3) and Ciliao (BL 32) can activate the *Qi* circulation of the urinary bladder channel. Qihai(RN 6) is combined with Sanyinjiao (SP 6) and Geshu(BL 17) to promote *Qi*, activate blood, and resolve blood stasis. The joint use of the above points may resolve the stagnant blood and regain the *Qi* transforming function of the urinary bladder.

Method: Apply filiform needles with reducing method and retain the needles for 20—30 minutes with three to four times of needling manipulation.

Alternative Treatment: Auricular Acupuncture

Prescription: Kidney　Urinary　Bladder　Urethra
　　　　　　　Subcortex　Sympathetic　Lung　Spleen

Method: Apply filiform needles at three to four points with mild stimulation and retain the needles for 15 minutes. Embedding of ear seeds is also applicable.

1.45　Retention of Urine

Retention of urine is a disease condition characterized by difficult urination, distending pain in the lower abdomen and even blockage of urine. It includes clinically the mild condition of difficult urinary discharge with dripping and obstructed urinary discharge with distending and urgent feeling in the severe case.

Retention of urine can be seen in uroschesis due to various causes.

Cause and Mechanism

Retention of urine is mostly due to poor body consitution in the aged or in patients survived lingering illness. The kidney deficiency and decline of life gate fire cause the dysfunction of the urinary bladder in controlling urination. Heat accumulation in the lower-*Jiao* and urinary bladder can impede the micturating function of the urinary bladder, resulting in urinary retention. Obstruction of the channels and collaterals as well as urethral obstruction due to traumatic injuries or surgical operation may also lead to retention of urine.

Differentiation

1. Kidney *Qi* Deficiency Type

The chief manifestations include forceless dribbling of urine, pallor complexion, listlessness, lumbar soreness, weakness of the four limbs, pale tongue proper, and deep thready pulse which is particularly weak in the kidney region.

2. Heat Retention in the Urinary Bladder

The chief manifestations include obstructed discharge of short scanty urine, distention in the lower abdomen, thirst with no desire for drinking, red tongue proper, yellow coating and rapid pulse.

3. Urethral Obstruction Type

The chief manifestations include dripping of urine, or obstruction of urine, pain and distention in the lower abdomen, red spots over the surface of the tongue, and rapid hesitant pulse.

Treatment

1. Kidney *Qi* Deficiency Type

Principle: Warm up *Yang Qi,* reinforce kidney and promote urinary dischrge by using points mainly from The Kidney Channel of Foot—*Shaoyin* and The Urinary Bladder Channel of Foot—*Taiyang.*

Prescription: Shenshu (BL 23)   Sanyinjiao (SP 6)

Yingu (KI 10)   Sanjiaoshu(BL 22)

Qihai (RN 6)   Weiyang(BL 39)

Explanation: Shenshu(BL 23) is combined with Yingu (KI 10), the *He*—sea point of the kidney channel, to invigorate the *Qi* mechanism of the kidney channel, and reinforce kidney *Qi*. Sanjiaoshu(UB 22)is combined with Weiyang(BL39), the Lwer *He*—sea point of the *Sanj iao* channel, to regulate the *Qi* mechanism of the *SanJiao* and the water passage. Sanyinjiao (SP 6), the point crossing the three *Yin* channels of the foot, may strengthen the spleen and kidney and promote urinary discharge. Qihai(RN 6) warms up the lower—*Jiao* and strengthens the *Yuan*—source *Qi*. The joint use of the above points can reinforce the *Qi* of the kidney, promote the function of the lower—*Jiao* and relieve urinary retention.

Point Modification: Add Yaoyangguan(DU 3) and Mingmen(DU 4) for soreness in the lumbar region

Method: Apply filiform needles with reinforcing method and retain the needles for 20–30 minutes, manipulating them two to three times. Shenshu(BL 23), Sanjiaoshu(BL 22) and Qihai (RN 6) can be applied with both acupuncture and moxibustion.

2. Heat Retention in the Urinary Bladder

Principle: Eliminate damp–heat by using points mainly from The Urinary Bladder Channel of Foot–*Taiyang* and The Spleen Channel of Foot–*Taiyin*.

Prescription: Pangguangshu(BL28)   Zhongji(RN 3)
                          Sanyinjiao (SP 6)   Yinlingquan (SP 9)

Explanation: Pangguangshu(BL28) and Zhongji(RN 3), known as the combination of Bask–*Shu* and Front–*Mu* points, are used to clear up the retention of heat in the urinary bladder, regulate the function of the urinary bladder and promote the *Qi* mechanism of the lower–*Jiao* Sanyinjiao (SP 6) is combined with Yinlingquan (SP 9), the *He*–sea point of the spleen channel, to eliminate the damp–heat in the lower–*Jiao* and strengthen the function of spleen in resolving water. The joint use of the above points may eliminate damp–heat and promote urinary discharge.

Method: Apply filiform needles with reducing method and retain the needles for 15–20 minutes, manipulating them two to three times.

3. Urethral Obstruction Type

Principle: Resolve stasis and promote urinary discharge by using mainly the Front–*Mu* and Back–*Shu* points of the urinary bladder, points from The Spleen Channel of Foot–*Taiyin*.

Prescription: Pangguangshu(BL28)   Zhongji(RN 3)
                          Sanyinjiao (SP 6)   Shuiquan(KI 5)
                          Shuidao (ST28)

Explanation: Pangguangshu (BL 28) and Zhongji(RN 3), the combination of the Back−*Shu* and Front−*Mu* points of the urinary bladder, regulate the *Qi* mechanism and promote urinary discharge. Sanyinjiao (SP 6) activate blood, resolve blood stasis, remove obstruction from the channels and collaterlas and promote urinary discharge. Shuiquan (KI 5), the *Xi*−cleft point of the kidney channel, promotes urinary discharge, relieve swelling and stop pain. The joint use of the above points may remove obstruction from the channels and collaterals, regulate *Qi* mechanism and promote urinary discharge.

Point Modification: Add Qihai(RN 6) for fullness and distention in the lower abdomen.

Method: Apply filiform needles with even or reducing method and retain the needles for 15−20 minutes, manipulating them two to three times.

Alternative Treatment:

1. Auricular Acupuncture

Prescription: Urinary bladder　Kidney　Urethra
　　　　　　SanJiao　Sympathetic　Subcortex

Method: Apply filiform needles at three to four points each time with moderate stimulation and retain the needles for 20−30 minutes. Embedding of ear seeds is also applicable.

2. Electric Stimulation

Prescription: Weidao(GB 28)

Method: Apply filiform needle at Weidao (GB 28) horizontally towards Qugu (RN 2) for about two to three *Cun* distance. This is then followed by electric stimulation with dense−sparse wave for 20−30 minutes.

1.46   Sweat Syndrome

Sweat syndrome is a condition of poor opening and closing of skin pores with heavy perspiration due to the imbalance of *Yin* and *Yang* of the body, and the dysharmony between the nutritive and defensive systems. This section mainly covers spontaneous sweating and night sweating. The former is characterized by perspiration that worsens by exertion while the latter characterized by perspiration during sleep at night that stops by itself when the patient is wakened.

Sweat syndrome can be seen in many diseases in modern medicine. The differentiation and treatment elaborated here can be referred to for both spontaneous sweating and night sweating as a symptom in such diseases as hyperthyroidism, vegetative nerve dysfunction, hypoglycemia, tuberculosis, rheumatic fever as well as spontaneous and night sweating seen in the acute and rehaibilitative stages of some infectious diseases.

Cause and Mechanism

There are many factors which may lead to sweat syndrome. Poor defensive *Yang* energy and dysharmony between the nutritive and defensive systems due to constitutional *Yang* deficiency with poor function of skin pores in opening and closing and invasion of exogenous pathengic wind; turbid dampness retention in the middle—*Jiao* turning into heat to steam the superficial portion of the body due to impairment and dysfunction of the spleen and stomach in transforming and transporting caused by either improper food intake or invasion of exogenous pathogenic dampness; or dormant heat in the interior with unrecovered *Yin Qi* of the body due to severe or lingering illness, may cause the sweat syndrome. Besides, over consumption of kidney essence due to excessive sexual indulgence or heat retention in the interior of the body due to the use of medicines that have heat property can also cause over consumption of *Yin* blood. Therefore, sweating appears when *Yin* does not match the hyperactive *Yang* in the body.

Differentiation

1. Spontaneous Sweating

The chief manifestations include contineous sweating without any exertion or worse by exertion, and cold limbs with cold sweat in the severe cases. It may be accompanied by palpitation, shortness of breath, lassitude, distention in abdominal and epigastric regions, white or slightly yellow tongue coating, and deficient feeble pulse.

2. Night Sweating

The chief manifestations include contineous sweating during sleep that stops when the patient is awake, red cheeks, feverish sensation in the palms and soles, red tongue proper with less coating than normal, and rapid thready pulse.

Treatment

1. Spontaneous Sweating

Principle: Reinforce *Yang,* and strengthen the superficial portion of the body by using points mainly from The Kidney Channel of Foot—*Shaoyin,* and The Large Intestine Channel of Hand—*Yangming.*

Prescription: Fuliu(KI 7)   Hegu(LI 4)
　　　　　　　Gaohuangshu(BL43)   Feishu(BL13)
　　　　　　　Pishi(BL20)   Zusanli(ST36)
　　　　　　　Qihai(RN 6)

Explanation: Hegu(LI 4), the *Yuan*—source point of the large intestine channel, dominates *Qi*. Fuliu(KI 7), the point from the kidney channel, dominates fluid. The combination of these two points may stop sweating. Feishu (BL 13) and Gaohuangshu(BL 43) reinforce lung *Qi* and strengthen the superficial defensive energy. Pishu (BL 20) and Zusanli (ST 36) strengthen the *Qi* of the spleen and stomach in order to promote the source for providing the acquired energy. Qihai(RN 6) regulates and reinforces the *Yuan*—source *Qi*. The joint use of the above points may refill the *Yuan*—source *Qi*, strengthen the defensive *Qi*, regulate the harmony between the nutritive and defensive systems so as to stop sweating.

Point Modification: Add Neiguan(PC 6) for palpitation and shortness of breath; and Zhongwan (RN12) for fullness and distention in the abdominal and epigastric regions.

Method: Apply filiform needles with both reinforcing and reducing methods and retain the needles for 15—20 minutes. Reduce Fuliu (KI 7) and reinforce the rest of the points, manipulating them one to two times.

2. Night Sweating

Principle: Nourish *Yin*, sedate fire and stop sweating by using points mainly from The Kidney Channel of Foot—*Shaoyin* and The Liver Channel of Foot—*Jueyin*.

Prescription: Taixi(KI 3)   Yinxi(HT 6)
                Sanyinjiao (SP 6)   Fuliu(KI 7)

Explanation: Taixi (KI 3), the *Yuan*—source point of the kidney channel, is used to nourish kidney *Yin* and sedate fire. Sanyinjiao (SP 6) disperses the deficient heat and nourish *Yin* blood. Yinxi(HT 6), the *Xi*—cleft point of the heart channel, may nourish heart *Yin* and sedate heart fire. Fuliu(KI 7) nourishes kidney *Yin* and reteats tidal fever. The joint use of the above points can nourish *Yin*, sedate fire and stop sweating.

Method: Apply filiform needles with even method and retain the needles for 15—20 minutes, manipulating once or twice.

Alternative Treatment: Auricular Acupuncture

Prescription: Lung   Heart   Sympathetic   Endocrine
             Adrenal   gland

Method: Apply filiform needles with moderate stimulation and retain the needles for 15—20 minutes. Embedding of ear seeds is also applicable.

1.47   Pulseless Syndrome

Pulseless syndrome refers to a weakness or disappearance of pulse at *Cunkou* that is one *Cun* distal to the end of the radial artery. Such a condition may also take place at the ulnar artery at the ankle. It can be seen in many diseases in modern medicine such as multiple aorto—arteritis, atherosclerosis obliterans, thromboangitis obliterans, arterial embolism, etc.

Cause and Mechanism

This condition is often caused by invasion of exogenous pathogenic wind—cold and dampness into the channels and collaterals, or *Yang* deficiency of the spleen and kidney that leads to poor circulation of *Qi* and blood and stasis of blood, resulting in the poor pulsating.

Differentiation

The Weakened or fainting pulse at *Cunkou* may be accompanied by dizziness, blurring of vision, lassitude, weakness of the arms, numbness, sorness and cold sensation in the arms, and purplish colour of the finger tips. Convulsions and loss of consciousness may also take place if the condition is severe. The symptoms and signs for pulseless syndrome involving the lower limbs are similar to those of the upper limbs.

Treatment

Principle: Regulate *Qi* and activate blood and resolve stasis to restore the normal pulsation.

Prescription: Taiyuan (LU 9)   Renying(ST 9)
                Daling (PC 7)   Neiguan (PC 6)
                Chize(LU 5)

Explanation: Taiyuan (LU 9) is both the *Yuan*−source point of the lung channel and Influential point of the vessel. Chize(LU 5) is the *He*−sea point of the lung channel. The combination of the two points can regulate the *Qi* circulation of the lung, activate blood and remove obstruction from the channels and collaterals. Renying (ST 9) is the merging place of the *Qi* of The Stomach Channel of Foot−*Yangming* and interescts the *Yangming* and *taiyang* channels. Yangming channel has more abundant *Qi* and blood puncturing Renying(ST 9) may regulate both *Qi* and blood and remove obstruction from the channels and collaterals. Daling (PC 7) and Neiguan(PC 6), respectively the *Yuan*−source and *Luo*−connecting points of the pericardium channel, may regulate blood circulation and resolve blood stasis because points of the pericardium channels can play the role of points from the heart channel. The joint use of the above points regulate *Qi* and blood, resolve blood stasis and restore normal pulsating.

Point Modification: Add Fengchi(GB20) and Baihui(DU 20) for dizziness; Jingming(BL 1) for blurring of vision; Quchi(LI 11)and Hegu(LI 4) for numbness and soreness of the arm; and add Zusanli (ST36), Yinbai(SP 1), Weizhong(BL40) and Chongyang(ST 42) for pulseless syndrome of the lower limbs.

Method: Apply filiform needles with even method and retain the needles for 15–20 minutes, manipulating them two to three times. It is better to produce some numbness sensation but out of too strong a needling stimulation. Needles are supposed to be retained over the time suggested.

Alternative Treatment: Auricular Acupuncture

Prescription: Ear–Shenmen Heart Kidney Spleen
               Subcortex Endocrine Upper limb
               Adrenal gland

Method: Apply filiform needles at four to five points with mild stimulation and retain the needles for 10–15 minutes. Ear needles are generally combined with the use of embedding of ear seeds.

1.48 Malaria

Malaria is an infectious disease characterized by shivering chills and strong fever at regular intervals. This condition can be divided into quotidian malaria, tertian malaria and quartan malaria according to the interval between every two attacks. There may be some palpable mass in the hyperchondriac region in the chronic case. And this is medically called malaria with splenomegaly.

Malaria, more common in summer and autumn, may also sporadically occur in other seasons.

Cause and Mechanism

Malaria is mainly caused by the invasion of pestilential factor and that of exogenous pathogenic heat, wind, cold and dampness dormant in the semi−exterior and semi−interior and wandering between the nutrient and defensive systems. Chills appear if such factors run into the nutrient system, and heat appears if they outwardly disturb the defensive system. The inbalance between nutrient and defensive systems and the struggle between the anti−pathogenic Qi and pathogenic Qi develop malaria.

Differentiation

Shivering chills and fever appear at regular intervals. They often start with yawning and forcelessness, and then with shivering chills, When the chills retreat, general fever takes place. In severe cases, there can be high fever, coma, delirium, deadly headache, red cheeks, fullness in the hypochondriac region, bitter taste and dryness in the mouth, thirst with desire for drinking, and sweating by the end of the attack. The body feels cool again when the fever stops. The tongue coating is thin, yellow and greasy, and the pulse is wiry and rapid.

There may also appear pallor complexion, lassitude, blurring of vision, dizziness, emaciation, and mass in the hypochondriac region if the malaria lasts for long period of time with irregular intervals.

Treatment

Principle: Regulate Qi of The Du Channel, eliminate the pathogenic factors from Shaoyang and stop malaria by using points mainly from The SanJiao Channel of Hand−Shaoyang.

Prescription: Dazhui(DU14)   Taodao(DU13)

Yemen (SJ 2)   Houxi (SI 3)   Jianshi(PC 5)

Explanation: Dazhui(DU 14), the converging point of Yang, may promote the circulation of Yang Qi and eliminate the pathogenic factor from the superficial portion of the body. It is used in combination with Taodao (DU 13) to promote *Qi* circulation of The *Du* Channel and regulate *Yin* and *Yang* in balance. It is an important point for halting malaria. Houxi(SI 3), the Confluent point communicating with The *Du* Channel, may disperse *Qi* the The *Du* Channel as well as the *Taiyang* channels to repel the pathogenic factors. Yemen (SJ 2) regulates *Qi* of the *Shaoyang* channel. Jianshi(PC 5), a point from The Pericardium Channel of Hand—*Jueyin* that form an external—internal relationship with The *Sanj iao* Channel of Hand—*Shaoyang,* is used to eliminate heat from the heart, promote the *Qi* mechanism of the *Sanj iao* and restore harmony between the interior and exterior. The joint use of these points may promote the *Yang Qi,* regulate nutrient and defensive systems, relieve pathogenic factors from the interior and exterior as well, and stop malaria.

Point Modification: Add the 12 *Jing*—well points with pricking for high fever, coma and delirium; Pishu(BL20) and Gaohuangshu (BL22) for lingering malaria; and Zhangmen(LR 13) and Pigen (Extra)for hypochondriac mass.

Method: Apply filiform needles with reducing method and retain the needles for 15—20 minutes, manipulating them three to four times. Treatment is given two to three hours in advance to the next attack of malaria when acupuncture is used to treat such a condition. Acupuncture may be combined with moxibustion if chills appears to be more prevailing than fever. Acupuncture is applied only without moxibustion if fever is more severe than cold. Taodao (DU 13) and Dazhui(DU 14) may be pricked with a three—edged needle to cause bleeding. Moxibustion can be applied at Pishu(BL 20), Gaohuangshu (BL 22) and Pigen (EX—B 4) for 15–20 minutes if the lingering malaria has already caused hypochondriac mass. Five to seven pieces of moxa cones can also be applied at the above points.

Alternative Treatment

1. Auricular Acupuncture

Prescription: Adrenal gland   Subcortex   Endocrine
                    Ear–Shenmen   Liver   Spleen
                    Gallbladder   Ear apex

Method: Apply filiform needles with strong stimulation at three to five points and retain the needles for 15–20 minutes. Ear apex is pricked with a three–edged needle to cause bleeding. Treatment is given two to three hours in advance of the next attack. Embedding of ear seeds or subcutaneous needles is also applicable.

2. Cupping

Prescription: Dazhui(DU14)   Taodao(DU13)
                      Zhiyang(DU 9)

Method: Prick these three points with a three–edged needle to cause bleeding. This is then followed by cupping. Treatment is given once every other day. This method can be applied independently or combined with other treatments which will help to produce a better therapeutic effect.

2 Surgical and Dermatological Diseases

2.1 Red—Streaked Infection

Red—streaked infection mostly occurs on the extremities and face marked by small deep—rooted furuncles as hard as pin nails that swiftly extend on an upward line, for which the name is given. It is similar to acute superficial lymphangitis in modern medicine.

Cause and Mechanism

Red—streaked infection is mainly caused by disturbance of heat in the *Zangfu* organs due to improper diet or intake of fatty spicy food. It may also be caused by invasion of exogenous pathogenic heat through a wound on the extremities, bringing out pathogenic heat transmitting into the meridians and ending in stagnation of both *Qi* and blood.

Differentiation

At the beginning, red—streaked infection starts as a miliary boil like a deep—rooted hard nail with itching, numbness and slight pain. This is then followed by local redness, swelling, increased pain, accompanied by chills, fever, nausea, vomiting and anorexia. If it happens on the body extremities, lesions on the upper extremity may extend to the elbow and armpit, and lesions on the lower extremity to the popliteal fossa or groin, There can be enlarged lymph nodes and tenderness in the affected areas. In severe cases, there are some general symptoms such as high fever, irritability, unconsciousness, delirium, dark urine, constipation, bright red tongue, and full rapid pulse. This kind of infection is known as carbuncle complicated by septicema in traditional Chinese medicine.

Treatment

Principle: Eliminate heat, cool the blood and relieve swelling by using points mainly from The *Du* Channel, The Large Intestine Channel of Hand—*Yangming* and The Stomach Channel of Foot—*Yangming*.

Prescription A: (for red—streaked infection on the head, face and upper extremities)Lingtai (DU10) Dazhui(DU14) Quchi (LI11) Quze (PC 3) Zhongchong (PC 9) Hegu (LI 4)

Explanation: Lingtai (DU10), a point from The *Du* Channel, is good for eliminating heat from the chest and superficial portion of the skin. Dazhui (DU14), the converging point of *Yang*, that dominates *Yang* and exterior, has the effect to eliminate heat from the superficial portion of the general body. Quze (PC 3) and Zhongchong (PC 9) eliminate heat from the *Sanjiao* relieve swelling and stop pain. Hegu (LI 4) and Quchi (LI11),points from The Large Intestine Channel of Hand—*Yangming*, respectively have the effect to ascend and disperse in an attempt to promote *Qi* circulation, and to remove stagnation in an attempt to activate blood and resolve stasis. The joint use of these two points may regulate defensive *Qi*, nutrient and blood systems, and eliminate pathogenic heat from the superficial portion of the body.

Prescription B: (For red—streaked infection on the lower limbs) Lingtai (DU10) Dazhui (DU14)

Weizhong (BL40) Xuanzhong (GB39)

Explanation: Lingtai (DU10) and Dazhui (DU14) are used for the same mechanism in prescription A. Weizhong (BL40), applied with reducing method, may eliminate heat, cool the blood and sedate fire. Xuanzhong (GB39), a point from The Gallbladder Channel of Foot—*Shaoyang*, may eliminate heat from the *Sanjiao* resolve dampness, relieve swelling and stop pain.

Point Modification Add Guanchong (SJ 1) for restlessness; and Shixuan (EX—UE11) and Renzhong (DU26) for high fever, loss of consciousness and delirium.

Method: Apply filiform needles with reducing method and continue to manipulate the needles for three to five minutes without further manipulation. Weizhong (BL40) and Zhongchong (PC 9) can be pricked with a three—edged needle to cause bleeding.

Alternative Treatment: Cupping

Prescription: Lingtai (DU10)

Method: After routine disinfection at Lingtai (DU10), prick the point with a three—edged needle to cause bleeding, then cupping is given. If red thread appears, disinfect the line routinely, prick the line from the beginning to the end every two to three centimetres away, then do cupping.

2.2   Scrofula

Scrofula refers to masses of irregular sizes without redness, feverish sensation, nor obvious pain in the posterior area of the ear, neck or nape. There can be one or several masses in line. The concept of scrofula in traditional Chinese medicine term the masses into big and small ones in size, respectively called *Li* and

Luo. It is similar to lymph tuberculosis in modern medicine.

Cause and Mechanism

Scrofula is usually due to phlegm—fire accumulating in the neck by the action of pathogenic fire consuming the body fluid, resulting from emotional upsets and prolonged stagnation of liver—qi, or due to rising of *Qi* with phlegm located in the neck resulting from dominant nation of liver—*Yang* and comsumption of body fluid, which is caused by deficiency of lung—*Yin* and kidey—*Yin*. The prolonged accumulation of phlegm and *Qi* may turn into excessive heat leading to erosion and discharge of pus. It is slow to heal and may require prolonged treatment.

Differentiation

1. Incipient Stage of Scrofula

Incipient scrofula does not obviously present general symtoms and signs. There are irregular sizes of masses similar to sizes of beans ranging from one to several pieces. These are fixed masses of hard quality without feverish sensation, pain or change of the skin colour.

2. Middle Stage of Scrofula

The masses are increasing in sizes, but still not moveable. There is some local pain and feverish sensation. The dark red masses are soft upon palpating. The condition is accompanied by tidal fever, red cheeks and lassitude.

3. Scrofula with Ulceration

Ulceration is usually developed from the middle stage when treatment given was not adequate. The ulcerated areas may appear to have purulent substance of dilute quality like bean curd residue. The ulcerated spots are hard to recover, and gradually form fistulas with lingering discharge of purulent fluid.

Treatment

1. Incipient Scrofula

Principle: Eliminate heat, resolve phlegm and soften the scrofula by using points mainly from The Pericardium Channel of Hand—*Jueyin,* The Liver Channel of Foot—*Jueyin* and The Galllbladder Channel of Foot—*Shaoyang.*

Prescription: Qimen (LR14)   Neiguan (PC   6)
　　　　　　Xingjian (LR 2)   Jianjing (GB21)
　　　　　　Foot—Linqi (GB41)   Tianjing (SJ10)
　　　　　　Jing bailao (EX—HN15)

Explanation: Points formed in this prescription are aimed at dealing with both the symptomatic *Biao* and root cause *Ben* at the same time. Qimen (LR14), the Front—*Mu* point of the liver, is combined with Neiguan (PC6), the *Luo*—connecting point of the pericardium channel, to strengthen the effect in soothing the liver and relieving stagnation of *Qi* in an attempt to deal with the root cause *Ben*. Xingjian (LR 2), the *Xing*—spring point of the liver channel, is combined with Jianjing (GB21), and Foot—Linqi (GB41), the *Shu*—stream point of the gallbladder channel, to eliminate heat and resolve phlegm, relieve swelling and soften the scrofula in an attempt to deal with symptomatic *Biao*. Jingbai Lao (EX—HN15) and Tianjing (SJ10) are empirical points for treating scrofula. These points in combination may strengthen the therapeutic effect.

Point Modification: Add Yifeng (SJ17) for scrofula in the nape; Binao (LI14), shousanli (LI10) for scrofula in the neck; and Zhoujian (EX—UE1) and Yangfu (GB38) for scrofula in the auxillary fossa.

Method: Apply filiform needles with reducing method and

retain the needles for 10–15 minutes, manipulating them two to three times. JingbaiLao (EX−HN15) and Tianjing (SJ10) are applied with five to seven pieces of small moxa cones.

Note: Acupuncture is generally suggested for treating scrofula in the first two stages, not for the advanced stage when ulceration has already taken place.

2.3　Herpes Zoster

Herpes zoster, known as heat rash belting the waist in traditional Chinese medicine since it mostly affects the lumbar region, refers to red−coloured blisters in line occurring in the lumbar or hypochondriac region. Herpes zoster is a term in modern medicine.

Cause and Mechanism

Emotional disturbance affecting the interior can cause hyperactive fire of the liver and gallbladder. The hyperactive wood overacts on the earth causing impaired function of the spleen and stomach with poor transforming and transporting. Therefore, the internal accumulation of damp−heat plus invasion of exogenous pathogenic damp−heat jointly lead to the onset of herpes zoster.

Differentiation

Prior to the onset of herpes zoster, patients may have general discomfort, slight fever, lassitude, and poor appetite. During the progression of herpes zoster, there often appears burning pain in the affected areas.

Herpes zoster starts with reddened skin. This is then followed by dense appearance of clusters of irregular sizes that soon develops into blisters in groups of three or five gathered in one or several places in line. The skin in between the blisters is normal. Herpes zoster mostly affects one side of the body, often in the hypochondriac region, throacic and abdominal region, but rarely on the facial region.

Herpes zoster in the lumbar and hypochondriac regions is characterized by redness of local skin, feverish sensation and burning pain. It is accompanied by bitter taste in the mouth, headache, dizziness, restlessness, shortness of temper, or congestion in the eyes, short scanty urine, red tongue proper with yellow coating, and rapid wiry pulse. This is mostly due to dormant wind—heat in the channels of the liver and gallbladder. Herpes zoster in the throacic region is characterized by a light colour of blisters, slight feverish sensation and flowing of fluid when the blisters are broken. It is accompanied by lassitude, poor appetite, yellow greasy tongue coating, and rapid slippery pulse. This is mostly due to retention of dampheat in the spleen and stomach.

Treatment

1.Wind—heat Type Herpes Zoster

principle: Soothe the liver, promote bile excretion and eliminate pathogenic heat by using points mainly from The Liver Channel of Foot—*Jueyin* and The Gallbladder Channel of Foot—*Shao Yang*.

Prescription: Lingtai(DU10) Zhigou(SJ 6) Xingjian(LR 2)

Foot—Linqi (GB41)   Taichong (LR 3)

Foot—Qiaoyin (GB44)   Zhentou (Extra)

Zhenwei (Extra)

Explanation:Lingtai (DU10), an important point for treating boils, can eliminate heat from the chest and the skin. Zhigou (SJ 6), Xingjian (LR 2), Foot—Linqi (GB41) and Taichong (LR 3) are points from the liver and gallbladder channels that have distributions in the hypochondriac regions. Puncturing these four points may sedate fire from the liver and gallbladder, regulate *Qi,* relive swelling and stop pain. Foot—Qiaoyin (GB44), the *Jing*—well point of the gallbladder channel, may eliminate heat, sedate fire and cool the blood. Zhentou (Extra)and Zhenwei (Extra), meaning the start and the end of the lined herpes zoster, are punctured to promote the *Qi* circulation in the local area in order to directly drive pathogenic heat out of the body.

Point Modification: Add Hegu (LI 4), Neiting (ST44) for herpes zoster in the head and facial region; and Guanchong (SJ 1) for excessive heat accumulation.

Method: Apply filiform needles with reducing method and retain the needles for 20—30 minutes, manipulating them three to five times.

2. Damp—heat Type Herpes Zoster

Principle: Eliminate heat, resolve dampness, strengthen spleen and relieve stagnation of *Qi* by using points mainly from The Stomach Channel of Foot—*Yangming* and The Spleen Channel of Foot—*Taiyin.*

Prescription: Local surrounding points Neiting (ST44)

                Gongsun (SP 4) Waiguan (SJ 5)

                Xiaxi (GB43) Weizhong (BL40)

                Zusanli (ST36)

Explanation: The local surrounding points are used to prevent further spreading of the zoster. Neiting (ST44), the *Xing*—spring point of the stomach channel, and Gongsun (SP 4), the *Luo*—connecting of the spleen channel, are combined to eliminate heat and resolve dampness. Waiguan (SJ 5), the *Luo*—connecting point of the *Sanjiao* channel, is combined with Xiaxi (GB43), the *Xing*—spring point of the gallbladder channel, to eliminate heat. Weizhong (BL40), known as the *Xi*—cleft point of blood, may cool the blood and eliminate heat. Zusanli (ST36), the *He*—sea point of the stomach channel, is used to strengthen the spleen, pacify the stomach, eliminate heat and resolve dampness.

Point Modification: Add Zhongwan (RN12) for poor appetite; Geshu (BL17) for herpes zoster appearing in areas above the waist; and Xuehai (SP10) and Yanglingquan (GB34) for herpes zoster appearing in areas below the waist.

Method: Apply filiform needles with reducing method and retain the needles for 20–30 minutes, manipulating them four to six times. Moxibustion can be applied at Zusanli (ST36) for 20 minutes.

Alternative Treatment: Auricular Acupuncture

Prescription: Adrenal gland Ear—Shenmen Subcortex Corresponding areas

Method: Apply filiform needles with strong stimulation for 15–20 minutes, manipulating them three to four times. Embedding of ear seeds is also applicable.

2.4 Erysipelas

Erysipelas is an acute contagious skin condition marked by sudden onset of local redness, swelling, feverish sensation and pain. The leison rises with clear—cut margins like scattered pieces of cloud.

Cause and Mechanism

Erysipelas is mostly caused by accumulation of damp—heat in the spleen and liver affecting the blood, or invasion of exogenous pathogenic wind—heat, dampness or fire when the defensive *Qi* is weak. The struggle between the endogenous heat and exogenous heat, when they meet each outwardly, affect in the skin. If this heat is not adeqautely dispersed from the skin portion, there will be onset of erysipelas.

Differentiation

Incipient erysipelas is characterized by general discomfort, aversion to cold, and fever. This is then followed by red—coloured erythema like pieces of cloud, feverish sensation, burning pain, and clear—cut margins of prominences that withdraw their colours upon pressing, but return to their original ones when hands are left from the prominences. Erysipelas soon extends to the surrounding areas while the colour in the central area turns into dark red. In several days, the skin gets recovered when the crusts fall off. Some of the affected areas may develop blisters that break with running fluid, itching sensation and pain. The accompanying symptoms and signs include restlessness, thirst, general feverish sensation, constipation and short scanty urine.

In general, erysipelas in the upper part of the body is mostly due to invasion of wind—heat, and that in the lower part of the body is mostly due to damp—heat.

Treatment

1. Wind—heat Type

Principle: Eliminate wind—heat and cool the blood by using points mainly from The *Du* Channel and The Large Intestine Channel of Hand—*Yangming*.

Prescription: Lingtai (DU10) Dazhui (DU14)

Zhongchong (PC 9) Quchi (LI11)

Hegu (LI 4) Quze (PC 3)

Explanation: Lingtai (DU 10) is used to eliminate heat from the chest and skin portion. It is an important point for treating skin eruptions. Dazhui(DU14), the converging point of *Yang,* is combined with Zhongchong (PC 9), the *Jing*–well point of the pericardium channel, to clear up wind, eliminate heat and sedate fire.Quchi(LI11), having the property of dominating blood and promoting blood circulation, is combined with Hegu(LI 4), having the property to dominate *Qi* and dispersing, to guide *Qi* to the the affected areas to dispel the pathogenic factors. Quze (PC 3) is good for eliminating heat and cooling the blood in order to clear the turbid *Qi* from the body.

Point Modification: Add Shaoshang (LU11) and Shangyang (LI 1) for strong fever; Taiyang (EX–HN5) and Yintang (EX–HN3) for headache; and Neiguan (PC 6) for restlessness and nausea.

Method: Apply filiform needles with reducing method and retain the needles for 25–20 minutes, manipulating them three to four times. Dazhui (DU14), Zhongchong (PC 9) and Quze (PC 3) can be applied with three–edged needle to cause bleeding.

2. Damp–heat Type

Principle: Eliminate damp–heat and cool the blood by using points mainly from The *Du* Channel and The Bladder Channel of Foot–*Taiyang*.

Prescription: Lingtai (DU10)　Weizhong (BL40)
　　　　　　　　　Xuanzhong (GB39)　Yinlingquan (SP 9)
　　　　　　　　　Sanyinjiao (SP 6)

Explanation: Lingtai (DU10) is used to eliminate pathogenic factors for skin eruptions. Weizhong (BL40) clears up heat and cools blood, eliminates wind, resolves dampness and relieves the turbid dampness. Xuanzhong (GB39), the Influential Point of marrow, relieves heat from the *Sanjiao* and resolves dampness. Yinlingquan (SP 9) and Sanyinjiao (SP 6) strengthen spleen and resolve dampness. The joint use of these five points may eliminate heat, resolve dampness and cool the blood.

Point Modification: Add Tianshu (ST25) and Guanyuan (RN 4) for diarrhea; Shixuan (EX−UE11) and Shuigou (DU26) for high fever.

Method: Apply filiform needles with reducing method and retain the needles for 15−20 minutes, manipulating them three to four times.

Alternative Treatment

1. Cupping

Prescription: Lingtai (DU 10)

Dazhui (DU14) for erysipelas in the upper part of the body; Weizhong (BL40) for erysipelas in the lower part of the body.

Method: Prick these points with a three−edged needle to cause bleeding after doing routine disinfection. This is then followed by cupping for 10−15 minutes.

2. Auricular Acupuncture

Prescription: Ear−Shenmen   Adrenal gland   Subcortex
                    Spleen Occipitus

Method: Apply filiform needles with strong stimulation and retain the needles for 10−15 minutes manipulating them once or twice. Embedding of ear seeds or subcutaneous needles is also applicable.

2.5　Eczema

Eczema, a common skin disease, is divided into acute and chronic types. Acute eczema is characterized by sudden onset of symmetric and polymorphic lesions in repeated attacks, and accompanied by erythma, edema, papule, vesiculation, oozing and intense itching. When cured, it presents decrustation without any traces. The chronic type eczema is transformed from the acute one and characterized by roughness of skin, dark red or grey colour of skin in the affected areas, scaled skin or lichen–like skin. Chronic eczema may often bring about acute attacks.

Cause and Mechanism

Eczema is mostly caused by invasion of exogenous pathogenic wind, heat and dampness at the superficial portion of the skin that halts the circulation of *Qi* and blood and brings about obstruction of channels and collaterals, resulting in dormant damp–heat on the surface of the body. However, dryness due to blood deficiency or malnutrition of the skin can also lead to chronic type of eczema.

Differentiation

1. Acute Eczema

The acute eczema is characterized by a rapid onset of erythma, subsequent papules that forms into groups of blisters in a few days. The clusters and flakes may break and effuse by scratching, which may also turn into ulceration with local redness and severe itching snesation. The tongue is red with thick sticky coating, and the pulse is slippery and rapid.

2. Chronic Eczema

Chronic eczema is related to lingering attacks of acute eczema. After repeated attacks of eczema in months or years, deficiency of blood causes dryness to form chronic eczema. The chief manifestations include roughness of skin, dark gray skin colour, deep sink creases, clear—cut margins of the affected skin, red tongue proper with less coating than normal, and rapid thready pulse. It keeps on bothering the patient and difficult to be cured.

Treatment

1. Acute Eczema

Principle: Eliminate wind and heat and resolve dampness by using points mainly from The Stomach Channel of Foot—*Yangming* and The Spleen Channel of Foot—*Taiyin*.

Prescription: Dazhui (DU14) Quchi(LI11) Sanyinjiao (SP 6)
Weizhong (BL40) Yinlingquan (SP 9)
Lingtai (DU10)

Explanation: Dazhui(DU 4), the converging point of *Ying,* is combined with Quchi (LI11) to eliminate pathogenic factors from the superficial portion of the body, wind and heat in particular.Sanyinjiao (SP 6), a point that crosses the three *Yin* channels of the foot, has the effect of promoting the *Qi* circulation of the three *Yin* channels in order to eliminate heat and resolve dampness. Weizhong (BL40) cools the blood, eliminates wind and resolves dampness. Yinlingquan (SP 9), the *He*—sea point of the spleen channel, may strengthen the spleen and resolve dampness. Lingtai (DU10) eliminates heat from the triple energizer and the skin portion.

Point Modification: Add Gongsun (SP 4) for abdominal pain; Tianshu (ST25) and Yanglingquan (GB34) for constipation;

Method: Apply filiform needles with reducing method and

retain the needles for 15—20 minutes, manipulating them two to three times Weizhong (UB40) can be pricked with a three—edged needle to cause bleeding. Lingtai (DU10)is applied with cupping after it is pricked.

2. Chronic Eczema

Principle: Mourish blood and eliminate wind by using points mainly from the three *Yin* channels of the foot.

Prescription: Taichong (LR 3) Sanyinjiao (SP 6)

Zusanli (ST36) Xuehai (SP10)

Geshu (BL17) Lingtai (DU10)

Expalantion: Taichong (LR 3) soothes the liver and nourishes blood. It also has the effect to remove stasis of blood. Sanyinjiao (SP 6), the crossing point of the three *Yin* channels of the foot, can strengthen spleen, reinforce the kidney and regulate the liver, It is also used in combination with Zusanli (ST36) to promote the source for providing the acquired energy. Xuehai (SP10), Geshu (SP10) clear up heat from the blood system, activate blood and stop itching sensation. Lingtai (DU10) relieves pathogenic heat from the skin portion.

Method: Aplly filiform needles with even method and retain the needles for 20—30 minutes, manipulating them two to three times.

Alternative Treatment Auricular Acupuncture

Prescription: Heart Lung Spleen Ear—Shenmen Adrenal
gland

Method: Apply filiform needles with moderate stimulation and retain the needles for 15—20 minutes. Embedding of ear seeds subcutaneous needles is also applicable.

2.6 Wind Wheal

Wind wheal refers to a sudden onset of skin eruption characterized by red or white rash and itching sensation without any pain. It comes and goes with aggravation by wind, hence the term wind wheal or hidden rash in traditional Chinese medicine. It is called urticaria in modern medicine.

Cause and Mechanism

Onset of wind wheal is often caused by wind invasion dormant in the skin portion due to the derangement of nutrient and defensive systems. Since wind often brings cold, heat and dampness to invade the body, in terms of etiology, wind wheal due to wind—heat affecting the blood system and wind wheal due to wind—cold and dampness affecting the *Qi* system are different. Also, the colour of the wind wheal can be white and red in nature. Nevertheless, improper diet characterized by intake of hot, spicy or greasy food, or sea food can cause internal retention of damp—heat in the gastrointestinal system to steam up the lung. Wind wheal will occur if the internal heat is not dispersed, but stays in the skin portion of the body.

Differentiation

Wind wheal always bears the features of rapid onset, redness of the skin and itching sensation without pain. Clinically, it is necessary to make it clear the actual colour and whether it is newly formed wheal or recurrence of the old one in addition to understanding the inducing factor. It is also important to know the complications. If wind—heat is more predominant, the wheals in prominence will appear red in colour with severe itching sensation and feverish sensation upon palpating. The condition is worse with heat and better with cold. The accompanying symptoms and signs include restlessness, thirst, red tongue proper with yellow coating, and superficial rapid pulse. If wind—cold is more predominant, the white—coloured wind wheals will become better with warmth, but worse with cold or wind. The accompanying symptoms and signs include aversion to cold, fever, pale tongue with thin coating, superficial slow pulse or superficial tense pulse. Wind wheal due to accumulation of heat in the stomach and intestines is often caused by improper food intake. It is accompanied by abdominal pain, diarrhea or constipation, nausea and vomiting, yellow greasy tongue coating, and rapid slippery pulse. If wind wheal appears in repeated attacks over a long period of time, it is mostly due to deficiency of *Qi* and blood. The attack can often be caused by tiredness. The accompanying symptoms and sings include dizziness, lassitude, pallor complexion, palpitation, shortness of breath, and spontaneous sweating

Treatment

1. Wind—heat Type

Principle: Eliminate wind and clear up heat, cool the blood, activate blood circulation and stop itching by using points mainly from The Large Intestine Channel of Hand—*Yangming*.

Prescription: Hegu (LI 4) Quchi (LI11) Dazhui (DU14)

                 Lingtai (DU10) Fengchi (GB20)

                 Weizhong (BL40) Geshu (BL17)

Explanation: Hegu (LI 4), Quchi (LI11) and Fengchi (GB20) are used to eliminate wind—heat from the superficial portion of the body, Geshu (BL17), Dazhui (DU14) and Weizhong (BL40) are used to regulate the nutrient and blood systems, eliminate heat from the *Qi* system, activate blood and cool the blood. They also can clear up wind and stop itching sensation. Lingtai (DU10) eliminates heat from the *Sanjiao* and that from the skin.

Method: Apply filiform needles with reducing method and retain the needles for 15—20 minutes, manipulating them two to three times. Dazhui (DU14) and Weizhong (UB40) can be pricked with a three—edged needle to cause bleeding.

2. Wind—cold Type

Principle: Eliminate wind, repel cold and regulate nutrient and defensive systems by using points mainly from The Large Intestine Channel of Hand—*Yangming* and The Gallbladder Channel of Foot—*Shaoyang*.

Prescription: Fengchi (GB20) Fengmen (BL12)

Quchi (LI11) Hegu (LI11) Dazhui(DU14)

Explanation: Fengchi (GB20) and Fengmen (BL12) are used to eliminate cold and disperse wind. Hegu(LI 4) has the effect of ascending and dispersing and Quchi (LI11) has the effect of activating. The joint use of these two points may relieve cold from the superficial portion of the body, eliminate wind and stop itching sensation. Dazhui (DU14), having the effect of promoting *Yang Qi,* is combined with Quchi (LI11) also to regulate the nutrient and defensive systems.

Method: Apply filiform needles with even method and retain the needles for 20—30 minutes. Moxibustion can be applied to Dazhui (DU14), Fengchi (GB20) and Fengmen (DU12) for 30—40 minutes.

3. Heat Accumulation in the Gastrointestinal System

Principle: Strengthen spleen, resolve dampness, eliminate heat from the nutrient system by suing points mainly from The Large Intestine Channel of Hand—*Yangming* and The Stomach

Channel of Foot—*Yangming*.

Prescription: Quchi(LI11) Zusanli(ST36) Xuehai(SP10)

Sanyinjiao(SP 6) Lingtai (DU10)

Explanation: Quchi (LI11) and Zusanli (ST36) are used to eliminate heat from the intestines according to the principle that He—sea points for disorders of the *Fu* organs. Xuehai (SP10) and Sanyinjiao (SP 6), respectively the sea of the blood and the crossing point of the three *Yin* channels of the foot, are able to strengthen the spleen, resolve dampness, eliminate heat and cool the blood. They also have the action to activate blood and stop itching sensation. Lingtai (DU10), the empirical point for the treatment of wind wheal, is used to strengthen the therapeutic effect.

Method: Apply filiform needles with reducing method and retain the needles for 15—20 minutes, manipulating them two to three times.

4. Deficiency of *Qi* and Blood

Principle: Reinforce *Qi* of the middle—*Jiao,* strengthen *Qi* and nourish blood.

Prescription: Qihai (RN 6) Zusanli (ST36)

Sanyinjiao (SP 6) Pishu (BL20) Hegu (LI 4)

Quchi (LI11) Geshu (BL17)

Explanation: Points formed in this prescription are used to strengthen the anti—pathogenic *Qi* and relieve pathogenic factors in an attempt to deal with the root cause. Therefore, Qihai (RN 6), Zusanli (ST36), Sanyinjiao (SP 6) and Pishu (BL20) are used to strengthen the spleen, pacify the stomach, reinforce *Qi* of the middle—*Jiao* and strengthen the source for providing the acquired energy. This is because the pathogenic *Qi* can be spontaneously relieved when anti—pathogenic Qi is strong. Hegu (LI 4) and Quchi (LI11), because of their ascending, dispersing and activating effect, are used in combination with Geshu (BL17) to promote Qi and blood circulation in the general body and activate Qi and blood in order to quench the wind and stop itching.

Method: Apply filiform needles with reinforcing method at Qihai (RN 6), Zusanli (ST36), Sanyinjiao (SP 6) and Pishu (BL20); with even method at Hegu (LI 4), Quchi (LI11) and Geshu (BL17), and retain the needles for 20—30 minutes, manipulating them two to three times. Direct moxibustion with 7—9 pieces of moxa cones can be applied at Zusanli (ST36) and Pishu (BL20). **Alternative Treatment:** Auricular Acupuncture

Prescription: Lung   Adrenal gland   Subcortex
Sympathetic   Uritcaria spot

Method: Apply filiform needles with moderate stimulation and retain the needles for 15—20 minutes. Embedding of ear seeds or subcutaneous needles is also applicable.

2.7   Psoriasis

Psoriasis is a modern medicine term to refer to a chronic skin condition characterized by repeated scaled dermatosis which is difficult to have a thorough cure. Some dry silver—white scales cover the affected areas and decrustate by scratching, hence the term white skin decrustation in traditional Chinese medicine.

Cause and Mechanism

Psoriasis is mostly caused by invasion of pathogenic wind, dampness and heat dormant in between the skin and muscles. Long term of Qi stagnation turning into heat will also over consume body fluid and blood. Dried blood can inturn cause internal disturbance of wind and poor nourishment of skin, resulting in roughness of skin, itching sensation and desquamation.

Differentiation

Psoriasis starts with intermittent itching sensation followed by flat papule. The papule gradually extends in areas of densely gathered groups. appearing in red colour of maculapule. There are several layers of silver white scale covering the affected areas. These layers of white silver scales fall off by scratching with intermittent attacks of severe itching. If wind, dampness and heat appear more predominant, there will be fresh redness of local skin, itching sensation, casting off of skin crusts, red tongue proper with yellow greasy tongue coating, and rapid soft pulse. If the psoriasis has a long past history, there will be dryness and thickness of the skin, casting off of skin scales, red tongue proper, thin white coating, and thready weak pulse. This is mostly due to blood deficiency with dry wind.

Treatment

1. Wind—damp—heat Type

Principle: Eliminate heat, resolve dampness, dispel wind and stop itching sensation by using points mainly from The Large Intestine Channel of Hand—*Yangming* and The Spleen Channel of Foot—*Taiyin*.

Prescription: Hegu (LI 4) Quchi (LI11) Taibai (SP 3) Yinlingquan (SP 9) Fengchi (GB20) Geshu (BL17) Renying (ST 9)

Explanation: Hegu (LI 4) and Quchi (LI11) are good for regulating *Qi* and blood and eliminate heat from the *Yangming* channel. The two in combination with Fengchi (GB20) also have the effect appeace the *Shaoyang* channels, relieve heat and wind from the skin portion and stop itching sensation. Taibai (SP 3) and Yinlingquan (SP 9), respectively the *Yuan*—source and *He*—sea points of the spleen channel, may strengthen the spleen and resolve dampness. Geshu (BL17), the Influential point of blood, is effective to activate blood, dispel wind and stop itching. Renying (ST 9) has the effect to regulate *Qi* and blood circulation and stop itching sensation.

Point Modification: Add Shaoze (SI 1) and Weizhong (BL40) for psoriasis in the neck; and Guanchong (SJ 1) and Zhigou (SJ 6) for psoriasis in the cheek.

Method: Apply filiform needles with reducing method and retain the needles for 15—20 minutes, manipulating them one to three times. Moxibustion is also applicable at Quchi (LI11) and Yinlingquan (SP 9).

2. Blood Deficiency Type with Dry Wind

Principle: Reinforce *Qi* and blood, eliminate wind and moisten the dryness by using points mainly from The Large Intestine Channel of Hand—*Yangming* and The Stomach Channel of Foot—*Yangming*.

Prescription: Hegu (LI 4) Quchi (LI11) Sanyinjiao (SP 6)
Zusanli(ST36) Xuehai(SP10) Renying(ST 9)

Explanation: Hegu (LI 4) and Quchi (LI11) eliminate wind—heat from the head and facial region. Sanyinjiao (SP 6) reinforces spleen and stomach as well as liver and kidney. The joint use of these three points may eliminate heat, cool blood, quench the wind and moisten the dryness. in an attempt to deal with the root cause. Sanyinjiao (SP 6) in combination with Zusanli (ST36) may also lift *Yang* and promote stomach, reinforce spleen and moisten the *Yin* in order to invigorate the source for manufacturing blood. Xuehai (SP10) regulates blood and moistens the dryness. Renying (ST 9) may activate blood, eliminate wind and stop itching.

Method: Apply filiform needles with even method and retain the needles for 15–20 minutes, manipulating them two to three times. Moxibustion is also applicable to Zusanli (ST36) and Sanyinjiao (SP 6)

Alternative Treatment: Auricular Acupuncture

Prescription: Lung   Ear–Shenmen   Adrenal gland
Kidney Heart Corresponding areas

Method: Apply filiform needles with moderate stimulation and retain the needles for 15–20 minutes, manipulating them once or twice.

2.8   Tinea Ungium

Tinea ungium is a modern medicine term referring to fungal infection of the hand characterized by irregular shapes of thickened skin on the palm with roughness and slight itching.

Cause and Mechanism

Tinea ungium is mostly caused by invasion of exogenous pathogenic dampness. Dampness invasion for a long time turns into either dryness or heat which further dry the blood and produce internal wind dormant at the skin portion leading to the condition.

Differentiation

Tinea ungium starts with itching in the hand and subsequent blisters which may extend to the whole palm without afftecting the dorsum of the hand. This is then followed by diminishing of blisters and casting off the withered skin. The skin on the palmar aspect of the hand thus turns thick and rough. In severe case, there will be severe itching and skin cracks with impaired flexing of the fingers. Tinea ungium often appears on one side of the hand or both hands at the same time. It is severe in the winter but less severe in the summer.

Treatment

Principle: Eliminate wind and heat, nourish *Yin* and moisten the dryness by using points mainly from The Pericardium Channel of Hand—*Jueyin* and The Kidney Channel of Foot—*Shaoyin*.

Prescription: Yongquan (KI 1) Laogong (PC 8)
Renying(ST 9) Jianshi(PC 5) Baxie(Extra)

Explanation: Yongquan (KI 1), the *Jing*—well point of the kidney channel, has the effect to eliminate heat, nourish Yin and moisten the dryness. Laogong (PC 8), the *Xing*—spring point of the pericardium channel, is good for eliminating heat from the *SanJiao* and an important point for treating tinea ungium. Renying (ST 9) may regulate the nutrient blood and relieve the fungal infection. Baxie (EX—UE9) may eliminate wind and heat. It is an empirical point for the treatment of tinea ungium.

Point Modification: Add Zhongwan (RN12) and Zusanli (ST36) for poor appetite; Shenmen (HT 7) and Neiguan (PC 6) for insomnia.

Method: Apply filiform needles with reducing method and retain the needles for 20—30 minutes, manipulating them two to three times.

2.9 Vitiligo

Vitiligo is a condition characterized by cutaneous patch of white colour without subjective symptoms.

Cause and Mechanism

Vitiligo is mostly due to poor nourishment of the skin caused by derangement of *Qi* and blood and stagnation of *Qi* and blood resulted from invasion of exogenous pathogenic wind into the skin portion.

Differentiation

Clinically, vitiligo is divided into local and scattered types. The former is a kind of vitiligo characterized by groups of irregular sizes of cutaneous leukoplakia with clear—cut margins and whitened patches, but neither itching nor pain. The scattered vitiligo may extend to the general body. Some the scattered patches in white colour may remain steady while others may disappear spontaneously. However, some of them may rapidly extend with irregular courses of affection.

Treatment

Principle: Regulate *Yin* and *Yang*, activate blood and eliminate wind by using points mainly from The Large Intestine Channel of Hand—*Yangming* and The Spleen Channel of Foot—*Taiyin*.

Prescription: Hegu(LI 4) Quchi (LI11) Fengchi (GB20)
                  Geshu (BL17) Ganshu (BL18)
                  Taichong (LR 3) Sanyinjiao (SP 6)
                  Yinbai (SP 1) Renying (ST 9)

Explanation: Hegu (LI 4), Quchi (LI11) and Fengchi (GB20) regulate the nutrient and defensive systems, and eliminate heat from the body organs involved. They also have the effect of repelling wind from the general body .Geshu (BL17), Ganshu (BL18) and Taichong (LR 3) nourish *Yin* and blood, activate blood and eliminate wind. Sanyinjiao (SP 6) strengthens spleen, reinforces liver and kidney and nourishes blood. Yinbai (SP 1) and Renying (ST 9) reinforce the *Qi* of the spleen and stomach and lift *Yang* energy.

Method: Apply filiform needles with even method and retain the needles for 15–20 minutes, manipulating them two to three times.

Alternative Treatment

1. Plum–blossom Needle Therapy

Prescription: Local points in the affected areas of the body

Method: After doing routine disinfection, tap with a plum–blossom needle until local redness of the skin appears. This is then followed by cupping.

2. Auricular Acupuncture

Prescription: Lung   Spleen   Heart   Ear–shenmen
             Subcortex Adrenal gland Corresponding points

Method: Apply filiform needles with strong stimulation and retain the needles for 10–15 minutes. Embedding of ear seeds is also applicable.

2.10 Alopecia

Alopecia refers to sudden regional loss of hair on the head. In traditional Chinse medicine, this is called oily–wind syndrome.

Cause and Mechanism

Alopecia is mostly caused by deficiency of liver and kidney with subsequent failure of deficient blood to go up nourishing the hair. The hair pores are open when the hair is poorly nourished and wind invades the pores on the occasion. Therefore, deficient blood with dry wind leads to hair loss. However, stagnation of liver *Qi* and impaired *Qi* mechanism will also result in hair loss because of the malnturition of hair due to stagnation of *Qi* and stasis of blood.

Differentiation

Alopecia patients often discover the hair loss accidentally without having subjective symptoms and signs. The incipient lesion appears round or irregular in shape with bright skin and clear—out margins. The hair loss may involve one or several areas on the scalp ranging from the size of finger nail to that of eye glasses. This is followed by more extended area of hair loss. In severe case, a major part or the whole hair can be lost.

If the hair falls off regionally with slight itching, dizziness, insomnia, tinnitus, slightly red tongue proper, thin white tongue coating, and weak thready pulse, this is mostly due to deficiency of liver and kidney and deficiency of blood with dry wind. If the patient has regional hair loss over a long period of time with dark greyish complexion, purplish stagnant spots on the edge of the tongue, and slow pulse, this is mostly due to stagnation of *Qi* and stasis of blood.

Treatment

1. Blood Deficiency Type

Principle: Nourish blood, eliminate wind, calm the mind and reinforce the kidney and liver by using points mainly from The Pericardium Channel of Hand—*Jueyin* and The Bladder Channel of Foot—*Taiyang*.

Prescription: Neiguan (PC 6)   Shenmen (HT 7)
　　　　　　　Baihui (DU20)   Dazhui (DU14)
　　　　　　　Ganshu (BL18)   Shenshu (BL23)
　　　　　　　Geshu (BL17)   Hegu (LI 4)
　　　　　　　Sanyinjiao (SP   6)

Explanation: Neiguan (PC 6) and Shenmen (HT 7) nourish blood and calm the mind. Baihui (DU20) and Dazhui (DU14) eliminate wind and heat, and stop itching. Ganshu (BL18), Shenshu (BL23) and Geshu (BL17) nourish liver and kidney, and regulate Qi and blood. Hegu (LI 4) and Sanyinjiao (SP 6) eliminate heat from the head, reinforce liver, spleen and kidney, and guid blood to follow Qi ascending to nourish the hair.

Point Modification: Add Shangxing (DU23) for dizziness; Zhongwan (RN12) and Zusanli (ST36) for poor appetite.

Method: Apply filiform needles with even method and retain the needles for 10–15 minutes, manipulating them once or twice. Moxibustion is also applicable to Dazhui (DU14) and Baihui (DU20) .

2. Blood Stasis Type

Principle: Soothe the liver Qi, activate blood and resolve blood stasis by using points mainly from The Pericardium Channel of Hand—Jueyin and The Gallbladder Channel of Foot—Shaoyang.

Prescription: Neiguan (PC 6)   Yanglingquan (GB34)

Geshu (BL17)   Fengchi (GB20)

Baihui (DU20)   Ganshu (BL18)

Renying (ST 9)

Explanation: Neiguan (PC 6) and Yanglingquan (GB34) soothe the liver Qi. The two are also used in combination with Geshu (BL17) to activate blood and resolve blood stasis. Fengchi (GB20) and Baihui (DU20) eliminate wind, eliminate heat and stop itching. Renying (ST 9) eliminates heat, cools the blood, activates blood and guides Qi to the affected part of the body in order to promote the growth of new hair.

Method: Apply filiform needles with reducing method and retain the needles for 15–20 minutes. Moxibustion is also applicable to the affected parts of the head for 20 minutes or until local redness of the skin.

Alternative Treatment: Auricular Acupuncture

Prescription: Lung   Liver   Kidney   Adrenal gland

Endocrine   Brain

Method: Apply filiform needles with mild stimulation and retain the needles for 15–20 minutes. Embedding of ear seeds or subcutaneous needles is also applicable.

2.11   Acne

Acne, also known as pulmonary wind acne, refers to papular nodule on the face, chest or back. White bodies like rice can be squeezed out, hence the Chinese name *Fenci*. It mostly occurs in adolescence and natural cure comes when the patient reaches adulthood.

Cause and Mechanism

Acne is mostly caused by dormant heat in the skin due to steaming of wind–heat from the lung meridian or retention of heat in the stomach and spleen due to over intake of hot spicy food. Derangement between The *Chong* and *Ren* Channels with poor opening and closing of the skin pores may lead to occurence of acne.

Differentiation

Acne in most cases affects the face, chest or back. It starts with scattered or dense papular nodules. Some of them will form acne which may release white bodies upon squeezing. This is then followed by the formation of small pustules with tidal feverish sensation on the face, itching sensation and pain. Scars may remain after the recovery of broken pustules.

Treatment

Principle: Eliminate wind and heat, activate blood, soften the pustules and regulate The *Chong* and *Ren* Channels by using points mainly from The Large Intestine Channel of Hand—*Yangming*, The Stomach Channel of Foot—*Yangming* and The *Du* Channel.

Prescription: Lingtai (DU10)　Hegu (LI 4)　Quchi (LI11)
　　　　　　　Fengchi (GB20)　Feishu (BL13)
　　　　　　　Sanyinjiao (SP 6)　Taichong (LR 3)

Explanation: Lingtai (DU10) is good for eliminating heat from the lung and the skin portion. Hegu (LI 4) and Quchi (LI11) regulate the circulation of *Qi* and blood and eliminate wind—heat from the skin portion. Fengchi (GB20) pacifies the *shaoyang* channel and clears up wind—heat from the head. Sanyinjiao (SP 6) is used in combination with Taichong (LR 3) to regulate The *Chong* and *Ren* Channels, activate blood, resolve stasis and soften the pustules.

Point Modification: Add Guanchong (SJ 1) and Weizhong (BL40) for itching sensation; and Dazhui (DU14) for fever.

Method: Apply filiform needles with reducing method and retain the needles for 15—20 minutes, manipulating them two to three times. Lingtai (DU10) may be pricked with a three—edged needle to cause bleeding and followed by cupping. Weizhong (UB40) may also be pricked with a three—edged needle to cause bleeding.

Alternative Treatment: Bleeding Therapy

Prescription: Ear apex

method: After routine disinfection, apply a pinch—pull action on the parts surrounding the ear apex, then puncture the point with a three—edged needle to cause bleeding of $2\sim3$ drops. Press the point for a while with a dry cotton ball after operation. Points on both ears are punctured alternately every $3\sim5$ days.

2.12   Flat Wart

Flat wart, a kind of small neoplasm at the superficial portion of skin, mostly affects the dorsum of hand and face without subjective symptoms and signs in general.

Cause and Mechanism

Emotional disturbance with liver *Qi* stagnation and *Yin* deficiency and dryness of blood plus invasion of exogenous pathogenic factors cause a struggle of the two in the skin portion, leading to stagnation of *Qi* and stasis of blood dormant at the skin to result in acne.

Differentiation

Acne mostly affects young people on the face, dorsum of hand or the back. The surface of the flat warts is smooth, but slightly high than the normal skin. The warts may be irregular in sizes, like rice particles or soya beans in slightly yellow or normal skin colour and clear—cut margins. The flat warts may be dense or scattered with local itching snesation but no subjective symptoms and signs. Some of the warts may withdraw by themselves while others may simply recur.

Treatment

Principle: Eliminate wind—heat, activate blood and relieve flat warts by suing points mainly from The Large Intestine Channel of Hand—*Yangming*.

Prescription: Hegu (LI 4)   Quchi (LI11)

Fengchi (GB20)   Hand−Zhongzhu (SJ 3)

Taichong (LR 3)

Expalantion: Hegu (LI 4) and Quchi (LI11) promote *Qi* and activate blood. They also have the effect of regulating nutrient and defensive systems, and eliminating wind−heat from the head and facial region. Fengchi (GB20) is good for eliminating pathogenic wind. Hand−Zhongzhu (SJ 3) and Taichong (LR 3) eliminate heat from the *SanJiao,* pacify the shaoyang channels, sedate liver fire, activate blood and relieve flat warts.

Method: Apply filiform needles with reducing method and retain the needles for 20−30 minutes, manipulating them two to three times. Three to five pieces of moxa cones are also applicable on the flat warts.

Alternative Treatment: Cauterized Needle Therapy

Prescription: Three to five pieces of flat warts

Method: After routine disinfection, puncture the flat warts with the cauterized needle to the base of the warts.

2.13   Clavus

Clavus refers to deep−rooted skin infections on the plantar region. Clavus looks like cock eyes, hence the name.

Cause and Mechanism

Clavus is often caused frequent squeezing or pressing frictions on the plantar region or toes.

Differentiation

Clavus mostly occurs on the sole due to frequent pressing or frictions. It starts with thickened skin in yellow or white colour with painful sensation. This is then followed by prominences of hard quality. These prominences are round, deep–rooted, and look like cock eyes. It is painful by pressing and may affect normal walking.

Treatment

Principle: Soften the clavus by using mainly the local points.

Prescription: Local points

Method: Apply filiform needles surrounding the clavus at the depth to the base of the clavus. Moxibustion is also applicable after needling.

Alternative Treatment: Cauterized Needle Therapy

Prescription: Local clavus point

Method: After routine disinfection, insert the cauterized needle to the center of clavus until reaching the base. Cauterized needles may also be used to puncture from the surrounding sides towards the center at the similar depth. Treatment is given once every two to three days until natural casting off of the clavus.

2.14   Tendon Cyst

Tendon cyst refers to vesicular swellings accompanied by local itching and weakness at places adjacent to joints. It is called tenosynovitis in modern medicine.

Cause and Mechanism

It is generally believed that tenosynovitis is mostly due to local overstrain that impairs tendons, or stagnation of *Qi* or stasis of blood in the channels and collaterals due to long time of standing.

Differentiation

Tenosynovitis, often appearing in the wrist and ankle, is more complained by patients in the thirties to fourties. The vesicular swellings are of irregular sizes ranging from the size of finger nails to that of walnuts. These smooth cysts that appear round or elliptic have very little mobility. Patients first feel the cysts by pressing. Over a long period of time, the surface of the cysts become hard. One or several cysts may form at the same time with local soreness, numbness and weakness.

Treatment

Principle: Activate blood and soften the cysts by using points mainly from the local area.

Prescription: Local points surrounding the cysts

Method: After routine disinfection in the local area, use a 26 gauge needle to insert first from the top to the bottom, then from the surrounding directions to the center of the cyst. Squeeze the points after withdrawing the needles until fluid flows out. This is followed by thirty minutes of moxibustion.

Alternative Treatment: Cauterized Needle Therapy

Prescription: Top of the cyst

Method: After routine disinfection, use a 26 gauge needle to insert quickly into the cyst after healing it on an alcohol lamp. After withdrawal of needle, press the inserted cyst to let the fluid come out. This is then followed by moxibustion for 20–30 minutes. Treatment is given once every other day.

2.15 Atheroma

Atheroma is also called wen in modern medicine. In traditional Chinese medicine, this conditon is referred as bean curd residue cyst, for inside the wen there exists some mat ter that looks like bean curd residue.

Cause and Mechanism

Atheroma is the consequence of phlegmatic *Qi* stagnant in the skin portion.

Differentiation

Atheroma mostly occurs in the head, facial region, ear, neck, back or hip areas. The cystic swellings are within the very superficial portion of the skin. These irregular cystic swellings appear soft and round in shape with clear—cut margins. These superficial swellings have no connection with the soft tissues in the deeper portion of the muscles. They are moveable and connected with skin with little depressions in the center slightly black in colour. Squeezing will force some substance similar to bean curd residue with a bad odour to come out. The growth of these swellings are generally slow without apparent objective symptoms.

Treatment

Refer the treatment description in 2.14.

2.16 Mastitis

Mastitis, or breast abscess, a kind of acute purulent infection of the breast, is mostly seen during lactation period,espe—cially in primiparae.

Cause and Mechanism

Mastitis is mostly caused by emotional disturbance and stagnation of liver *Qi* that leads to dysfunction of liver in maintaining free flow of *Qi* and stagnant lactation, or by improper diet such as over indulgence of greasy food that leads to dysfunction of spleen *Qi* in ascending and descending *Qi* of stomach as well as heat retention in the stomach. However, broken nipple with exogenous invasion that encounters the internal heat can also cause stagnant lactation. Stagnant lactation in a long run will also turn into heat with excessive heat retenion in the local area that develops into mastitis.

Differentiation

Mastitis is chiefly manifested by redness of the breast, swelling breast, feverish sensation, lactation deficiency, infection, fever with aversion to cold, general discomfort and distention and palpating pain.

1. Stagnation of Liver *Qi*

In addition to the main manifestations, the accompanying symptoms and signs of this type of mastitis include fullness and distending pain in the hypochondriac region, abdominal distention, bitter taste, restless, shortness of temper, poor appetite, thin yellow tongue coating, and rapid wiry pulse.

2. Heat Rentention in The Stomach

In addition to the main manifestations, the accompanying symptoms and signs of this type of mastitis include thirst with desire to drink, nausea, poor appetite, foul mouth, constipation, yellow tongue coating, and rapid full pulse.

Treatment

1. Liver *Qi* Stagnation Type

Principle: Soothe the liver *Qi*, eliminate heat and relieve stagnation by using points mainly from The Liver Channel of Foot—*Jueyin,* The Stomach Channel of Foot—*Yangming* and The Gallbladder Channel of Foot—*Shaoyang*.

Prescription: Qimen (LR14)   Neiguan (PC 6)

Danzhong (RN17)   Zusanli (ST36)

Xingjian (LR 2)   Jianjing (GB21)

Explanation: The Stomach Channel of Foot *Yangming* distributes also in the breast region and The Liver Channel of

Foot–*Jueyin* passes through the nipple. Therefore, Qimen (LR14), the Front–*Mu* point of the liver, Neiguan (PC 6), the *Luo*–connecting point of the pericardium channel, and Danzhong (RN17), the Influential point of *Qi,* are used to relieve fullness in chest, soothe the liver *Qi* and relieve *Qi* stagnation. Zusanli (ST36), the *He*–sea point of the stomach channel, is combined with Xingjian (LR 2), the *Xing*–spring point of the liver channel, to eliminate heat from the stomach, relieve *Qi* stagnation and swelling, and stop pain. Jianjing (GB21) is added to produce a better therapeutic effect because this an experience point for the treatment of mastitis.

Point Modification: Add Rugen (ST18) for breast distention; Shaoze (SI 1) for poor lactation; and Dazhui (DU14) and Fengchi (GB20) for fever and headache.

Method: Apply filiform needles with reducing method and retain the needles for 15–20 minutes, manipulating them two to three times.

2. Stomach Heat Retention Type

Principle: Eliminate heat, disperse the mass, relieve swelling and promote lactation by using points mainly from The Stomach Channel of Foot–*Yangming*.

Prescription: Rugen (ST18)　Yingchuang (ST16)
　　　　　　　Shaoze (SI 1)　Zusanli (ST36)
　　　　　　　Liangqiu (ST34)　Neiting (ST44)

Explanation: The Stomach Channel of Foot–*Yangming* runs down from supraclavicular fossa to the nipple. Therefore, Rugen (ST18), and Yingchuang (ST16) are used to clear up heat from the stomach and remove obstruction that disturbs lactation. Zusanli (ST36), the *He*–sea point of the stomach channel, is combined with Liangqiu (ST34), the *Xi*–cleft point of the stomach channel, and Neiting (ST44), the *Xing*–spring point of the stomach channel, to eliminate heat, relive swelling and stop pain. Shaoze (SI 3) is added to help promote lactation. The joint use of these points may eliminate heat, relieve swelling and promote lactation.

Point Modification: Add Danzhong (RN17) and Jianjing (GB21) for stagnant lactation; and Dazhui (DU14), Hegu (LI 4) and Fengchi (GB20) for fever with aversion to cold.

Method: Apply filiform needles with reducing method and retain the needles for 15–20 minutes, manipulating them two to three times. Shaoze (SI 1) can be treated with a three–edged needle to cause bleeding.

Alternative Treatment: Auricular Acupuncture

Prescription: Liver Stomach Chest Internal ear
                      Endocrine Mammary gland
                      Ear apex

Method: Apply filiform needles with strong stimulation and retain the needles for 10–15 minutes. Ear apex can be applied with three–edged needle to cause bleeding.

Note: Acupuncture is appropriate for treating the early stage of mastitis when purulent substance has not yet been formed.

2.17 Intestinal Abscess

Intestinal abscess refers to accumulation of heat in the intestines producing purulent substance. Clinically, the patient may have fever with aversion to cold, palpable mass in the lower lateral abdomen and pain that worse by pressing, or pain with difficulty in extending the leg. This is called appendicitis in modern medicine.

Cause and Mechanism

The onset of appendicitis is mostly caused by sudden over eating of hot, spicy, greasy or oily food that leads to food retention in the middle—*Jiao* and accumulation of damp—heat in the intestines, or impairment of intestinal collaterals due to fast running immediately after meal, or obstruction of *Qi* mechanism due to emotional disturbance. All these factors can cause stagnation of *Qi* and stasis of blood in the interior to turn into heat affecting the intestinal tissues to develop appendicitis.

Differentiation

1. Stasis Type

At this stage, the purulent substance has not been formed. The chief manifestations include paroxysmal pain in the abdomen that is worse with pressing, slight tenseness of abdominal wall, abdominal distention, belching, poor appetite, nausea, vomiting, slight fever with aversion to cold, constipation or normal stools, dark red or normal tongue proper, thin white or yellow tongue coating, and wiry tense pulse.

2. Heat Retention Type

At this stage, the purulent substance has just been formed, but not yet spreaded. The chief manifestations include abdominal colic, tenseness of abdominal wall, pain in the lower right abdomen that do not respond to pressing, difficult extending of the leg, strong fever, spontaneous sweating, constipation, short scanty urine, red tongue proper, yellow greasy tongue coating, and rapid slippery pulse of a wiry nature.

Treatment

1. Stasis Type

Principle: Regulate *Qi* circulation, stop pain, relieve swelling and resolve stasis by using points mainly from The Stomach Channel of Foot—*Yangming* and The Spleen Channel of Foot—*Taiyin*.

Prescription: Tianshu (ST25) Dachangshu (BL25) Zusanli (ST36) Xuehai (SP10) Diji (SP 8)

Explanation: Tianshu (ST25), the Front—*Mu* point of the large intestine, is combined with Dachangshu (BL25), its Back—*Shu* point, known as the combination Front—*Mu* and Back—*Shu* points, to promote the circulation of intestinal *Qi* and regulate the *Qi* mechanism of large intestine. Zusanli (ST36) is combined with Xuehai (SP10) for its related channel to promote *Qi* circulation, activate blood and resolve stasis. Diji(SP 8), the *Xi*—cleft point of the spleen channel, is used to regulate *Qi* and stop pain. The joint use of these five points ensure a remarkable effect.

Point Modification: Add Fujie (SP14) for abdominal distention; Hegu(LI 4), Quchi (LI11) and Neiting (ST44) for fever; and Neiguan (PC 6) and Guanchong (PC 9) for vomiting.

Method: Apply filiform needles with reducing method and retain the needles for 15—20 minutes, manipulating them two to three times.

2. Heat Retention Type

Principle: Eliminate heat, resolve dampness, promote *Qi* circulation and relieve stagnation of *Qi* by using points mainly from The Stomach Channel of Foot—*Yangming* and The Large Intestine Channel of Hand—*Yangming*.

Prescription: Shangjuxu (ST37) Tianshu (ST25) Quchi (LI11)

Explanation: Large intestine is mainly an organ to do transporting of waste and this function is better performed with no obstruction. Therefore, in the treatment of intestinal disorder, Shangjuxu (ST37), the Lower−*He*−sea point of the large intestine, is combined with Tianshu (ST25), the Front−*Mu* point of the large intestine, to eliminate heat from the intestine, promote the *Qi* mechanism of the intestines, resolve dampness and promote bowel movement. Shangjuxu (ST37) is selected in accordance with the principle that *He*−sea points are best for dealing with *Fu* disorders . Quchi (LI11) is a special point for regulating *Qi* of the large intestine, eliminate heat and store fluid.

Point Modification; Add Hegu (LI 4) and Neiting (ST44) for fever; Neiguan (PC 6) for vomiting; Fujie (SP14) and Dachangshu (BL25) for abdominal distention; and Zusanli (ST36) and Yanglingquan (GB34) for constipation.

Method: Apply filiform needles with reducing method and retain the needles for 15−20 minutes, manipulating them three to four times.

Alternative Treatment: Auricular Acupuncture

Prescription: Appendix   Lower portion of rectum

               Large intestine   Sympathetic

               Ear−Shenmen

Method: Apply filiform needle with strong stimulation and retain the needles for 15−20 minutes, manipulating them three to four times. Embedding of ear seeds or subcutaneous needles is also applicable.

Note: Acupuncture is good for treating simple appendicitis in early stage or appendicitis involving no forming of pus.

2.18   Hemorrhoids

Hemorrhoids refers to swollen or twisted veins in the anus and lower rectum . Hemorrhoids is a common disease of the anus and rectum, mostly seen in adults. Therefore, there is a saying in China that every nine out of ten suffer from hemorrhoids. This condition is also called hemorrhoids in modern medicine. According to the different location, hemorrhoids can be divided into internal, external and mixed types of hemorrhoids among which the internal type is most common. This condition is also called hemorrhoid boil because the swollen and twisted veins can cause anus pain, sinking and distending sensation, itching, and bleeding.

Cause and Mechanism

Hemorrhoids is often caused by internal dry heat due to improper intake of greasy, spicy, hot food and over indulgence alcohol, or impairment of collaterals due to forceful bowel excretion in case of constipation. Occupational sitting, long time walk, carrying heavy load and deficiency of *Zangfu* organs can cause invasion of exogenous pathogenic wind—damp and retention of heat in the interior, leading to downward flowing of damp—heat accumulated in the anus with stasis to result in hemorrhoids.

Differentiation

Early internal hemorrhoids involves sinking pain in the anus, and small soft swollen veins in fresh red or purplish green colour. Bleeding is often caused by pressing during bowel excretion charcterized by dripping of bleeding in the mild case and shooting of blood in the severe case. Hemorrhoids are mostly due to retention of damp—heat if accompanied by feverish sensation in the anus, permeating fluid, constipation, thirst, red tongue proper, and rapid pulse. The hemorrhoids is mostly due to sinking of *Qi* if accompanied by pallor complexion, shortness of breath, reluctant speech, poor appetite, poor energy, prolapse of swollen veins, pale tongue proper, and weak thready pulse. Such patients have poor body constitution and repeated hemorrhoids attack. Their deficiency of *Qi* and blood is due to excessive loss of blood.

External hemorrhoids is mainly characterized by visible swollen veins that increase in size and become hard in nature. It is usually caused by long sitting, long standing or anus friction. In general external hemorrhoids does not involve bleeding.

Treatment

1. Damp–heat Retention Type

Principle: Eliminate heat, resolve dampness, promote *Qi* circulation and resolve stasis by using points mainly from The Bladder Channel of Foot–*Taiyang*, The Lung Channel of Hand–*Taiyin* and The Pericardium Channel of Hand–Jueyin.

Prescription: Kongzui (LU 6) Ximen (PC 4)

Chengshan (BL57) Erbai (EX–UE2)

Hegu (LI 4) Quchi (LI11)

Explanation: Kongzui (LU 6) is the *Xi*–cleft point of the lung channel that is internally–externally related to the large intestine channel. It has the effect of helping descend lung *Qi* and eliminating heat and dampness from the large intestine. It is also good for promoting *Qi* circulation and activating blood. Ximen (PC 4) may eliminate heat from the blood and promote *Qi* of the *Sanj iao,* promote *Qi* circulation, resolve stasis and stop pain. Chengshan (BL57) may guide *Qi* to the affected part of the body because its pertaining channel communicates with the anus so that the effect of the above will be even better. Quchi (LI11) and Hegu (LI 4) are used to promote *Qi* circulation of the large intestine, activate *Qi* and blood, and eliminate heat from the large intestine.

Point Modification: Add Shiqizhui (Extra) and Baihui (DU20) for internal hemorrhoids with prolapsing; and Shangqiu (SP 5) for lingering swollen veins.

Method: Apply filiform needles with reducing method and retain the needles for 15–30 minutes, manipulating them three to four times.

2. *Qi* Deficiency Type with Sinking

Principle: Reinforce *Qi* of the middle–*Jiao,* activate blood and resolve hemorrhoids by using points mainly from The Bladder Channel of Foot–*Taiyang,* The *Ren* Channel and The *DU* Channel.

Prescription: Baihui (DU20)   Qihai (RN 6)

      Baihuanshu (BL30)   Chengshan (BL57)

      Kongzui (LU   6)   Ximen (PC   4)

Explanation: Baihui (DU20) can lift the sunk *Yang Qi.* Qihai (RN   6) warms up kidney *Qi* in order to assist Baihui (DU20) in lifting *Qi.* Baihuanshu (BL30) may promote *Qi* circulation for the channels in the anus region. At the same time, it activates *Yang Qi.* Kongzui (LU 6) helps the lung perform descending of *Qi ,* eliminates heat from the intestines, activates the circulation of *Qi* and blood and stops pain. Chengshan (BL57) is used to guide *Qi* mechanism in the anus because its pertaining channel diverges into it. Ximen (PC 4) clears up heat from the heart, promotes the *Qi* transforming of the *Sanj iao,* promotes circulation of *Qi* and stops pain.

Method: Apply filiform needles with reinforcing method and retain the needles for 20—30 minutes, manipulating them two to three times. Qihai (RN 6) and Baihui (DU20) may also be treated with moxibustion for 30—40 minutes.

Alternative Treatment

1. Pricking

Prescription: Tender points on the back, viz, the dark red spot without changing its colour when pressed, or the stagnant spots on the upper labial frenulum.

Method: After routine disinfection, use a three—edged needle to prick the subcutaneous tissue or stagnant spots on the upper labial frenulum to cause a tiny amount of bleeding. Treatment is given once every three days.

2. Auricular Acupuncture

Prescription: Lower rectum Large intestine Pile spot
Subcortex Spleen Adrenal gland

Method: Apply filiform needles with strong stimulation and retain the needles for 15 minutes. Embedding of ear seeds or subcutaneous needle is also applicable.

3. Laser Therapy

Prescription: Hemorrhoids spot

Method: Radiate the hemorrhoids spot with He—Ne laser beams for 15—20 minutes once or twice daily.

2.19 Neck Sprain

Neck sprain is characterized by soreness and pain with diffi-cult turning or limited movement on one side of the neck. It may be similar to rheumatic pain in the neck or chronic cervical disc injury in modern medicine.

Cause and Mechanism

Neck sprain is mostly caused by invasion of wind—cold into the local channels and collaterals, or derangement of *Qi* and blood due to awkward sleeping position, leading to poor nourishing of tendons and tendon spasm.

Differentiation

Most patients feel neck rigidity and muscular soreness and pain when get early in the morning. They have limited movement and difficulty to turn to either side or backward. The soreness and pain may also radiate towards shoulder and arm. There will be obvious tenderness, but no swelling nor redness of the local skin. Both stools and urine appear normal, with thin white tongue coating and wiry tense pulse.

Treatment

Principle: Eliminate wind—cold and ease the tendons and collaterals by using points mainly from The *Du* Channel, The Small Intestine Channel of Hand—*Taiyang* and The Bladder Channel of Foot—*Taiyang*.

Prescription: Fengchi (GB20) Dazhui (DU14)

Tianzhu (BL10) Jianwaishu (SI14)

Jianjing (GB21) Houxi (SI 3)

Explanation: Fengchi (GB20), Dazhui (DU14), Tianzhu (BL10), Jianwaishu (SI14) and Jianjing (GB21) may promote the circulation of *Qi* in the local area and eliminate wind—cold. Houxi (SI 3), communicating with The Du Channel and one of the eight Confluent points, has the effect to ease the tendons, eliminate wind and stop pain. The Small Intestine Channel passes through the shoulder region curving on the scapula and crossing on the shoulder. This is another reason why Houxi (SI 3) is used to treat such a problem.

Method: Apply filiform needles with even method and retain the needles for 15–20 minutes, manipulating them two to three times. Moxibustion can also be applied at Fengchi (GB20) and Dazhui (DU20) for 15–20 minutes.

Alternative Treatment

1. Cupping

Prescription: Tenderness

Method: After routine disinfection, prick the tender point with a three–edged needle and then quickly cup the tender point for five to ten minutes.

2. Auricular Acupuncture

Prescription: Neck   Occipitus   Urinary bladder

Tender point   Subcortex   Ear–Shenmen

Method: Apply filiform needles with strong stimulation and retain the needles for 10–15minutes. Embedding of ear seeds is also applicable.

2.20   Frostbite

Frostbite refers to local pallor, cyanosis, itching, burning pain, edema, vesicles or even necrosis or ulceration on the local cutaneous lesion due to severe winter cold affection. It mostly occurs on the hand, foot, facial region or external ear, pertaining to local chilblain in terms of modern medicine.

Cause and Mechanism

Severe cold is the main causative factor of frostbite. Constitutional deficiency of *Qi* and blood, lack of physical exercise, hunger, tiredness, long time resting, or long time of use tourniquet, plus severe cold invasion may easily cause poor circulation of *Qi* and blood, leading to blood stasis and frostbite.

Besides, being in the severe cold weather with sudden exposure heat or vice versa may also lead to the onset of frostbite.

Differentiation

Mild frostbite is characterized by pallor, cyanosis, cold pain with numbness, subsequent fever, burning sensation and itching, and local blisters. If there is no infection involved, the affected areas will gradually become dry with scar until final recovery. Generally, there is no remaining scar.

Severe frostbite is characterized by pallar, cold pain, numbness, poor sensation, subsequent dark red skin, swelling and forming of blisters. After the breaking of the blisters, the skin will turn purplish in colour with ulceration. This is then followed by flowing of purulent fluid and slow healing by itself. In the very severe case, the muscles, tendons and even bones will be affected with motor and sensory disturbance. There will also be some general symptoms such as high fever and chill when secondary affection takes place.

Treatment

1. Mild Frostbite

Principle: Warm up the channels and collaterals, eliminate cold, activate blood and stop pain by using mainly local points.

Prescription: (1)Hegu (LI 4) Dazhui (DU14)

Renying (ST 9) Fengchi (GB20)

Baihui (DU20) for the head

(2)Baxie (EX−UE9) Hegu (LI 4)

Waiguan (SJ 5) Houxi (SI 3) for the hand

(3)Bafeng (EX−LE10) Taichong (LR 3)

Foot—Lingqi (GB41) Yongquan (KI 1)
Zusanli (ST36) Yinbai (SP 1) for the foot.

Explanation: The *Yangming* channels have some branches in the facial region. Therefore, Renying (ST 9) and Hegu (LI 4) are used to promote *Qi* and blood in the facial region. Moxibustion at Dazhui (DU14), the converging of all *Yang*, may warm up the channels and collaterals. Fengchi (GB20) and Baihui (DU20) may promote the *Qi* and blood in the head region in order to eliminate wind and cold, activate blood and stop pain. Baxie (Extra) has the effect of eliminating wind and cold. Hegu (LI 4), Houxi (SI 3) and Waiguan (SJ 5) regulate *Qi* and blood in the *Yang* channels of the hand in order to warm up channels, eliminate cold, remove obstruction from the channels and collaterals, and stop pain. Bafeng (EX—LE10) and Yongquan (KI 1) may eliminate wind—damp and warm up the channels and collaterals. Taichong (LR 3) and Foot—Lingqi (GB41) promote *Qi* circulation in the channels, regulate *Qi* and stop pain. Zusanli (ST36) and Yinbai (SP 1) reinforce spleen *Qi* and lift *Yang* energy.

Method: Apply filiform needles with reinforcing method and retain the needles for 20—30 minutes, manipulating them two to three times. Moxibustion is also applicable at Dazhui (DU14), Baihui (DU20), Zusanli (ST36), Yongquan (KI 1), Yinbai (SP 1) and Fengchi (GB20).

2. Severe Frostbite

Principle: Warm up the channels and collaterals. Promote the warming of *Yang* energy, activate blood and resolve stasis by using points mainly from The *Ren* Channel, The *Du* Channel and The Kidney Channel of Foot—*Shaoyin*.

Prescription: Dazhui (DU14) Shuigou (DU26)

Guanyuan (RN 4)   Qihai (RN 6)

Mingmen (DU 4)   Yongquan (KI 1)

Hegu (LI 4)   Zusanli (ST36)

Explanation: The joint use of Dazhui (DU14), Shuigou (DU26), Guanyuan (RN 4) and Qihai (RN 6) may warm up the channels and collaterals, eliminate cold and promote the warming of *Yang* energy. Mingmen (DU 4) and Yongquan (KI 1) warm up kidney *Yang* and reinforce essence and blood. Hegu (LI 4) and Zusanli (ST36) may regulate the *Qi* of the middle—*Jiao* in order to promote the source for providing the acquired energy to resolve stasis and produce new organic tissue.

Point Modification: Add Hand—zhongzhu (SJ 3) for frostbite on the dorsum of the hand and Kunlun (BL60) for frostbite on the dorsum of foot.

Method: Apply filiform needles with reinforcing method and retain the needles for 20—30minutes. Moxibustion is also applicable at Guanyuan (RN 4), Dazhui (DU14), Yongquan (KI 1) and Zusanli (ST36) for 15—20 minutes.

2.21   Tetanus

Tetanus refers to a condition characterized by stiffness of and back, opisthotonos, trismus, murmuring speech, severe spasm of tendons and muscles, painful limbs and deviation of the eye and month due to exogenous pathogenic wind on a previous wound.

Cause and Mechanism

Tetanus starts with invasion of exogenous pathogenic wind into the channels and collaterals through a wound. And, the exogenous wind induces disturbance of endogenous wind in the body to cause impaired circulation of nutrient and defensive *Qi* and poor nourishment of tendons and vessels, leading to spasm, convulsions, or vital reverse flow of *Qi* of *Zangfu* organs.

Differentiation

Pre—attack Stage is chiefly manifestated by lassitude, headache, profuse sweating, restlessness or stretching sensation in the wound.

The attack stage is characterized by locked jaws, difficulty for food intake, murmuring speech, sad smile complexion, neck rigidity, opisthotonos, repeated convulsions of the four limbs, high fever, mental confusion, deep rapid or wiry rapid pulse. If the patient also has loss of consciousness, deep, profuse sweating, severe irritability, this mostly indicates a crutial condition of reverse flow of *Qi*.

Treatment

Principle: Soothe the liver, quench the wind, eliminate heat and sedate the convulsion by using points mainly from The *Du* Channel, The Large Intestine Channel of Hand—*Yangming* and The Stomach Channel of Foot—*Yangming*.

Prescription: Dazhui (DU14)   Fengfu (DU16)

                      Jinsuo (DU 8)   Renzhong (DU26)

                      Hegu (LI 4)   Weizhong (BL40)

                      Taichong (LR 3)   Shenmai (BL62)

Explanation: It is held in traditional Chinese medicine that sudden onset of body rigidity all belongs to wind factor. Excessive *Yang* will produce heat while excessive heat will produce wind. Therefore, Dazhui (DU 14), the converging of *Yang,* is used in combination with Fengfu (DU16) and Jinsuo (DU 8) in order to promote *Qi* circulation of The *Du* Channel, eliminate heat and sedate convulsions. Shuigou (DU26) is used to relieve patient from back rigidity. Hegu (LI 4) is used in combination with Taichong (LR 3), known as the four−gate points, attempting to soothe the liver, quench the wind and resuscitate the patient so as to relieve trismus, sad smile complexion, etc. Weizhong (BL40) is used in combination with Shenmai (BL62) to regulate the *Qi* of The Urinary Bladder Channel of Foot−*Taiyang* and relieve back rigidity. The joint use of these eight points may eliminate heat, sedate convulsion, soothe the liver and quench the wind.

Point Modification: Add Houxi (SI 3) for neck rigidity; Xiaguan (ST 7) for locked jaws; and Yanglingquan (GB34) for convulsion of the four limbs.

Method: Apply filiform needles with reducing method and retain the needles for 20−30 minutes, manipulating them two to three times.

Alternative Treatment

1. Cupping

Prescription: Dazhui (DU14) and the points respectively one cm anterior, posterior, left and right to Dazhui (DU14)

Method: Prick the five points to cause bleeding after routine disinfection. This is followed by a quick cupping on this area focusing Dazhui (DU14) as the center for ten minutes approximately until there is no blood coming out.

2. Auricular Acupuncture

Prescription: Liver Chest Ear−Shenmen Spinal coloumn

Method: Apply filiform needles with strong stimulation and retain the needles for 15−20 minutes. Embedding of ear seeds is also applicable.

2.22   Ascarid Colic

Ascarid colic refers to a kind of paroxysmal colic or a sudden upward drilling pain in the upper abdomen due to upward movement of ascarid in the intestine running into the biliary duct. The pain makes the patient turn from side to side on the bed, cry, feel nausea, vomit, sweat or even suffer from rigidity of the limbs, hence the name ascarid colic. The pain can soon be relieved and the patient becomes normal when the ascarid withdraws from the biliary duct. This condition is called biliary ascariasis in modern medicine.

Cause and Mechanism

Onset of ascarid colic is mostly due to ascaris in the intestines. Ascaris is very active in running into intestinal passeges. Whenever there is a dysfunction of the *Zangfu* organs due to invasion of cold or heat into the stomach, the ascarid will go upward to run into the biliary duct.

Differentiation

Most of these patients have had ascarid either from the stools or from occasional vomiting. Clinically, patient feels a sudden onset of paroxysmal pain below the xyphoid process. It is characterized by tossing in bed with flexed knees, turnings of the body, cryings, pale complexion, sweating and limb convulsion. The pain can sometimes radiate to shoulder and lumbar region at irregular time intervals ranging from several minutes to hours. The attack may at least appear once a day or several times daily. The patient feels normal as soon as the ascarid withdraws from the biliary duct. The accompanying symptoms and signs during the attack include nausea, vomiting, white greasy tongue coating, and wiry rapid pulse.

Treatment

Principle: Soothe the liver and gallbladder, regulate *Qi* circulation, stop pain and dispel ascarid by using points mainly from The Gallbladder Channel of Foot—*Shaoyang*, The Stomach Channel of Foot—*Yangming* and The *Ren* Channel.

Prescription: Yanglingquan(GB34)　Neiguan(PC 6)

　　　　　　　Zhigou (SJ　6)　Zusanli (ST36)

　　　　　　　Riyue (GB24)　Jiaji (EX—B20)

Explanation: Yanglingquan (GB34), the *He*—sea point of the gallbladder channel, is combined with Riyue (GB24), the Front—*Mu* point of the gallbladder, to soothe the *Qi* of the liver and gallbladder, dispel ascarid and stop pain. Neiguan (PC 6), the Confluent point communicating with The Yinwei Channel, is combined with Zhigou (SJ 6) to regulate *Qi* circulation of the *Zangfu* organs in order to dispel ascarid and stop pain. Zusanli (ST36) may regulate the *Qi* circulation of the stomach and intestine, relieve spasm and stop pain. Jiaji points from T8—T10 may promote the *Qi* circulation of the liver and gallbladder, relieve spasm and dispel ascarid so that the pain relieving effect is far better.

Method: Apply filiform needles with reducing method and retain the needles for 20—30 minutes, manipulating them three to four times.

Alternative Treatment: Auricular Acupuncture

Prescription: Sympathetic　Ear--Shenmen　Liver

　　　　　　　Gallbladder　Duodenum　Pancreas

Method: Apply filiform needles with strong stimulation and retain the needles for 15—20 minutes. Embedding of ear seeds or subcutaneous needles is also applicable.

2.23   Intestinal Obstruction

Intestinal obstruction is characterized by abdominal pain, vomiting, abdominal distention, passing wind and difficult bowel evacuation due to impeded intestinal transportation caused by stagnation and obstruction of intestines. It is included in intestinal obstruction in modern medicine too.

Cause and Mechanism

Intestinal obstruction is mostly due to over eating, fierce physical exercices, or cold stagnation, or retention of heat, dampness accumulation in the middle—*Jiao,* or constipated intestines or obstruction of intestines due to ascarid, etc, leading to obstruction of intestines, accumulation of either heat or cold resulting in obstructed *Qi* mechanism of the middle—*Jiao*

Differentiation

Incipient intestinal obstruction is characterized by severe abdominal pain, vomiting and abdominal distention. There will be constipation and painful mass in the lower abdomen without passing wind. The tongue coating is dry yellow and the pulse is tense and wiry, but slippery and rapid as well.

Treatment

Principle: Remove obstruction from the intestines, relieve accumulations and guide *Qi* circulation by using points mainly The Stomach Channel of Foot—*Yangming*.

Prescription: Tianshu (ST25) Shangjuxu (ST37)

Xiajuxu (ST39) Zhigou (SJ 6)

Dachangshu (BL25) Zusanli (ST36)

Fenglong (ST40)

Explanation: Tianshu (ST25) is the Front–*Mu* point of the large intestine channel; Zusanli (ST36), the lower *He*–sea a point of the stomach channel; Shangjuxu (ST37), the lower *He*–sea point of the large intestine channel; Xiajuxu (ST39), the lower *He*–sea a point of the small intestine channel; and Dachangshu (BL25), the Back–*Shu* point of the large intestine. The joint use of the five points may promote the *Qi* circulation of the gastrointestinal system, relieve accumulations and guide *Qi* circulation. Zhigou (SJ 6) in combination with Fenglong (ST40) may eliminate heat from the middle–*Jiao,* moisten the intestines and promote bowel movement.

Method: Apply filiform needles with reducing method and retain the needles for 20–30 minutes, manipulating them three to four times.

Alternative Treatment

Auriculotherapy

Prescription: Large intestine Small intestine Stomach
Abdomen Ear–Shenmen Subcortex
Sympathetic

Method: Apply filiform needles with reducing method and strong stimulation. Retain the needles for 15–20 minutes. Embedding of subcutaneous needles is also applicable.

Note: Acupuncture treatment is suitable for intestinal obstruction only in the early stage.

3 Gynecology

3.1 Irregular Menstruation

Irregular menstruation refer to abnormal menstrual flow concerning the cycle, duration, colour, quantity and quality. They are mainly related to the climatic and environmental changes or emotional disturbances.

Cause and Mechanism

1. Preceded Menstrual Flow: The flow in this case comes earlier than the expected cycle due to mainly the failure of spleen to govern the blood, dysharmony between the *Chong* and *Ren* Channels, and *Qi* deficiency, or pathogenic heat in blood causing disturbance in the sea of blood so that the flow appears in advance.

2. Delayed Menstrual Flow: This condition may ascribe to either deficiency or excess factors. The former is caused by deficiency of nutrient blood or that of *Yang Qi;* the latter by obstruction of the *Chong* and *Ren* Channels due to stagnation of *Qi* and blood, or blood stasis formed by cold retention, and impaired circulation of *Qi* and blood between The *Chong* and *Ren* Channels, leading to delayed menstrual flow.

3. Disorderly Menstrual Flow: This condition is mostly caused by impaired circulation of *Qi* and blood due to stagnation of liver *Qi,* deficiency of kidney *Qi.* Common factors such as emotional depression. excessive anger, over consumption of kidney *Qi* due to excessive sex or grand multiparity may all lead to

dysharmony between The *Chong* and *Ren* Channels, resulting in a disorderly menstrual flow.

Differentiation

1. Precede Mentrual Flow: The flow is advanced at least more than seven days. There may appear massive periods of fresh red or purplish red colour within one month. The accompanying symptoms and signs include irritability, flushed face, dry mouth with desire for cold drinks, or afternoon fever, night sweating, feverish palms and soles, red tongue proper with yellow or less coating, slippery rapid or rapid thready pulse.

2. Delayed Menstrual Flow: The scanty flow in dark red or light red colour is late usually by more than seven days. It is dilute in quality mixed with clots. The accompanying symptoms include cold pain in the lower abdomen, relieved with hot packing, aversion to cold, pale complexion, dizziness and vertigo, blurred vision, dull pain in the lower abdomen responding to pressing, pale tongue proper with thin white coating, and deep slow pulse.

3. Disorderly Menstrual Flow: The flow appears in alternating cycles either in advance or in procrastination which can be massive or scanty. Such an uneven flow in purplish or light red colours is often accompanied by distending pain in the breast and hypochondriac region, restlessness with irritability, frequent belching, or dizziness, tinnitus, weakness in lumbus and knees, pale tongue proper with white coating, wiry or deep pulse.

Treatment

1. Precede Menstrual Flow

Principle: Invigorate *Qi,* nourish blood and regulate the *Chong* and *Ren* Channels by using points mainly from The Bladder Channel of Foot—*Taiyang* and *Ren* Channel.

Prescription: Yinbai (SP 1) Sanyinjiao (SP 6)
Qihai (RN 6) Zusanli (ST36)

Explanation: Yinbai (SP 1), the base of The Spleen Channel of Foot—*Taiyin*, can invigorate spleen *Qi* and elevate general *Yang* of the body, and help spleen control *Qi* and blood. Sanyinjiao (SP 6) tonifies spleen, liver and kidney, regulates the function of The *Chong* and *Ren* Channels, nourish the blood and promotes the blood circulation. It is the principal point for the treatment of gynecological diseases. Zusanli (ST36) regulates the function of spleen and stomach so as to enrich the source of *Qi* and blood. Qihai (RW 6) reinforces *Yuan Qi*, tonifies the essence and blood, and warm up the lower—*Jiao* as well as uterus.

Method: Apply filiform needles with reinforcing method and retain needles for 20 minutes. Moxibustion can be applied to Yinbai (SP 1) for 30 minutes.

2. Delayed Menstrual Flow

Principle: Promote the circulation of *Qi* and blood, expel pathogenic cold from the channels by using points mainly from The Bladder Channel of Foot—*Taiyang* and The *Ren* Channel.

Prescription: Sanyinjiao (SP 6) Hegu (LI 4)
Guanyuan (RN 4) Diji (SP 8)
Geshu (BL17)

Explanation: Diji (SP 8), th *Xi*—cleft point of the Spleen Channel of Foot—*Taiyin*, in combination with Geshu (UB17) can promote blood circulation and restore normal menstruation. Sanyinjiao (SP 6) promotes the flow of *Qi* and blood, removes blood stasis, replenishes *Qi* and blood, reinforces *Yuan Qi*, and eliminates cold. Hegu (LI 4), the point from The Large Intestine Channel of Hand—*Yangming*, can also promote the flow of *Qi* and blood. Guanyuan (RN 4) warms up the lower *Jiao* and uterus, nourishes essence and blood, and removes cold from the lower abdomen.

Method: Apply filiform needles with reinforcing method and retain needles for 20–30 minutes. Moxibustion can be applied to Guanyuan (RN 4) for 30–40 minutes each time.

3. Disorderly Menstrual Flow

Principle: Soothe the liver *Qi* and regulate the function of The *Chong* and *Ren* Channels by using points mainly from The Liver Channel of Foot–*Jueyin* and The *Ren* Channel.

Prescription: Taichong (LR 3) Sanyinjiao (SP 6)
               Zhongji (RN 3) Ganshu (BL18)

Explanation: Taichong (LR 3) can regulate liver *Qi*, promote the menstruation by removing blood stasis. Ganshu (BL18) may soothe the liver *Qi* and nourish *Yin* and blood. Zhongji (RN 3), a point from the *Ren* Channel, can harmonize the *Chong* and *Ren* Channels. This point in combination with Sanyinjiao (SP 6) may strengthen spleen and tonify the liver and kidney, so as to nourish the uterine collaterals and regulate the function of The *Ren* and *Chong* Channels.

Method: Apply filiform needles with reasonable reinforcing or reducing method and retain the needles for 15–20 minutes.

Alternative Treatment: Auricular Acupuncture

Prescription: Uterus, endocrine, liver, kidney, spleen and ovary.

Method: Apply filiform needles with moderate stimulation and retain the needles for 15–20 minutes.

3.2   Dysmenorrhea

Dysmenorrhea refers to the periodic pain, intolerable in severe case, involving the lower abdomen or affecting the lumbosacral region prior to, post or during the menstrual flow. It is mostly complained of by young women.

Cause and Mechanism

The etiology of dysmenorrhea concerns with the impaired circulation of *Qi* and blood due to either the deficiency of *Qi* and blood or stagnation of *Qi* and blood, leading to the dysharmony between The *Chong* and *Ren* Channels and blood stasis in the uterus in the consequence of dysmenorrhea.

The Excess Type: The onset is caused by cold–damp retention in The *Chong* and *Ren* Channels, and blood stasis in the uterus due to factors such as catching cold, intake of cold food or dwelling in damp places during the menstrual period. Liver *Qi* stagnation with subsequent stagnant *Qi* and blood stasis may also impede the normal menstrual flow and develop dysmenorrhea by means of obstruction.

The Deficiency Type: Deficiency of the liver and kidney, grand multiparity, or surviving some prolonged illness can cause the deficiency of both *Qi* and blood, insufficiency of The *Chong* Channel and poor nourishment of uterine collaterals, leading to the pain during menstrual flow.

Differentiation

1. Retention of cold–damp

The cold pain in the lower abdomen, paggravated by pressing but alleviated by warming, appears prior to or during the menstrual flow. It is accompanied by scanty flow of dark red colour with clots. The tongue coating is white and sticky, and the pulse is deep and tight.

2. Stagnation of *Qi* and Stasis of Blood

The distending pain of lower abdomen together with the distention in the breast and the hypochondriac region takes place before or during the menstrual flow. It is accompanied by dripping of scanty dark purplish flow with clots. The pain alleviates soon after the discharge of the clots. The tongue proper is dark purplish with spots and the pulse is wiry.

3. *Yin* Deficiency of the Liver and Kidney

The slight pain in the lower abdomen relieved by pressing occurs during or post the menstrual flow. The scanty flow of a less red colour is also accompanied by dizziness, tinnitus, soreness in the lumbar region and knees. The tongue proper is less red than normal with thin white coating, and the pulse is deep and thready.

4. Insufficiency of *Qi* and Blood

Some dull pain in the abdomen, relieved by pressing, bothers the patient prior to or post the menstrual flow. The flow is of a less fresh colour and dilute quality. It is accompanied by the general weakness, palar complexion, poor appetite, and loose stool. The tongue proper is pale with thin coating, and the pulse is weak and thready.

Treatment

1. Retention of Cold–damp

Principle: Expel pathogenic cold by warming the channels and collaterals and resolve dampness and blood stasis by using points mainly from The *Ren* Channel and The Spleen Channel of Foot–*Taiyin*.

Prescription: Qihai (RN 6)   Tianshu (ST25)
Mingmen (DU 4)   Sanyinjiao (SP 6)
Ciliao (BL32)

Explanation: Qihai (RN 6) is used for its effect of reinforcing the kidney *Qi*; Tianshu (ST25) for its warming effect. These two points in combination with Mingmen (DU 4) may invigorate the *Yang Qi* and eliminate cold. Sanyinjiao (SP 6) strengthens the spleen in particular, but the liver and kidney as well. It also has the effect to eliminate dampness, resolve blood stasis and promote the circulation of blood. Ciliao (BL32) is an empirical point for dysmenorrhea.

Method: Apply filiform needles with reinforcing method and retain the needles for 20–30 minutes. Moxibustion should be applied after acupuncture.

2. Stagantion of *Qi* and Stasis of Blood

Principle: Regulate the circulation of *Qi*, activate blood, resolve blood stasis and relieve pain by using points mainly from The *Ren* Channel and The Liver Channel of Foot—*Jueyin*.

Prescription: Taichong (LR 3)   Sanyinjiao (SP 6)
Hegu (LI 4)

Explanation: Taichong (LR 3), the source point of the liver channel, can soothe the stagnant liver *Qi* and regulate the circulation of *Qi* and blood. Sanyinjiao (SP 6), the coalescent point of the three *Yin* channels of the foot, is combined with Hegu (LI 4) to regulate the circulation of *Qi* and blood and relieve the pain.

Point Modification: Add Neiguan (PC 6) and Yanglingquan (GB34) for suffocating sensation in the chest and pain in the hypochondriac region.

Method: Apply filiform needles with reducing method and

retain the needles for 15−20 minutes. Moxibustion is also applicable.

3. *Yin* Deficiency of the Liver and Kidney

Principle: Reinforce the liver and kidney and regulate the harmony between The *Chong* and *Ren* Channels by using points mainly from The *Ren* Channel and some back−*Shu* points from The Bladder Channel of Foot−*Taiyang*.

Prescription: Ganshu (BL18)   Shenshu (BL23)

Guanyuan (RN   4)   Sanyinjiao (SP   6)

Explanation: Ganshu (BL18) and Shenshu (BL23) are used to reinforce the liver and kidney. Guanyuan (RN 4), the point of The *Ren* Channel, tonifies the kidney *Qi* and warms up the uterus. Sanyinjiao (SP 6) strengthens the spleen together with the liver and kidney. It also replenishes the vital energy and blood, and harmonizes The *Chong* and *Ren* Channels.

Point Modification: Add Taixi(KI 3) for dizziness and tinnitus.

Method: Apply filiform needles with reinforcing method and retain the needles for 15−20 minutes.

4. Insufficiency of *Qi* and Blood

Principle: Replenish *Qi* and blood by using points mainly from The *Ren* Channel and The Stomach Channel of Foot−*Yangming*.

Prescription: Guanyuan (RN   4)   Shenshu (BL23)

Zusanli (ST36)   Sanyinjiao (SP   6)

Explanation: Guanyuan (RN 4), the point of The *Ren* Channel, can warm up the lower−*Jiao*, reinforce the primordial *Qi*, eliminate cold from the uterus and regulate the harmony between The *Chong* and *Ren* Channels. Shenshu (BL23) invigorates the *Qi* of kidney. Sanyinjiao (SP 6), combined with Zusanli (ST36), strengthens the spleen and stomach, tonify *Qi* and blood, reinforces the liver and kidney, and regulates the harmony between The *Chong* and *Ren* Channels.

Method: Apply filiform needles with reinforcing method and retain the needles for 15–20 minutes. Moxibustion can also be applied after acupuncture.

Alternative Treatment: Auricular Acupuncture

Prescription: Ear—Shenmen Sympathetic Uterus

Endocrine Kidney

Method: Apply filiform needles with noderate stimulation and retain the needles for 15–20 minutes. Two to three ear points are selected for use each time. Embedding of ear seeds is also applicable.

3.3 Amenorrhea

Amenorrhea refers to any female who does not experience the first menstrual flow at the age of 18, or an adult woman who ceased to have menstrual flow over a period of more than three months. The former is called the primary amenorrhea while the latter the secondary amenorrhea in modern medicine.

Cause and Mechanism

Amenorrhea is clinically divided into deficiency and excess types. The former is related to deficinecy of blood in which there is no flow to be released because of the emptiness of The *Chong* and *Ren* Channels. The latter is due to the obstruction of The *Chong* and *Ren* Channels by stagnation of *Qi* and stasis of blood which blocks the menstrual flow. Specifically, over consumption of blood due to deficiency of the liver and kidney, chronic illness with weak constitution, or poor nourishment of The *Chong* and *Ren* Channels due to deficiency of the spleen and stomach and subsequent insufficiency of the acquired energy, can both lead to the deficient type of amenorrhea. Emotional disturbances with subsequent disorderly *Qi* mechanism ,or retention of pathogenic factors in the uterus due to invasion of exogenous pathogenic wind—cold and over intake of cold or raw food can both cause the blockage of *Qi* and blood of the The *Chong* and *Ren* Channels, resulting in excess type of amenorrhea.

Differentiation

1. Amenorrhea due to Blood Deficiency

This type of amenorrhea is characterized by the absence of menses over the age of 18, or delayed menstrual period with a decreasing flow until there is no flow at all. It is accompanied by soreness in the lumbar region and knees, dizziness and vertigo, or anorexia, loose stool, palpitation, shortness of breath, reluctant speech, or feverish sensation in the palms and soles, palar complexion or tidal fever. The tongue proper is red or pale with white or thin coating, and the pulse is thready and weak.

2. Amenorrhea due to Blood Stasis

This type of amenorrhea is characterized by an abscence of menses and irritability, distending sensation in the chest and hypochondriac region, or distending or cold pain in the lower abdomen which is aggravated by pressing but relieved by warmth. The edge of the tongue appears purplish dark and the pulse is wiry or deep uneven.

Treatment

1. Amenorrhea due Blood Deficiency

Principle: Nourish *Qi* and blood by using points mainly from

The *Ren* Channel and some back–*Shu* points of The Bladder Channel of Foot–*Taiyang*.

Prescription: Pishu (BL20) Shenshu (BL23) Qihai (RN 6)
               Zusanli (ST36)

Explanation: Points formed in this prescription have the effect to promote both the spleen and stomach, nourish *Qi* and blood, and replenish The *Chong* and *Ren* Channels. The spleen and stomach are the foundation of the acquired energy as well as the source of reproduction of *Qi* and blood. Only when both *Qi* and blood from the source are abundant can the menstruation appears normal. Therefore, Pishu (BL20) and Zusanli (ST36) are chosen to strengthen the spleen and stomach. The kidney is the foundation of the congenital energy. Only when the physiological function of the kidney is normal can the essence and blood be sufficient. Shenshu (BL23) and Qihai (RN 6) are thus used to replenish kidney *Qi* and warm up the lower–*Jiao*

Point Modification: Add Tianshu (ST25) for anorexia and loose stool; and Neiguan (PC 6) for palpitation.

Method: Apply filiform needles with reinforcing method, and retain the needles for 20–30 minutes. Moxibustion should be applied after needling.

2. Amenorrhea due to Blood Stasis

Principle: Soothe the liver, regulate the circulation of *Qi* and expel the pathogenic cold from the channels by using points mainly from The *Ren* Channel and The Spleen Channel of Foot–*Taiyin*.

Prescription: Zhongji (RN 3) Hegu (LI 4) Ganshu (BL18)
               Danshu (BL19) Sanyinjiao (SP 6)
               Taichong (LR 3)

Explanation: Zhongji (RN 3), the point of The *Ren* Channel, can regulate the function of The *Chong* and *Ren* Channels, and promote the function of the lower—*Jiao* Taichong (LR 3) can regulate the liver *Qi* and tonify the blood and remove blood stasis. Ganshu (BL18) and Danshu (BL19) relieve the stagnation of liver *Qi*. Sanyinjiao (SP 6), the coalescent point of the three *Yin* channels of the foot, is combined with Hegu (LI 4) to promote the circulation of *Qi* and blood for normalizing the menstrual flow.

Point Modification: Add Neiguan (PC 6) for distention and fullness sensation in the chest and hypochondriac region.

Method: Apply filiform needles with reducing method and retain the needles for 15—20 minutes. Treatment is given once a day. Moxibustion may be applied to Zhongji (RN 3) after needling, if amanorrhea is caused by the pathogenic cold.

Alternative Treatment: Auricular Acupuncture

Prescription: Endocrine Uterus Liver Kidney Spleen Stomach Ear—Shenmen

Method: Apply filiform needles to 3—4 points each time with moderate stimulation. Treatment is given once every other day for 10 times in one course. Embedding of ear seeds is also applicable.

3.4 Prolapse of Uterus

Prolapse of uterus refers to different degrees of lapse of uterus, or even uterus lapsing out of the vaginal orifice in severe cases. It includes the same prolapse of uterus and distention of vaginal wall in modern medicine.

Cause and Mechanism

The main cause of proplaspe of uterus concerns with the sunken *Qi* of the middle—*Jiao* and poor consolidation over uterus due to kidney *Qi* deficiency, both of which may lead to impairment of the uterine collaterals failing to keep the uterus in normal position. Over exhaustion of energy in delivery and early physical labour after delivery may cause deficiency of the spleen *Qi* and sunk *Qi* of the middle—*Jiao* which fails to do its normal lifting. Multiple pregnancy and labours and over sexual indulgence with over consumption of kidney *Qi* can result in dysfunction of The *Dai* Channel in restricting and the disharmony between The *Ren* and *Chong* Channels, causing prolapse of uterus.

Differentiation

1. *Qi* Deficiency

The uterus descends into the vagina or even out of the vaginal orifice aggravated by overstrain. It is accompanied by a sinking sensation in the lower abdomen, general lassitude, shortness of breath, pale complexion, heavy white leukorrhea of dilute quality, pale tongue proper with thin white coating, and weak pulse.

2. Kidney Deficiency

Prolapse of uterus is accompaniedby sinking sensation in the lower abdomen, dizziness, tinnitus, soreness in the lower back and knees, frequent urination especially at night, slight red tongue proper and deep weak pulse.

Treatment

1. *Qi* Deficiency

Principle: Lift *Qi* and consolidate the uterus by using points mainly from The *Du* Channel, The Spleen Channel of

Foot–*Taiyin* and The Stomach Channel of Foot–*Yangming*.

Prescription: Baihui (DU20) Qihai (RN 6) Weidao (GB28)

Guilai (ST29) Zusanli (ST36)

Sanyinjiao (SP 6)

Explanation: Baihui (DU20), the point of *Du* Channel, is used to lift the *Yang Qi*. Qihai (RN 6), Weidao (GB28) and Guilai (ST29) reinforce *Qi* and consolidate the uterus. Zusanli (ST36) and Sanyinjiao (SP 6) replenish spleen *Qi*. The combination of all these points can serve for the purpose of invigorating *Qi*, elevating *Yang* and consolidating the uterus.

Point Modification: Add Yinlingquan (SP 9) for leukorrhea.

Method: Apply filiform needles with reinforcing method and retain the needles for 20–30 minutes. Moxibustion may be applied after needling.

2. Kidney Deficiency

Principle: Tonify kidney *Qi* and consolidate the uterus by using points mainly from The *Ren* Channel and The Kidney Channel of Foot–*Shaoyin*.

Prescription: Guanyuan (RN 4) Shenshu (BL23)

Ciliao (BL32) Quyuan (LR 8)

Explanation: Guanyuan (RN 4) and Shenshu (BL23) can warm up the kidney *Yang* and reinforce the vital energy. Ciliao (BL32) is used as a local point for relieving soreness in the lower back. Quyuan (LR 8), the *He*–sea point of The Liver Channel of Foot–*Jueyin*, nourishes the blood and eases the uterus.

Point Modification: Add Baihui (DU20) for dizziness and tinnitus.

Method: Apply filiform needles with reinforcing method and retain the needles for 20–30 minutes. Treatment is given once a day. Moxibustion can be applied after needling.

Alternative Treatment: Scalp Acupuncture

Prescription: Bilateral reproductive regions Motor sensory region of the foot

Method: Retain the needles for 15—20 minutes with intermittent needling stimulations.

3.5 Metrorrhagia

Metrorrhagia refers to the type of uterine bleeding irrelevant to the normal menses. In traditional Chinese medicine, metrorrhagia is divided into the profuse and dripping ones. The former is characterized by a sudden onset of massive bleeding while the latter by a gradual dripping of blood from the uterus, occurring alternately. It is one of the common gynecological conditions, pertaining to dysfunctional uterine bleeding in modern medicine, and more complained of by women in their adolescence and climaterium.

Cause and Mechanism

The chief cause of metrorrhagia is concernd with the impairement of The *Chong* and *Ren* Channels that fails to restrict the blood in the uterus. Such an impairement is often due to the damage of the spleen by over worry with subsequent deficiency of *Qi* of the middle—*Jiao* that is unable to control the blood, or due to deficiency of kidney *Qi*. Besides, invasion of exogenous pathogenic heat, or emotional disturbance with stagnation of liver *Qi* turning into fire can both cause retention of heat in the lower—*Jiao* forcing the blood to flow outside of the normal channel.

Differentiation

1. Spleen Deficiency

The sudden profuse metrorrhagia is followed by continuous scanty bleeding in light red colour, general lassitude, palar complexion, shortness of breath, reluctant speech, poor appetite, loose stool, pale tongue proper with thin white coating, and weak thready pulse.

2. Kidney Deficiency

The symptoms of kidney deficiency include profuse of dripping uterine bleeding of light red colour and dilute quality, cold limbs, darkish complexion, soreness in the lower back and knees, frequent urinary discharge, pale tongue proper with thin white coating, and deep thready pulse. The patients with kidney *Yin* deficiency have symptoms such as palpitation,. insomnia, soreness in the lower back and knees, afternoon fever, red tongue proper with less coating, and rapid thready pulse.

3. Blood Heat Retention

The sudden onset of profuse or prolonged uterine bleeding in deep red colour and sticky quality is followed by restlessness, thirst, constipation straw urinary discharge, red tongue proper with yellowish or yellow greasy coating, and rapid full pulse.

Treatment

Principle: Arrest the bleeding, control blood and reinforce vital energy by selecting points mainly from The *Ren* Channel and The Spleen Channel of Foot—*Taiyin*.

Prescription: Guanyuan (RN 4) Sanyinjiao (SP 6)
Yinbai (SP 1)

Point Modification: Add Xuehai (SP10) and Xingjian (LR 2) for heat in the blood; Pishu (BL20)and Zusanli (ST36) for spleen deficiency; and Shenshu (BL23) and Taixi (KI 3) for kidney deficiency.

Explanation:

Yinbai (SP 1), the *Jing*—well point of The Spleen Channel of Foot—*Taiyin,* can invigorate the spleen *Qi* and help to ascend the lucid *Yang* to dominate both *Qi* and blood. Guanyuan (RN 4), the point meeting the three *Yin* channels of the foot, The *Chong* and *Ren* Channels, can promote *Qi* of The *Chong* and *Ren* Channels, warm up the lower—*Jiao* and the uterus, invigorate the vital energy and nourish blood. Sanyinjiao (SP 6), the coalescent point of the three *Yin* channels of the foot, and the main point for treating gynecological diseases, can strengthen the function of the spleen in dominating the blood. Xuehai (SP10) and Xingjian (LR 2) are used to clear up heat in the blood. Pishu (BL20) and Zusanli (ST36) are added to strengthen the spleen *Qi*. Shenshu (BL23) and Taixi (KI 3) are applied to nourish the kidney *Yin* and reduce heat.

Point Modification: Add Tianshu(ST25) and Shangjuxu (ST37) for anorexia and loose stool; and Zhigou (SJ 6) for constipation.

Method: Apply filiform needles with reducing method for heat retention in the blood without using moxibustion and with reinforcing method for kidney deficiency. Moxibustion is added after for kidney deficiency type. Needles are retained for 15—20 minutes each time.

Alternative Treatment: Auricular Acupuncture

Prescription: Uterus Endocrine Ovary Kidney spleen
Ear—Shenmen Liver

Method: Use 2—4 points each time with moderate stimulation for 30 minutes once a day or once every other day.

3.6 Leukorrhea

Leukorrhea refers to the increasing vaginal discharge of an abnormal colour, quality and odour. It is also called white leukorrhea because of the predominant white colour seen in the clinic. This disease is common in gynecology.

Cause and Mechanism

Leukorrhea is often due to over thinking, impairement of the spleen and stomach with subsequent poor transforming and transporting and retention of dampness and water which flow downward to the lower—*Jiao,* or due to over sexual indulgence, multiple labour with subsequent deficiency of kidney *Qi* and vital essence, leading to the poor restriction of The *Dai* Channel. It may also be caused by the downward flow of damp—heat along The Liver Channel of Foot—*Jueyin* to the lower—*Jiao*

Differentiation

1. Spleen Deficiency

Persistent white or slight yellowish leukorrhea of sticky quality without a foul smell. It is accompanied by sallow complexion, general lassitude, anorexia, loose stool pale tongue proper with white sticky coating and slow weak pulse.

2. Kidney Deficiency

The massive vaginal discharge of white colour and dilute quality is accompanied by soreness in the lumbar region, loose stool, cold sensation in the lower abdomen, frequent and excessive urination, pale tongue proper with white coating ,and deep slow pulse.

3. Damp—heat Retention

The yellowish discharge of massive quantity and bad odour

from the vagina resembles purulent substance. It is accompanied by itching in the vagina, sinking pain in the lower abdomen, bitter taste in the mouth, thirst, dry stool, scanty urination, sticky yellowish tongue coating, and rapid slippery pulse.

Treatment

1. Spleen Deficiency

Principle: Reinforce spleen *Qi*, resolve dampness and check leukorrhea by using points mainly from The *Ren* Channel, The Gallbladder Channel of Foot–*Shaoyang* and The Spleen Channel of Foot–*Taiyin*.

Prescription: Daimai (GB26) Baihuanshu (BL30)
Qihai (RN 6) Sanyinjiao (SP 6)

Explanation: Daimai (GB26) consolidates the *Qi* of The Dai Channel. Baihuanshu (BL30) and Qihai (RN 6) regulate the *Qi* circulation of The *Ren* Channel and The Urinary Bladder Channel of Foot–*Taiyang* for the purpose of removing dampness. Sanyinjiao (SP 6) is used to strengthen the spleen, resolve dampness and regulate the liver and kidney.

Point Modification: Add Zhongwan (RN12), Tianshu (ST25) and Zusanli (ST36) for poor appetite and loose stool.

Method: Apply filiform needles with reinforcing method and retain the needles for 15–20 minutes, once a day. Moxibustion may be applied after needling.

2. Kidney Deficiency

Principle: Reinforce kidney *Qi* and stabilize the function of The *Ren* and *Dai* Channels by using points mainly from The *Ren* Channel and The Kidney Channel of Foot–*Shaoyin*.

Prescription: Guanyuan (RN 4) Daimai (GB26)
Shenshu (BL23) Ciliao (BL32) Zhaohai (KI 6)

Explanation: Guanyuan(RN 4), Shenshu(BL23) and Zhaohai (KI 6) are used to warm up the lower−*Jiao*, replenish the vital energy, warm up the uterus and nourish the blood. Daimai (GB26) and Ciliao (BL32) are the effective points for treating leukorrhea.

Point Modification: Add Shangjuxu (ST37) for loose stool.

Method: Apply filiform needles with reinforcing method for 15−20 minutes daily. Moxibustion should be applied after needling.

3. Damp−heat Retention

Principle: Clear up heat, resolve dampness and check leukorrhea by using points mainly from The Gallbladder Channel of Foot−*Shaoyang* and The Spleen Channel of Foot−*Taiyin*.

Prescription: Daimai (GB26) Ciliao (BL32)

Yinlingquan (SP 9) Xuanzhong (GB39)

Xingjian (LR 2)

Explanation: Daimai (GB26) regulates the *Qi* of the *Dai* Channel. Giliao(BL32) clears up damp−heat from the lower−*Jiao*. Xingjian (LR 2), the *Ying*−spring point of The Liver Channel of Foot−*Jueyin*, eliminates heat from its pertaining channel. Yinlingquan (SP 9) clears heat and dampness from the spleen channel. Xuanzhong (GB39) clears up heat from the *Sanjiao* resolves dampness.

Point Modification: Add Zhigou (SJ 6) for dry stool.

Method: Apply filiform needles with reducing method for 15−20 minutes once a day.

Alternative Treatment: Auricular Acupuncture

Prescription: Ear−Shenmen Uterus Kidney

Urinarybladder Spleen

Method: Puncture 2–3 points each time with filiform needles and moderate stimulation for 15–20 minutes once every other day. Embedding of ear seeds is also appliceble.

3.7 Morning Sickness

Morning sickness, also know as pregnant vomiting, is symptomized by nausea, vomiting, dizziness, anorexia or vomiting right after food intake. It is virtually the early reaction of pregnancy which gradually subsides during the first three months of pregnancy.

Cause and Mechanism

Morning sickness is mainly caused by the adverse rising of Qi in The *Chong* Channel with subsequent poor descending of stomach Qi. Two types of the condition viz, deficiency of the spleen and stomach and in coordination between the liver and stomach, are commonly seen in the clinic. Constitutional deficiency of the spleen and stomach plus no relief of menses during pregnancy gives rise to an easy attack of Qi of The *Chong* Channel into the stomach. And deficiency of stomach Qi fails to perform its descending. Therefore, the ascending part of the stomach Qi together with the rising of Qi of The *Chong* Channel leads to nausea and vomiting. The dysfunction of the spleen in transforming and transporting causes phlegmdamp retaining in the middle–*Jiao*. Part of the phlegm–damp retained in the middle–*Jiao* may also ascend together with the rising Qi of The *Chong* Channel to cause nausea and vomiting. Besides, blood deficiency during pregnancy may cause the hyperactive liver Qi to be likely to attack the stomach, leading to the incoordination between the liver and stomach. Such an incoordination causes poor descending of the stomach

Qi which eventually leads to vomiting.

Differentiation

1. Deficiency of The Spleen and Stomach

The morning sickness is characterized by distention in the hypochondriac region with nausea, dislike of food, or even instant vomiting with food intake. It is accompanied by tastelessness in the mouth, vomiting of clear fluid, lassitude and sluggishness, palpitation, shortness of breath, pale tongue proper with white sticky coating, and slow slippery pulse of a weak nature.

2. Incoordination Between the Liver and Stomach

The morning sickness is characterized by vomiting of bitter or sour fluid in the early period of pregnancy. It is accompanied by fullness in the chest, pain the hypochondriac region, belching, sighing, low spirit, dizziness, head distention, excessive thirst, bitter taste in the mouth, pale tongue proper with slight yellowish coating, and wiry slippery pulse.

Treatment

1. Deficiency of the Spleen and Stomach

Principle: Strengthen the spleen and stomach, halt the ascending *Qi* and arrest nausea by using points mainly from The *Ren* Channel, The stomach Channel of Foot−*Yangming* and The Spleen Channel of Foot−*Taiyin*.

Prescription: Zhongwan (RN12)   Zusanli (ST36)

Gongsun(SP 4) Pishu(BL20)

Weishu(BL21) Neiguan (PC   6)

Explanation: Zusanli (ST36), having the function to pacify the stomach, halts the ascending *Qi* and arrests the nausea. It is used in combination with Gongsun (SP 4) to regulate the *Qi* mechanism of the stomach and spleen in order to soothe the aggresive *Qi* of The *Chong* Channel as well as the adverse flow of stomach *Qi*. Neiguan (PC 6) relieves stuffiness in the chest, regulates *Qi* circulation, halts the adverse flow of *Qi* and stops vomiting. Pishu (BL20) and Weishu (BL21) are used in combination with Zhongwan (Ren12), known as the method of combing the Back—*Shu* and Front—*Mu* points, to strengthen the function of the stomach and the spleen, and regulate their *Qi* circulation.

Method: Apply filiform needles with reinforcing method for 15—20 minutes each treatment.

2. Incoordination Between the Liver and Stomach.

Principle: Soothe the live, pacify the stomach, descend the adverse flow of *Qi* and stop vomiting by using points mainly from The Liver Channel of Foot—*Jueyin* and The Stomach Channel of Foot—*Yangming*.

Prescription: Neiguan (PC 6) Zhongwan (RN12)

Zusanli (ST36) Taichong (LR 3)

Explanation: Neiguan (PC 6) soothes the *Qi* circulation in the chest. Taichong (LR 3) in combination with Zusanli (ST36) may soothe the liver and strengthen the spleen, so that the spleen will not further counteract on the liver. Zhongwan (RN12) pacifies the stomach and checks the upward adverse flow of *Qi* and stops nausea and vomiting.

Point Modification: Add Fenglong (ST40) for turbid phlegm obstruction in the middle—*Jiao*

Method: Apply filiform needles with reducing method and retain the needles for 15—20 minutes once a day. Acupuncture is contraindicated in women with nervousness or habitual miscarriage in order to avoid abortions.

Alternative Treatment: Auricular Acupuncture

Prescription: Ear—Shenmen Liver Stomach Sympathetic
Spleen

Method: Apply filiform needles with mild stimulation once a day. Ten treatments consist of one course. Embedding of ear seeds is also applicable.

3.8 Malposition of Fetus

Malposition of fetus refers to the abnormal fetal position in uterus in 28 weeks of gestation. It is an asymptomatic condition commonly seen in multipara or those with lax abdominal wall. Complications will appear when the parturient is not adjusted. Malposition of fetus related to structure of constricted pelvis or uterine deformity is beyond the therapeutic scope of acupuncture discussed here.

Treatment

Prescription: Zhiyin (BL67)

Explanation: Zhiyin (BL67) is the point where the *Qi* of The Bladder Channel of Foot—*Taiyang* originates. The *Qi* of both The Urinary Bladder Channel of Foot—*Taiyang* and The Kidney Channel of Foot—*Shaoyin* merges here since these two channels are internally—externally related. Moxibustion applied at Zhiyin (BL67) may also help to maintain the coordination of the internally—externally related two channels so as to make the position of fetus return normal.

Method: Ask the pregnant woman to offer a sitting or lying posture with the belt loosened. Apply moxibustion at bilateral Zhiyin (BL67) for 15—20 minutes, once or twice daily. The same treatment is repeated till the fetal position is adjusted to normal status. According to some source of report, the success ratio is over 80%. It is more effective for multipara than primiparae and most effective in women with seven months of gestation.

3.9 Protracted Labour

Protracted labour refers to a delivery with parturition of more than twenty—four hours. It is often due to abnormal contraction of the womb or malposition of the fetus. However, protracted labour caused by other factors such as uterine deformity and cephalopelvic disproportion is not suggested for treatment by means of acupuncture.

Cause and Mechanism

Protracted labour is often caused by weak constitution with poor energy, exhaustion of *Qi* and blood due to premature contraction of the womb. It is also due to a lack of ante partum exercises, parturient nervouness, or invasion of pathogenic cold that causes poor circulation of *Qi*, stagnation of *Qi* and blood stasis, bring on protracted labour.

Differentiation

1. Difficiency of *Qi* and Blood

This type of protracted labour is characterized by some dull paroxysmal pain with slight heavy and distending sensation and prolonged course of delivery. It is accompanied by profuse bleeding of light colour, pallor complexion, palpitation, shortness of breath, lassitude, pale tongue proper with thin coating, and deficient type of full pulse or deep thready pulse that is weak in nature.

2. Stagnation of *Qi* and Stasis of Blood

This type of protracted labour is characterized by some

paroxysmal pain in the lower back and abdomen, scanty bleeding of dark red colour. It is accompanied by protracted labour, bluish complexion, nervousness, distention and fullness in the chest and epigastrium, repeated nausea, dark red tongue, and deep, forceful, rapid but uneven pulse.

Treatment

1. Deficiency of *Qi* and Blood

Principle: Nourish *Qi* and blood and strengthen the labour energy by using points mainly from The Spleen Channel of Foot—*Taiyin* and The Kidney Channel of Foot—*Shaoyin.*

Prescription: Qihai (RN 6)　Sanyinjiao (SP 6)

　　　　　　　Fuliu (KI　7)　Zhiyin (BL67)

Explanation: Qihai (RN 6) warms up the kidney *Yang.* and invigorates the *Qi* of the three *Yin* channels of the foot. Fuliu (KI 7) tonifies *Qi* of the kidney. Zhiyin (BL67) , the *Jing*—well point of The Bladder Channel of Foot—*Taiyang,* is an effective point for quickening the delivery.

Point Modification: Add Neiguan (PC 6) for palpitation and shortness of breath.

Method: Apply filiform needles with reinforcing method. Moxibustion should be applied to Qihai (RN 6) at the same time.

2. Stagnation of *Qi* and Stasis of Blood

Principle: Regulate *Qi,* activate and quicken the delivery by selecting points mainly from The Large Intestine Channel of Hand—*Yangming* and The Spleen Channel of Foot—*Taiyin.*

Prescription: Hegu (LI 4)　Sanyinjiao (SP 6)

　　　　　　　Zhiyin (BL67)　Duyin (EX—LE11)

Explanation: The application of reinforcing method at Hegu (LI 4), the *Yuan*—source point of The Large Intestine Channel of

Hand—*Yangming,* and reducing method at Sanyinjiao (SP 6), the intersecting point of the three *Yin* channels of the foot, has the effect to reinforce *Qi,* nourish blood and speed up delivery. Both Zhiyin (BL67), the *Jing*—well point of The Urinary Bladder Channel of Foot—*Taiyang,* and Duyin (EX—LE11) are empirical points for speeding up the delivery. These four points in combination may serve the purpose to quicken the delivery.

Point Modification: Add Neiguan (PC 6) and Zhigou (SJ 6) for distention and fullness in the chest and hypochondrium.

Method: Apply filiform needles with reducing method.

Alternative Treatment: Auricular Acupuncture

Prescription: Uterus endocrine kidney Subcortex

Method: Apply filiform needles with moderate stimulation. Manipulate the needles every three to five minutes during the treatment.

3.10   Retention of Placenta

Retention of placenta refers to the delayed relief of placenta 30 minutes after the delivery.

Cause and Mechanism

Retention of placenta is mostly due to weak constitution, deficiency of vital energy, prolonged labour course which over—consumes both *Qi* and blood. Invasion of pathogenic cold and stagnation of *Qi* and blood with subsequent stagnation of *Qi* and blood, and weakening of the uterine activity may also lead to retention of placenta.

Differentiation

1. *Qi* Deficiency

Placenta is retained after labour. It is accompanied by mild distention in the lower abdomen, soft palpable masses with no pain even by pressing, vaginal bleeding of light colour, palar complexion, lassitude, cold limbs, pale tongue proper with thin white coating, and weak pulse.

2. Blood Stasis

The retention of placenta is accompanied by cold pain in the lower abdomen aggravated by pressing, hard masses, scanty vaginal bleeding of dark red colour, purplish tongue proper, and deep hesitant pulse.

Treatment

1. *Qi* Deficiency

Principle: Reinforce *Qi* and enrich blood by using points mainly from The *Ren* Channel and The Spleen Channel of Foot—*Taiyin*.

Prescription: Guanyuan (RN　4)　Sanyinjiao (SP　6)
　　　　　　　Duyin (EX—LE11)

Explanation: Guanyuan(RN 4), the point of The *Ren* Channel, communicates with uterus. Sanyinjiao (SP 6) is the intersecting point of the three *Yin* channels of the foot. These two points in combination with both acupuncture and moxibustion may reinforce *Qi* and nourish blood. Duyin (EX—LE11) is an empirical point for dealing with retention of placenta.

Point Modification: Add Yinbai (SP 1) with moxibustion for profuse vaginal bleeding.

Method: Apply filiform needles with reinforcing method, plus moxibustion after needling.

2. Blood Stasis

Principle: Promote blood circulation and resolve blood stasis by using points mainly from The *Ren* Channel, The Large Intestine Channel of Hand—*Yangming* and The Spleen Channel of Foot—*Taiyin*.

Precription: Zhongji (RN 3) Hegu (LI 4) Sanyinjiao (SP 6) Jianjing (GB21) Duyin (EX—LE11)

Explanation: Zhongji (RN 3), point of The *Ren* Channel communicating with the uterus, may activate blood and resolve blood stasis if it is punctured with reducing method. Neddling Hegu (LI 4) with reinforcing method and Sanyinjiao (SP 6) with reducing method may promote *Qi* circulation and activate blood. Their combination with Duyin (EX—LE11) is particularly indicated in retention of placenta. Jianjing (GB21), though normally contraindicated in pregnancy, is used here to force the placenta to come out because the point offers a sinking effect.

Method: Apply filiform needles with reducing method. Moxibustion may be applied after needling.

Alternative Treatment: Electric Stimulation

Prescription: Hegu (LI 4) Sanyinjiao (SP 6)

Method: Apply electric stimulation for 30 minutes, after the patient feels the needling sensation.

3.11   Lochia

Lochia refers to vaginal discharge of cellular debris, mucus and blood following childbirth. The complete discharge needs three weeks of time. Persistent vaginal discharge over three weeks after delivery is called lochiorrhea.

Cause and Mechanism

Lochia may be due to weak constitution with deficiency of anti—pathogenic *Qi,* or over consumption of both *Qi* and blood during delivery, early physical labour after childbirth which results in sinking of *Qi* and poor consolidation of The *Chong* and *Ren* Channels so as to fail to govern the blood. Excessive loss of *Yin* fluid with subsequent *Yin* deficiency causes heat in the interior. Invasion of exogenous pathogenic heat or heat transformed from liver *Qi* stagnation may all stay in the interior. Such factors may disturb The *Chong* and *Ren* Channels impending a disorderly blood circulation that develops into lochia. Nevertheless, invasion of exogenous pathogenic cold encountering blood in the body may produce blood stasis in the uterus, which also results in the incoordination of The *Chong* and *Ren* Channels. and lochiorrhea.

Differentiation

1. *Qi* Deficiency

Lingering lochiorrhea of profuse of scanty quantity marked by light red colour and dilute quality without a bad odour. It is accompanied by a hollow, sinking sensation in the lower abdomen, general lassitude pllor complexion, pale tongue with white thin coating, and weak slow pulse.

2. Blood Heat

The Lochia which procedes the normal period of time is rather heavy in quantity with dark red colour, sticky quality and a bad odour. It is accompanied by redness in the cheeks, thirst, red tongue proper, and rapid thready pulse.

3. Blood Stasis

The dripping lochia is characterized by a slow unsmooth discharge of scanty quality and dark purplish colour with clots. The accompanying symptoms and signs include pain the lower abdomen that is aggravated by pressing, purplish tongue, and wiry uneven pulse.

Treatment

1. *Qi* Deficiency

Principle: Strengthen *Qi* and arrest bleeding by selecting points mainly from The *Ren* Channel, The Spleen Channel of Foot—*Taiyin* and The Stomach Channel of Foot—*Yangming*.

Prescription: Yinbai (SP 1) Guanyuan (RN 4)

Zusanli (ST36) Sanyinjiao (SP 6)

Explanation: Yinbai (SP 1), the origin of The Spleen Channel of Foot—*Taiyin,* may replenish the spleen *Qi* and consolidate the circulation of *Qi* and blood. Guanyuan (RN 4), the place where the primordial *Qi* of the general body merges, reinforces the primordial *Qi*. Zusanli (ST36) and Sanyinjiao (SP 6) are used together to strengthen the middle—*Jiao* and promote the function of spleen in governing the blood circulation.

Point Modification: Add Pishu (BL20) for profuse lochia.

Method: Apply filiform needles with reducing method and retain the needles for 20—30 minutes, once a day. Moxibustion may be applied after acupuncture.

2. Blood Heat

Principle: Replenish *Yin,* clear up heat and cease bleeding by using points mainly from The *Ren* Channel and the three *Yin* channels of the foot.

Prescription: Qihai (RN 6) Xuehai (SP10)

Zhongdu (LR 6) Taixi (KI 3)

Explanation: Qihai (RN 6), the point of The *Ren* Channel communicating with the uterus, has the function to regulate and invigorate *Qi*. Reducing method applied at this point can clear up heat in the lower—*Jiao* Xuehai (SP10), the point of The Spleen Channel of Foot—*Taiyin,* may regulate blood circulation and normalize the menstruation. Reducing method applied at this point may remove heat from the blood. Zhongdu (LR 6), the Xi–cleft point of The Liver Channel of Foot–*Taiyin*, has the function to soothe the liver and clear up heat. Taixi (KI 3) is used to tonify kidney *Yin* and clear up the deficient heat.

Point Modification: Add Zhaohai (KI 6) for thirst in the mouth.

Mothod: Apply filiform needles with reducing method and retain the needles for 15–20 minutes once a day.

3. Blood Stasis

Principle: Activate blood circulation and resolve blood stasis by using points mainly from The *Ren* Channel and The Spleen Channel of Foot–*Taiyin*.

Prescription: Zhongji (RN 3)　Taichong (LR 3)
　　　　　　Sanyinjiao (SP 6)

Explanation: Zhongji (RN 3), the point of The *Ren* Channel, harmonizes The *Chong* and *Ren* Channels, activates blood circulation and resolves blood stasis. Taichong(LR 3), the *Yuan*–source point of The Liver Channel of Foot–*Jueyin*, soothes the liver *Qi*, nourishes its blood and clears away the blood stasis from the channels. Sanyinjiao (SP 6), the intersecting point of the three *Yin* channels of the foot, has the effect to promote the circulation of *Qi* and blood, activate and replenish blood, and resolve blood stasis.

Point Modification: Add moxibustion at Guanyuan (RN 4) for cold pain in the lower abdomen.

Method: Apply filiform needles with reducing method and retain the needles for 15–20 minutes, once a day. Moxibustion should be applied in case of blood stasis due to exogenous pathogenic cold.

Alternative Treatment: Auricul Acupuncture

Prescription: Ear—Shenmen Sympathetic Uterus Endocrine
Spleen Kidney Liver Subcortex

Method: Apply filiform needles with moderate stimulation
and retain the needles for 15–20 minutes, once a day. Select two
or three points for auricular acupuncture each time. Embedding
of ear seeds is also applicable.

3.12　Lactation Deficiency

Lactation deficiency refers to low or no production of milk
after childbirth. The nomenclature for lactation deficiency in traditional Chinese medicine is lack of milk of halted milk flow.

Cause and Mechanism

Traditional Chinese medicine holds the view that milk is
transformed from *Qi* and blood. Either constitutional deficiency
of spleen and stomach with insufficiency of the source of acquired
energy, or heavy loss of blood during delivery may result in over
consumption of *Qi* and blood which can not manufacture enough
milk. Emotional depression after delivery may cause the liver to
lose its maintaince over the free flow of *Qi* with subsequent
impairment of *Qi* mechanism and obstructed *Qi* circulation, leading to halted milk production.

Differentiation

1. Deficiency of *Qi* and Blood

This kind of lactation deficiency is characterized by small
amounts of milk production of dilute quality of even no production of milk after the childbirth. The breasts feel soft with no
distention. The accompanying symptoms and signs include palar

complexion, lassitude, anorexia, loose stools, pale tongue proper with less coating, and weak thready pulse.

2. Stagnation of Liver *Qi*

There is insufficiency or absence of milk production after labour but distention and fullness in the chest and hypochondriac region, and distending pain in the breasts. Such a kind of lactation deficiency also involves with emotional depression, or slight fever, irritability, poor appetite, thin yellow tongue coating, and wiry or rapid wiry pulse.

Treatment

Principle: Tonify *Qi* and blood in case of deficiency of *Qi* and blood; and promote the circulation of liver *Qi* in case of stagnation of liver *Qi*. The secondary principle of treatment in either case is to promote milk secretion.

Prescription: Danzhong (RN17)   Shaoze (SI 1)

　　　　　　　Rugen (ST18)

On the basis of the above principal prescription, plus Pishu (BL20) and Zusanli (ST36) for lactation deficiency due to deficiency of *Qi* and blood; and Neiguan (PC 6) and Qimen (LR14) for that due to stagnation of liver *Qi*.

Explanation: Danzhong (RN17) is used to regulate *Qi* circulation because blood can circulate well only when *Qi* is regulated normally. The normal *Qi* and blood circulation makes it sure that there is sufficient substantial source for milk production. Since The Stomach channel of Foot—*Yangming* passes through the breast, Rugen (ST18) is used to regulate the *Qi* circulation of its pertaining channel in the breast area so that the channel *Qi* in that area can travel smoothly, thus promoting the milk secretion. Shaoze (SI 1), the *Jing*—well point of The Small Intestine Channel of Hand–*Taiyang* may promote the circulation of both *Qi* and blood when it is punctured shallowly with filiform needle. It is an empirical point for promoting milk secretion. In case of deficiency of *Qi* and blood, Pishu (BL20) and Zusanli (ST36) are added in order to strengthen the spleen and stomach as well as the source for manufacturing *Qi* and blood. In the case of stagnation of liver *Qi*, Neiguan (PC 6) and Qimen (LR14) are chosen to soothe the liver *Qi* and relieve fullness sensation in the chest. Blood circulates normally only when *Qi* does in the same way.

Point Modification: Add Tianshu (ST25) for poor appetite and loose stool; and Yanglingquan (GB34) for distention and fullness sensation in the chest and hypochondriac region.

Method: Apply filiform needles with reinforcing method for insufficient lactation due to the deficiency of both *Qi* and blood. Moxibustion may be applied at Pishu (BL20), Zusanli (ST36) and Tianshu (ST25) after needling for 20–30 minutes. But, apply filiform needles with reducing method for lactation deficiency due to the stagnation of liver *Qi*. Needles in either case are retained for 15–20 minutes once a day.

Alternative Treatment: Auricular Acupuncture

Prescription: Chest Endocrine Liver Kidney

Method: Apply filiform needles with moderate stimulation and retain the needles for 15–20 minutes once a day. Embedding of ear seeds is also applicable.

3.13   Puerperal Pain

Puerperal pain refers to the pain in the lower abdomen in puerperium. It is mostly complained by multipera and within 1–2 days after the delivery. This condition is also called baby pillow pain in traditional Chinese medicine.

Cause and Mechanism

Heavy loss of blood during labour with subsequent emptiness of The *Chong* and *Ren* Channels causes malnutrition of the uterine collaterals or deficiency of both *Qi* and blood, resulting in the poor blood circulation and stagnant pain in the lower abdomen. The asthenia of uterine collaterals after labour gives rise to exogenous pathogenic cold invasion. Blood stasis due to the cold can cause obstruction in the uterine collaterals. Emotional depression with subsequent stagnation of liver and poor *Qi* mechanism brings on the uterine retention of blood stasis and causes abdominal pain if the stasis is not relieved timely.

Differentiation

1. Puerperal Pain due to Blood Deficiency

Some dull pain that responds to pressing in the lower abdomen is accompanied by scanty lochia of light red colour, dizziness, tinnitus, general lassitude, severe constipation, pale red tongue proper with thin coating, and thready pulse of the deficient type.

2. Puerperal Pain due to Blood Stasis

The distending pain aggravated by pressing is felt in the lower abdomen after delivery. The scanty lochia that is difficult to be released is of dark purplish colour with clots, or accompanied by some distending pain in the hypochondriac region. The tongue proper appears dark purplish or dark purplish with stagnant spots. The pulse is wiry and hesitant.

3. Puerperal Pain due to Cold Stagnation

The cold pain in the lower abdomen is aggravated by pressing and alleviated by warmth. It is accompanied by scanty lochia with clots, pale greenish complexion, cold limbs, dark purplish tongue proper with white coating, and deep tense pulse.

Treatment

1. Puerperal Pain due to Blood Deficiency

Principle: Tonify *Qi* and blood by using points mainly from The *Ren* Channels, The Stomach Channel of Foot–*Yangming* and The Spleen Channel of Foot–*Taiyin*.

Prescription: Guanyuan (RN 4) Zusanli (ST36)

Sanyinjiao (SP 6)

Explanation: Guanyuan(RN 4), the point of The *Ren* Channel, can warm up the lower–*Jiao* invigorate the primordial *Qi,* replenish essence and blood and eliminate cold pain the lower abdomen. Zusanli (ST36) and Sanyinjiao (SP 6) may strengthen the function of the spleen and stomach, and reinforce the source for providing the acquired energy.

Point Modifications: Add Baihui (DU20) for dizziness; and Zhaohai (KI 6) for constipation.

Method: Apply filiform needles with reinforcing method. Moxibustion may be applied after needling.

2. Puerperal Pain due to Blood Stasis

Principle: Promote blood circulation, remove blood stasis from the channels and relieve the pain by using points mainly from The *Ren* Channel, The Spleen Channel of Foot–*Taiyin* plus one Back–*Shu* point.

Prescription: Zhongji (RN 3) Guilai (ST29)

Geshu (BL17) Xuehai (SP10)

Sanyinjiao (SP 6) Hegu (LI 4)

Explanation: Zhongji (RN 3) and Guilai (ST29) are selected to remove obstruction from the channels and collaterals, promote the circulation of *Qi* and blood, and cease pain. Geshu (BL17), the Influential Point of the blood, is paired with Xuehai (SP10) to activate blood and resolve blood stasis. Sanyinjiao (SP 6) tonifies the spleen as well as the liver and kidney. It is also used to regulate The Chong and *Ren* Channels, activate and nourish blood. Hegu (LI 4) is good for promoting *Qi* circulation because of its ascending effect and dispersing function. It assists the rest of the points to activate blood, resolve stasis and stop pain.

Point Modification: Add Taichong (LR 3) for stagnation of *Qi* and stasis of blood.

Method: Apply filiform needles with reducing method and retain the needles for 20 minutes. Needles are manipulated every 3–5 minutes.

3. Puerperal Pain due to Cold Stagnation

Principle: Warm up the channels, expel cold and relieve pain by using points mainly from The *Ren* Channel and The Spleen Channel of Foot–*Taiyin*.

Prescription: Guanyuan (RN 4) Shenshu (BL23)
                    Sanyinjiao (SP 6)

Guanyuan (RN 4), the point of The *Ren* Channel, can warm up the Lower–*Jiao* and uterus, invigorate the primordial *Qi*, replenish essence and blood, and cure cold pain in the lower abdomen. Shenshu (BL23) can warm up the kidney and dispel cold. Sanyinjiao (SP 6) may tonify the liver and kidney, replenish The *Chong* and *Ren* Channels, regulate and nourish *Qi* and blood, promote blood circulation, and relieve pain.

Point Modification. Add Ciliao (BL32) for severe abdominal pain.

Alternative Treatment: Auricular Acupuncture

Prescription: Uterus Endocrine Ear—Shenmen Liver Kidney

Method: Apply the needles with moderate stimulation and retain the needles for 15—20 minutes once a day. Embedding of ear seeds is also applicable.

3.14   Eclampsia Gravidarm

Eclampsia gravidarm may occur in the third trimester of pregnancy, eutopic parturient or even after childbirth. It is a condition characterized by sudden fainting, loss of consciousness, convulsions, general lassitude, trismus, general rigidity and upward staring of the eyes. This condition ends up with a self—recovery in a few minutes, which is then followed by another similar attack, resembling epileptic attacks. Therefore, it is referred as pregnant epilepsy, similar to the severe type of pregnant toxication.

Cause and Mechanism

Eclampsia is mainly caused by constitutional *Yin* deficiency of the liver and kidney and consequent hyperactivity of liver *Yang*. During pregnancy, a considerable portion of blood is assembled in the uterus to nourish the fetus. This leads to a more severe condition of *Yin* deficiency of the liver and kidney and hyperactivity of liver *Yang,* which eventually results in the attacks mentioned above.

Differentiation

The pregnant woman who is likely to develop eclampsia, in several months of pregnancy, sometimes feels dizziness, palpitation, shortness of breath, worsening edema of the lower limbs, flushed face, bitter taste in the mouth and thirst. When the attack starts, she may suddenly fall faint with loss of consciousness, have convulsions of the four limbs, trismus, upward staring of eyes, or a mouthful of whitish foam. The tongue proper is dark red, and the pulse is rapid wiry. The attack may take place intermittently.

Treatment

Principle: Nourish *Yin,* tonify blood and quench the liver wind by using points mainly from The *Du* Channel, The Liver Channel of Foot—*Jueyin,* The Pericardium Channel of Hand—*Jueyin* and The Kidney Channel of Foot—*Shaoyin.*

Prescription: Shuigou (DU26) Neiguan (PC 6)
　　　　　　　Fengchi (GB20) Taichong (LR 3)
　　　　　　　Sanyinjiao (SP 6) Zhaohai (KI 6)
　　　　　　　Yongquan (KI 1)

Explanation: Shuigou (DU26)is selected to expel wind and resuscitat. Neiguan (PC 6) is used to soothe the suffocating sensation in the chest and calm the heart and mind. Fengchi (GB20) and Taichong (LR 3) are needled to soothe the liver, nourish the blood, quench wind and calm the convulsions. Sanyinjiao (SP 6) and Zhaohai (KI 6) may strengthen the spleen, replenish the *Yin* of the liver and kidney, moisten *Yin* and nourish blood, regulate The *Chong* and *Ren* Channels. Yongquan (KI 1) is chosen to tonify the kidney essence, nourish *Yin* and sedate the abnormal ascending *Qi*.

Method: Apply filiform needles with reducing method for Shuigou (DU26), Neiguan (PC 6), Fengchi (GB20) and Taichong (LR 3), but reinforcing method for Sanyinjiao (SP 6), Zhaohai (KI 6) and Yongquan (KI 1). Retain the needles for 15—20 minutes.

Alternative Treatment: Auricular Acupuncture

Prescription: Ear—Shenmen Liver Kidney Brain Stem

Method: Apply filiform needles with moderate stimulation and retain the needles for 15—20 minutes.

3.15 Infertility

A married woman who fails to become pregnant in two consecutive years of time, while the reproductive function of her marriage partener is medically proved normal, is considered to suffer from infertility. It was called no offspring in the ancient times.

Cause and Mechanism

A great majority of infertility cases are due to congenital deficiency of kidney *Qi* or insufficiency of essence and blood, leading to the deficiency of The *Chong* and *Ren* Channels and malnutrition of the uterus with consequent infertility. However, the invasion of exogenous pathogenic cold retained in the uterus may cause stagnation of cold and blood stasis as well as the obstruction of the uterine collaterals. Furthermore, poor function of the spleen in transporting and transforming as well as the habitual diet of oily greasy food brings on retention of phlegm—damp in the interior, leading to the impaired *Qi* mechanism and obstruction of the uterine collaterals. Obstruction is thus the main obstacle for pregnancy.

Differentiation

1. Infertility due to Kidney Deficiency

This kind of infertility involves irregular menstruation, and scanty flow of light red colour. It is accompanied by general lassitude, dizziness, tinnitus, soreness in the lumbar region and knees, pale tongue proper with white coating, and deep thready or deep slowly pulse.

2. Infertility due to Blood Deficiency

This kind of infertility involves scanty flow of light red menses in delayed cycles. It is accomapnied by emaciation, sallow complexion, dizziness, palpitation, general lassitude, pale tongue proper with little coating, and deep thready pulse.

3. Infertility due to Cold in Uterus

This kind of infertility may still have normal menses though sometimes the cycle is prolonged with dark red flow with clots. The flow is often dilute. It is accompanied by cold limbs, cold pain in the lower abdomen alleviated by warmth, frequent discharge of profuse urine, pale tongue proper with white coating, and deep slow pulse.

4. Infertility due to Phlegm—damp Retention

This kind of infertility involves an obese constitution, prolonged menstrual cycle or even amenorrhea and profuse discharge of sticky leukorrhea. It is accompanied by pallid complexion, dizziness, palpitation, white sticky tongue coating, and soft slippery pulse.

Treatment

1. Infertility due to Kidney Deficiency

Principle: Tonify kidney *Qi* and regulate The *Chong* and *Ren* Channels by using points mainly from The Spleen Channel of Foot—*Taiyin* and The Kidney Channel of Foot—*Shaoyin*.

Prescription: Shenshu (BL23) Mingmen (DU 4)
Sanyinjiao (SP 6) Taixi (KI 3)

Explanation: Shenshu (BL23), Mingmen (DU 4) and Taixi (KI 3) tonify kidney essence and blood, warm up the kidney *Yang* and invigorate the primordial *Qi.* Sanyinjiao (SP 6), the intersecting point of the three *Yin* channels of the foot, can strengthen the spleen and regulate menstruation and reinforce the liver and kidney.

Point Modification: Add Yonquan (KI 1) for dizziness and vertigo.

Method: Apply filiform needles with reinforcing method and retain the needles for 20—30 minutes once a day.

2. Infertility due to Blood Deficiency

Principle: Tonify *Qi* and blood and regulate The *Chong* and *Ren* Channels by using points mainly from The *Ren* Channel, The Stomach Channel of Foot—*Yangming* and The Spleen Channel of Foot—*Taiyin*.

Prescription: Qihai (RN 6) Zusanli (ST36)
　　　　　　　Sanyinjiao (SP   6) Zigong (EX—CA1)

Explanation: Qihai (RN 6), the intersecting point of The *Ren* Channel and the three *Yin* channels of the foot, can invigorate the primordial *Qi* and warm up kidney *Yang*. Zusanli (ST36) and Sanyinjiao (SP 6) may strengthen the spleen and stomach, the source for providing the acquired energy, replenish the liver and kidney in order to promote the function of The *Chong* and *Ren* Channels. Zigong (EX—CA1), meaning the uterus, is an empirical point for treating infertility.

Point Modification: Add Shenmen (HT 7) and Neiguan (PC 6) for dizziness and palpitation.

Method: Apply filiform needles with reinforcing method and retain the needles for 15—20 minutes, once a day.

3. Infertility due to Cold in Uterus

Principle: Warm up the channels and collaterals and expel cold by using points mainly from The *Ren* Channel, The *Du* Channel and The Stomach Channel of Foot—*Yangming*.

Prescription: Guanyuan (RN 4) Zigong (Extra)

Zusanli (ST36)   Mingmen (DU 4)

Explanation: Guanyuan (RN 4) is selected to warm up the lower—*Jiao* and uterus, invigorate the primordial *Qi* and tonify essence and blood in order to expel the pathogenic cold from the abdomen. Zusanli (ST36) can strengthen the spleen and stomach for the purpose to promote the source for providing the acquired energy. Ming—men (DU 4) warms up the kidney *Yang* and regulates menstruation. Zigong (EX—CA1) is an empirical point for treating infertility.

Point Modification: Add Guilai(ST 29) for delayed menstrual flow.

Method: Apply filiform needles with reinforcing method and retain the needles for 20—30 minutes, once a day. Moxibustion may be applied after needling.

4. Infertility due to Phlegm—damp Retention

Principle: Eliminate dampness, resolve phlegm, promote *Qi* circulation and regulate menstruation by using points mainly from The *Ren* Channel, The Spleen Channel of Foot—*Taiyin* and The Stomach Channel of Foot—*Yangming*.

Prescription: Zhongji (RN 3)   Qichong (ST30)   Diji (SP 8)
Fenglong (ST40)   Sanyinjiao (SP 6)

Explanation: Zhongji (RN 3) and Qichong (ST30) are selected to promote *Qi* and regulate menstruation. Diji(SP 8) may strengthen the spleen and eliminate dampness. Fenglong (ST40), the *Luo*—connecting point of The Stomach Channel of Foot—*Yangming*, has the effect to strengthen spleen, remove dampness and resolve phlegm. Sanyinjiao(SP 6), the crossing point of the three *Yin* channels of the foot, has the function to strengthen the spleen, replenish the liver and kidney, regulate *Qi* and promote The *Chong* and *Ren* Channels. The use of the above points may jointly achieve the purpose of removing dampness and phlegm and regulating *Qi* and menstruation.

Point Modification: Add Neiguan(PC 6) for dizziness and palpitation.

Method: Apply filiform needles with even method and retain the needles for 15−20 minutes, once a day. Moxibustion may be applied after needling.

Alternative Treatment: Auricular Acupuncture

Prescription: Endocrine Uterus Kidney Ovary
                 Subcortex

Method: Apply the needles with moderate stimulation. Select 2−3 points each time for ten consecutive treatments in one course. Embedding of ear seeds is also applicable.

3.16   Hysteria

Hysteria in terms of traditional Chinese medicine refers to a condition characterized by a series of mental symptoms and signs such as emotional depression or unrest, abnormal cry or laughing. The causative factor of the condition is related to emotional disturbances such as depression, excessive joy, anger or grief. It is similar to hysterial emotional outburst in modern medicine.

Cause and Mechanism

Excessive anger can impair the function of liver in maintaining free flow of *Qi,* causing derangement of *Qi* mechanism and emotional unrest. Habitual depression with over thinking and sorrow cause the liver to over−act the spleen, the source for providing the acquired energy. This over−acting process may lead to a physical status that the heart is poorly nourished by the blood and the mind is poorly nourished by the mind, resulting in onset of hysteria.

Differentiation

1. Liver *Qi* Stagnation

This type of hysteria is charcterized by mental depression, irritability, restlessness, fullness and distention in the chest and hypochondriac region, frequent yawnings, poor self–control, dry mouth, constipation, red tongue with less coating, and wiry pulse.

2. Emotional Depression.

This type of hysteria is chacterized by low spirit, trance, emotional unrest, constant cries with grief or sorrow, pale tongue proper with white coating, and thready pulse.

Treatment

1. Liver *Qi* Stagnation

Principle: Soothe the liver *Qi*, tranquilize the heart and bring back normal consciousness by using points mainly from The *Du* Channel, The Liver Channel of Foot–*Jueyin,* The Pericardium Channel of Hand–*Jueyin* and · The Heart Channel of Hand–*Shaoyin.*

Prescription: Shuigou (DU26) Jianshi (PC 5)

Shenmen (HT 7) Fenglong (ST40)

Taichong (LR 3)

Explanation: Shuigou (DU26), the point of The *Du* channel, has the effect to tranquilize the heart and bring back normal consciousness. Jianshi (PC 5) and Shenmen (HT 7) are needled to clear up heart fire and tranquilize the mind. Fenglong (ST40), the *Luo*–connecting point of The Stomach Channel of Foot–*Yangming,* is effective to expel pathogenic wind, resolve phlegm, promote the bowel movements and eliminate damp—heat in the gastrointestinal system. Taichong (LR 3) may nourish the liver blood, to soothe the liver *Qi* and relieve stagnation.

Point Modification: Add Zhigou (SJ 6) for constipation.

Method: Apply filiform needles with reducing method and retain the needles for 15—20 minutes, once a day.

2. Emotional Depression

Principle: Soothe the liver, regulate the flow of *Qi,* nourish the heart and calm the mind by using points mainly from The Pericardium Channel of Hand—*Jueyin* and The Kidney Channel of Foot—*Shaoyin.*

Prescription: Daling (PC 7)   Shenmen (HT 7)

Sanyinjiao (SP 6)   Taichong (LR 3)

Hegu (LI 4)   Shangwan (RN13)

Explanation: Daling (PC 7) and Shenmen (HT 7) are used to tranquilize the heart and mind. Sanyinjiao (SP 6), the crossing point of the three *Yin* channels of the foot, strengthens the spleen, nourishes heart blood and tonifies the liver and kidney. Taichong (LR 3) in combination with Hegu (LI 4) soothes the depressed liver *Qi* and nourishes the blood. Shangwan (RN13) is selected to relieve fullness sensation in the chest, pacify the stomach, promote the function of the middle—*Jiao* and clear away heat from the heart and stomach.

Point Modification: Add Laogong (PC 8) for trance.

Method: Apply filiform needles with even method and retain the needles for 15—20 minutes, once a day.

Alternative Treatment: Auricular Acupuncture

Prescription: Ear—Shenmen   Heart   Kidney   Stomach

Liver   Occipital   Brain   Stem

Method: Apply filiform needles with strong stimulation and retain the needles for 15 minutes, once a day. Puncture 2−3 points each time. Embedding of ear seeds is also applicable.

4　Pediatric Diseases

4.1　Whooping Cough

Whooping cough, known as pertusis in modern medicine, is one of the common respiratory infectious diseases suffered by infants. It is characterized by paroxysmal cough with spasm accompanied by a wheezing sound in the throat. Children mostly under the age of five may develop the condition all year around, especially in winter and spring.

Cause and Mechanism

The main causative factor of whooping cough is ascribed to the seasonal epidemic invasions that produce turbid phlegm in the interior of the body, obstructing the *Qi* passage. Such an obstruction causes dysfunction of the lung to perform its normal dispersing and descending. Therefore, the abnormal ascending of lung *Qi* leads to this type of lingering cough.

Differentiation

1. Incipient Stage:

Early pertusis is manifested by cough, running nose, sneezing, or aversion to cold with fever similar to that in common cold. The cough aggravates with loss of voice in two to three days and worsens with time. The accompanying symptoms and signs include white sputum with foams, thin white tongue coating, and superficial pulse.

2. Paroxysmal Stage

Spasmodic cough in this stage is mainly in paroxysmal attacks with loud noise. Wheezing sounds still remain in the throat when the attack is over. Patient feels better in the daytime and worse at night with difficulty to expectorate the sticky sputum. Nausea follows cough immediately. Vomiting helps relieve the spasm. The accompanying symptoms and signs include dry mouth, straw urine, constipation, or bloody sputum and epistaxis, yellow tongue coating, and slippery rapid pulse.

3. Rehabilitating Stage

The paroxysmal cough lessens day by day marked by a reduced frequency of attacks. The accompanying symptoms and signs include low spirits, spontaneous sweating, shortness of breath, weak cough, hoarseness of voice, red tongue proper with thin or peeled coating, and thready rapid pulse.

Treatment

1. The Incipient Stage

Principle: The exogenous pathogenic invasion attacks first the superficial portion of the body that is dominated by the lung. The principle of treatment is to relieve the exterior syndrome, disperse the lung *Qi* and stop cough by using points mainly from The Lung Channel of Hand—*Taiyin* and The Large Intestine Channel of Hand—*Yangming*.

Prescription: Fengmen(BL12) Feishu(BL13)

Lieque(LU 7) Hegu(LI 4)

Explanation: Fengmen(BL12) is used to eliminate the superficial wind. Lieque (LU7), the *Luo*—connecting point of the lung channel in combination with Hegu(LI4), the *Yuan*—source point of the large intestine channel, can help the lung disperse *Qi* and stop cough. Feishu(BL13) assists the above points to achieve a better effect in dispersing lung *Qi* and stopping cough.

Point Modification: Add Dazhui(DU14) for aversion to cold with absence of sweating; and Shaoshang(LU11) for congestion in the throat with itching sensation.

Method: Apply filiform needles with reducing method. Treatment is given once daily without retention of needles. Moxibustion is also applicable to Fengmen(UB12) and Dazhui(DU14).

2. Paroxysmal Stage

Principle: Eliminate heat from the lung, resolve phlegm and stop cough by selecting points mainly from The *Du* Channel and The Lung Channel of Hand—*Taiyin*.

Prescription: Dazhui(DU14)　Shenzhu(DU12)
　　　　　　　Chize(LU 5)　Fenglong(ST40)
　　　　　　　Neiguan(PC6)

Explanation: Dazhui(DU14) and Shenzhu(DU12) are used to clear up pathogenic heat. Chize(LU5), the *He*—sea point of the lung channel, and Fenglong(ST40), the *Luo*—connecting point of the stomach channel, are used to disperse the abnormal ascending of lung *Qi* , resolve phlegm and stop cough. Neiguan(PC6), the *Luo*—connecting point of the pericardium channel communicating with The *Yinwei* Channel, may soothe the chest disorder by vigorating the flow of lung *Qi* , and eliminate the internal heat.

Point Modification: Add Quchi(LI11) for general fever; Tianfu (LU3) and Shangxing(DU23) for hemoptysis and epistaxis.

Method: Apply filiform meedles with reducing method. Treatment is given once daily without retention of needles.

3. Rehabilitating Stage

Principle: Moisten the lung, relieve cough and strengthen the lung and spleen by using points mainly from The Lung Channel of Hand—*Taiyin* and The Stomach Channel of Foot—*Yangming*.

Prescription: Feishu(BL13)   Pishu(BL20)

Taiyuan(LU 9)   Zusanli(ST36)

Lieque(LU 7)   Zhaohai(KI 6)

Explanation: Feishu(BL13), Pishu(BL20) and Zusanli(ST36) are applied to strengthen the spleen and lung. Taiyuan(LU9), the *Yuan*—source point of the lung channel, has the function of to reinforce lung and relieve cough. Lieque(LU7), the *Luo*—connecting point of the lung channel, communicates with the *Ren* Channel. Zhaohai(KI 6), the *Shu*—stream point of the kidney channel, communicates with The Yinqiao Channel. These two points in combination, known as the combination of the Eight Confluent Points, have the effect to benefit the *Yin* and moisten the dryness.

Point Modification: Add Gaohuangshu(BL43) for weakness of the body; Zhongwan(RN12), Tianshu(ST25) and Qihai(RN6) for poor appetite and loose stools; and Guanyuan(RN4) for cold limbs.

Method: Apply filiform needles with reinforcing method. Moxibustion is also applicable to Feishu(BL13), Pishu(BL20) and Zusanli(ST36) for 20—30 minutes. Treatment is given once a day without needling retention.

Alternative Treatment: Auricular A cupuncture

Prescription: Bronchus Lung Ear—Shenmen Sympathetic

Method: Apply filiform needles with moderate stimulation. Points on both ears are punctured alternately with 2—3 points being selected each time. Treatment is given once daily. Embedding of ear seeds is also applicable for independent use. Furthermore, ear seeds implanting can be applied in combination with the filiform needles, which can improve the therapeutic effects.

4.2　Infantile Diarrhea

Infantile diarrhea, chiefly manifested by frequent bowel movement of loose or watery feces or feces like egg yellow, is a common gastrointestinal disease in children. Those who are mostly under the age of two may develop it all year around, especially in winter and spring. It is similar to infantile indigestion in modern medicine.

Cause and Mechanism

Children may be easily attacked by damp–cold invasion due to their tender *Zangf u* organs and weakness of the spleen and stomach. Irregular food intake, over eating of raw or cold food or unclean food may impair the stomach and spleen. Congenital defiency with decline of the vital gate fire causes excessive cold retention in the interior. The above three main factors cause the dysfunction of the spleen and stomach in transforming, transporting and digestion so that food is poorly nourished and the food essence can not be normally separated from the turbid substance, resulting in infantile diarrhea.

Differentiation

1. Cold–damp Diarrhea

The stool is watery with foam, borbory gmus and abdominal pain.It is accompanied by general aversion to cold with preference for warmth, but no thirst, pale tongue proper with thin white coating, and thin deep pulse.

2. Damp–heat Diarrhea

The yellowish stool is watery with bad odour, abdominal colic, general feverish sensation with thirst, burning sensation in the anus, scanty straw urine, yellow and greasy tongue coating, and slippery rapid pulse.

3. Diarrhea due to Food Retention

The epigastric distension and pain are alleviated by bowel movement with stool of bad odour. It is accompanied by poor appetite, vomiting, disturbed sleep, thick greasy tongue coating in yellow colour, and full slippery pulse.

4. *Yang* Deficiency Diarrhea

The lingering diarrhea characterized by watery stool or that like egg yellow occurs fairly frequently, shortly after meals. It is accompanied by cold limbs, poor spirit, difficulty to fall into sleep, prolapse of rectum, pale tongue with white coating, and slightly thready pulse.

Treatment

1. Cold−damp Diarrhea

Principle: Warm up *Yang*, eliminate cold, strengthen the spleen and resolve dampness by puncturing points mainly from the *Ren* Channel and The Stomach of Foot−*Yangming*.

Prescription: Zhongwan(RN12) Tianshu(ST25)

Zusanli(ST36) Guanyuan(RN 4)

Shenque(RN 8)

Explanation: Zhongwan(RN12), the Influential point of the Fu organs, and Tianshu(ST25), the Front−*Mu* point of the large intestine, are used to regulate the gastrointestinal functions and pacify the middle−*Jiao* Zusanli(ST36), the inferior *He*−sea point of the stomach, is used to strengthen the spleen and pacify the stomach and resolve dampness. Guanyuan(RN 4) and Shenque(RN8) are used to warm up the *Yang* and resolve dampness.

Point Modification: Add Gongsun(SP4) for severe abdominal pain.

Method: Apply filiform needles with even method, but without needle retention. Moxibustion is also applicable to Zhongwan(RN12), Tianshu(ST25), Zusanli(ST36) and Guanyuan(RN4) for 20−30 minutes. Shenque(RN8) is only suggested for moxibustion. Treatment is given once daily.

2. Damp−heat Diarrhea

Principle: Clear up heat and resolve dampness by puncturing points mainly from The Stomach Channel of Foot−*Yangming*.

Prescription: Zhongwan(RN12) Tianshu(ST25)
Zusanli(ST36) Quchi(LI11)
Neiting(ST44)

Explanation: Zhongwan(RN12) is the Front−*Mu* point of the stomach. Tianshu(ST25) is the Front−*Mu* point of the large intestine. The combination of both may regulate the gastrointestinal functions and pacify the middle−*Jiao* so that the normal transporting and transforming can be restored. Zusanli(ST36), in inferior *He*−sea point of the stomach, is used to descend stomach *Qi* and help resolve dampness. Quchi(LI11) and Neiting(ST44) can eliminate damp−heat in the gastrointestinal system.

Point Modification: Add Chize(LU5), Weizhong(BL40) for severe heat; and Yinlingquan(SP9) for severe dampness.

Method: Apply filiform needles with reducing method but without needle retention. Weizhong(BL40) may be pricked to cause bleeding with a three−edged needle.

3. Diarrhea due to Food Retention

Principle: Promote digestion by puncturing points mainly from The *Ren* Channel and The stomach Channel of Foot—*Yangming*.

Prescription: Zhongwan(RN12) Tianshu(ST25)
            Qihai(RN 6) Zusanli(ST36)
            Neiting(ST44)

Explanation: Zhongwan(RN12), Tianshu(ST25) and Zusanli(ST36) are used for regulating the function of stomach and intestines, and promote digestion. Qihai(RN 6) is used to regulate *Qi* and relieve pain. Inner Neiting(ST44) has good effect for promoting digestion.

Point Modification: Add Neiguan(PC6) for vomiting.

Method: Apply filiform needles with reducing method, but without needle retention.

4. Yang Deficiency Diarrhea

Principle: Strengthen the spleen and warm up the kidney by puncturing points of The Stomach Channel of Foot—*Yangming* plus some Back—*Shu* points;

Prescription: Pishu(BL20) Shenshu(BL23)
            Zhangmen(LR13) Zhongwan(RN12)
            Zusanli(ST36) Baihui(DU20)

Explanation: Pishu(BL20) is the Back—*Shu* point of the spleen, Zhangmen(LR13), the Front—*Mu* point of the spleen, and Zhongwan(RN12), the Front—*Mu* point of the stomach, These three points in combination may invigorate spleen *Yang*, strengthen the transporting function of the spleen and stop diarrhea. Shenshu(BL23) is used to warm up the kidney *Yang*. Baihui(DU20) has the function to reinforce *Qi* and stop diarrhea because it can help the sunk *Qi* to ascend.

Point Modification: Add Guanyuan(RN4) for cold limbs.

Method: Apply filiform needles with reinforcing method, but without needle retention. Moxibustion is also applicable to Pishu(BL20), Shenshu(BL23), Zusanli(ST36), Baihui(DU20) and Guanyuan(RN4) for 20−30 minutes. The Treatment is given once daily.

4.3 Infantile Malnutrition

Infantile malnutrition is related to either improper nursing or the affect of various illnesses which weaken the function of the spleen and stomach, and over consumption of *Qi* and blood. It is mainly characterized by general deficiency and emaciation, bothering children mostly under the age of five. It includes dystropia, vitamin deficiency in modern medicine.

Cause and Mechanism

Improper feeding and irregular food intake may impair the spleen and stomach, causing their dysfunction in transporting and transforming. Such a dysfunction gives rise to dilute watery stool, poor distribution of food essence, and malnutrition of the body. Further, intestinal parasitosis and other chronic illnesses may over−consume *Qi*, blood and body fluid, causing malnutrition in a long run.

Differentiation

Infantile malnutrition is characterized by emaciation, loose muscles, scaled skin, sparse hair, listlessness, sallow complexion, or outstanding blue veins in the severe case.

Infantile malnutrition due to deficiency of spleen and stomach is accompanied by loose watery stool with undigested food, poor appetite, poor sleep, pale tongue proper, and weak thready pulse.

Infantile malnutrition due to parasites may involve the eating of unclean food, paroxysmal abdominal pain, brygmus in sleep, pale tongue proper, and thready wiry pulse.

Treatment

1. Weakness of the Spleen and Stomach

Principle: Reinforce the spleen and stomach, and aid recovery from malnutrition by puncturing points mainly from The Spleen Channel of Foot—*Taiyin* and The Stomach Channel of Foot—*Yangming*.

Prescription: Zhongwan(RN12)   Zhangmen(LR13)
Pishu(BL20)   Weishu(BL21)
Zusanli(ST36)   Sifeng(EX—UE10)

Explanation: Zhongwan(RN12) is the Front—*Mu* point of the stomach; Zhangmen(LR13), the Front—*Mu* point of the spleen; Pishu(BL20), the Back—*Shu* point of the spleen;and Weishu (BL21), the Back—*Shu* point of the stomach. These four points in combination, known as the combining of the Back—*Shu* points and Front—*Mu* points, together with Zusanli(ST36), the inferior *He*—sea point of the stomach, have the effect to build up the spleen, replenish the *Qi* of the middle in order that the source for providing the acquired energy may flourish again. Abundant *Qi* of the middle—*Jiao* helps patient solve malnutrition. Sifeng(EX—UE10) has an excellent effect of removing food retention. It is held in traditional Chinese medicine that food retention due to poor digestion is the preliminary cause for infantile malnutrition. Food retention must be relieved in an attempt to treat infants for malnutrition. Therefore, Sifeng(EX—UE10) is used here to eliminate food retention for the purpose to treat malnutrition.

Point Modification: Add Xiawan(RN10), Tianshu(ST25) for abdominal distention and loose stools; Guanyuan(RN4) for cold limbs; and Shenmen(HT7) for disturbed sleep;

Method: Apply filiform needles with reinforcing method once a day. A shallow insertion is done without needling retention. Sifeng(EX—UE10) is pricked with a three—edged needle to cause discharge of a little bit of yellowish fluid of sticky quality by means of squeezing. Pricking is applied once every other day.

2. Parasitic Infection

Principle: Remove food retention and expel intestinal parasites by puncturing points mainly from The *Ren* Channel and The Stomach Channel of Foot—*Yangming*.

Prescription: Zhongwan(RN12)   Tianshu(ST25)
                     Zusanli(ST36)   Baicongwo(Extra)

Explanation: Zhongwan(RN12) and Tianshu(ST25) relieve food retention in the gastrointestinal system. Zusanli(ST36), the inferior *He*—sea point of the stomach channel, may build up the spleen and replenish the *Qi* of the middle—*Jiao* Baichongwo (EX—LE3) is an essential point for treating parasitosis.

Point Modifications Add Qihai(RN 6) for abdominal distention.

Method: Apply filiform needles with reducing method, which should be soon followed by reinforcing method without needling retention. The treatment is given once daily.

Alternative Treatment: Plum—blossom Needle Therapy

Prescription: Pishu(BL20)   Weishu(BL21)
                     Zusanli(ST36)   Sanjiaoshu(BL22)
                     Sifeng(EX—UE10)   Huatuojiaji(V7—V17)

Method: Apply plum—blossom needle tapping with moderate stimulation until local redness with moisture.

4.4   Infantile Convulsion

Infantile convulsion, also known as epileptic convulsion, is a disease often seen in infants. This disease may be caused by various factors or illnesses. Its main manifestations include convulsive limbs, neck rigidity, opisthotonos, or mental confusion in the severe cases. It ails children mostly under the age of five. The younger the child is, the higher incidence tends to be.

The onset of infantile convulsions may take place in any season. It is mainly caused by high fever, central nerve system disease, or metabolic dystrophy. as seen in case pneumonia, bacillary dysentery, cerebrititis, tetanus, etc. Since the onset can be either sudden or slow, and convulsion be either strong or weak, infantile convulsion is divided into deficiency, excess, cold and heat types. It is clinically divided into acute and chronic types.

4.4.1   Acute Infantile Convulsion

Cause and Mechanism

Physically, infants are not fully developed. Their defensive system against exogenous pathogenic invasion is weaker than that of adults, so are their internal *Zangf u* organs. They are also mentally weak in response to unexpected frightening. Therefore, infants can easily suffer from seasonal pathogenic invasions which may run into the interior of the body to form heat. Heat further transforms into fire. Excessive fire produces phlegm while extreme heat leads to internal disturbance of wind. Improper food intake may cause impairment of the spleen and stomach, and internal retention of turbid phlegm which may turn into heat gives rise to wind disturbance. Sudden fright or fear may simply disturb the mental state, leading to mental confusion. All the above factors may result in onset of infantile convulsion.

Differentiation

The acute type of infantile convulsion is characterized by a sudden onset, high fever, flushed face, restlessness, head shaking, excessive tongue movement, and somnolence with frequent fright. These are followed by mental confusion, upward staring, contraction of the limbs, neck rigidity, locked jaws and shortness of breath.

1. Seasonal Pathogenic Invasions

This type of acute infantile convuslion is accompanied by fever, headache, cough, congested throat, or nausea and vomiting, thin yellow tongue coating, and rapid superficial pulse.

2. Phlegm—Heat

This kind of infantile convulsion is accompanied by distending pain in the abdomen, vomiting, poor appetite, sputum gurgling in the throat, constipation, or bloody stool with stinking odour and pus, yellow greasy tongue coating, and wiry slippery pulse.

3. Sudden Fright

This kind of infantile convulsion is characterized by intermittent cyanotic or blushed complexions, cold limbs, disturbed sleep with frequent fright, cyanotic stool, and irregular rapid pulse.

Treatment

1. Seasonal Pathogenic Invasion

Principle: Eliminate wind and heat, bring back resuscitation and relieve convulsions by puncturing points mainly from The Liver Channel of Foot—*Jueyin*, The *Du* Channel and the twelve

Jing—well points.

Prescription: Dazhui(DU14)   Hegu(LI 4)

Taichong(LR 3)   Yanglingquan(GB34)

12 *Jing*—well points

Explanation: Dazhui (DU14), the converging point of the *Yang*, can promote the *Yang Qi* of the general body and expel the pathogenic factors from the superficial portion of the body. Hegu (LI 4) and Taichong (LR 3), respectively the *Yuan*—source points of the large intestine channel and the liver channel, are effective in combination to clear the mind and bring back resuscitation, sedate convulsion and quench the wind. This is a kind of method known as opening the four gates for the purpose to soothe the liver and quench the wind. Pricking the twelve *Jing*—well points can help to eliminate heat from the channels involved. YanglingQuan(GB34) is used to relax the tendons and stop convulsions.

Point Modification: Add Quchi(LI11) for high fever; and Neiguan(PC 6) for vomiting.

Method: Apply filiform needles with reducing method, but without needling retention. Dazhui(DU14) and the twelve *Jing*—well points are pricked with a three—edged needle to cause bleeding.

2. Phlegm—Heat

Principle: Clear away heat, eliminate phlegm, quench wind and bring back resusciation by puncturing points mainly from The *Ren* Channel, The *Du* Channel, The Stomach Channel of Foot—*Yangming* and The Liver Channel of Foot—*Jueyin*.

Prescription: Shuigou(DU26)   Zhongwan(RN12)

Fenglong(ST40)   Daling(PC 7)

Taichong(LR 3)

Explanation: Shuigou(DU26), a point of the *Du* Channel communicating with the brain, is used to promote resuscitation. Zhongwan(RN12) and Fenglong(ST40) can remove stagnant *Qi* and resolve phlegm. Daling(PC 7) clears away heat from the heart so as to calm the mind. Taichong(LR 3), the *Yuan*—source point of the liver channel, is used to soothe the liver and quench the wind.

Point Modification: Add Jiache(ST 6) and Hegu(LI 4) for locked jaws; and Tianshu(ST25) for abdominal pain.

Method: Apply filiform needles with reducing method, but without needling retention.

3. Sudden Fright

Principle: Relieve convulsions and calm the mind by puncturing points mainly from The *Du* Channel, The Heart Channel of Hand—*Shaoyin* and The Kidney Channel of Foot—*Shaoyin*.

Prescription: Yintang(EX—HN2) Shenmen(HT 7)
                 Taixi(KI 3) Taichong(LR 3)

Explanation: Yintang(EX—HN2) is effective to relieve convulsions. Shenmen(HT 7), the *Yuan*—source point of the heart channel, can reinforce the heart *Qi* and calm the mind. The combination of Taixi (KI 3), the *Yuan*—source point of the kidney channel, and Taichong(LR 3), the *Yuan*—source point of the liver Channel, may regulate the liver, nourish blood, moisten *Yin* and sedate the hyperactive *Yang*. The harmony between *Yin* and *Yang* makes for sound sleep and spontaneous calm from convulsions.

Point Modification: Add Luxi(SJ19) for protracted convulsions; and Shuigou(DU26) for continuous soporous state.

Method: Apply filiform needles with reducing method, but without needling retention.

Alternative Treatment: Auricular Acupuncture

Prescription: Ear—Shenmen sympathetic Brain Stem Heart
Subcortex

Method: Apply filiform needles with strong stimulation. The needles are retained for 30 minutes with needling manipulation done every ten minutes.

4.4.2 Chronic Infantile Convulsion

Cause and Mechanism

Chronic infantile convulsion is mostly seen after severe disease or lingering illness. Constitutional deficiency of the spleen and stomach may lead to a poor source for providing the acquired energy. Subsequent kidney *Yin* deficiency and liver blood insufficiency may result in internal wind disturbance. Nevertheless, acute infantile convulsion if treated improperly or inadequately may develop into the chronic type.

Differentiation

Chronic infantile convulsion is marked by a slow onset with occasional convulsions, pallor complexion, emaciation, listlessness, disturbed sleep with eyes opened, and cold limbs. Chronic convulsion involving spleen and stomach deficinecy is accompanied by loose stool of greenish colour, occasional borborygmus, pale tongue proper with white coating, and deep weak thready pulse. Chronic convulsion involving *Yin* deficiency of the liver and kidney is accompanied by restlessness due to deficient heat, tidal fever, peeled tongue coating with slight coating on the edge of the tongue. and rapid thready pulse.

Treatment

Principle: Reinforce the spleen and kidney with a secondary principle of treatment to quench the liver wind by puncturing points mainly from The *Du* Channel and The Stomach Channel of Foot—*Yangming*, plus some Back—*Shu* points.

Prescription: Pishu(BL20)   Weishu(BL21) Shenshu(BL23)
Qihai(RN 6)   Zusanli(ST36)
Taichong(LR 3)   Baihui(DU20)

Explanation: Pishu(BL20), Weishu(BL21) and Shenshu (BL23), respectively the Back—*Shu* points of the spleen, stomach and kidney, are able to tonify the spleen and kidney. Qihai(RN6) builds up the premordial *Qi* so as to strengthen the spleen in transforming. Zusanli(ST36), the inferior *He*—sea point of the stomach channel, is the essential point for strengthening the spleen and stomach, the source for providing the acquired energy. Taichong(LR3) is effective for soothing liver *Yin*, tonify blood, quench wind and sedate convulsions. Baihui(DU20) has the function to elevate the spleen *Yang* and clear away the wind.

Point Modification: Add Tianshu(ST25) for loose stools.

Method: Apply filiform needles with reinforcing method, but without needling retontion, once daily. Moxibustion is also applicable for 20—30 minutes after needling.

Alternative Treatment: Auricular Acupuncture

Prescription: Ear—Shenmen Sympathetic Kidney Spleen
Stomach Liver Brain Stem Subcortex

Method: Apply filiform needles at 3—4 points each time with moderate stimulation. Bilateral ear points are used alternately, and treatment is given once daily. Embedding of ear seeds either independently or in combination with needling is applicable. However,the combined approach improves the therapeutic effects.

4.5 Infantile *Wei* Syndrome

Infantile *Wei* syndrome, also known as infantile paralysis, is a kind of acute infectious disease caused by the invasion of seasonal epidemics. Its incipient manifestations are similar to those of common cold such as fever, headache, and congestion in the throat. These may be accompanied by cough, nausea, vomiting, diarrhea and general muscle pain. The incipient symptoms and signs are then followed by muscular flaccidity, acroparalysis, myophagism and dyscinesia. It mostly affects the unilateral lower limb in children predominantly under the age of five. The incidence of infantile paralysis is high in summer and autumn, similar to the sequela of poliomyelitis in modern medicine.

Cause and Mechanism

The pathogenic heat as the seasonal epidemics initially invades the lung and stomach, causing over—consumption of lung fluid and derangement of stomach *Qi* in descent. This is then followed by the retained damp—heat steaming the *Yangming* channel. The flowing of pathogenic damp—heat in the channels causes derangement of *Qi* and blood circulation and poor nourishment of vessels and tendons. Hence, the lingering looseness of tendons fails to control bones, muscles and joints, gradually developing into the *Wei* syndrome.

Differentiation

The affected infants suffer from weakness of the general body, pallor or sallow complexion, and unilateral paralysis of the body especially affecting the lower limb. A small number of mild cases may gradually have a complete recovery within three months, while the majority seem to develop muscular atrophy, flaccidity and weakness with motor impairment, or even articular deformation in severe cases.

Treatment

Principle: Nourish the blood and remove obstruction from channels and collaterals by puncturing points mainly from The Large Intestine Channel of Hand—*Yangming* and The Stomach Channel of Foot—*Yangming*.

Prescription: (1)Upper Limb Paralysis

Jianyu(LI15) Quchi(LI11)

Shousanli(LI10) Hegu(LI 4)

(2)Lower Limb Paralysis

Huantiao(GB30) Biguan(ST 31)

Futu(ST32) Zusanli(ST36)

Yanglingquan(GB34) Sanyinjiao(SP 6)

Explanation: Jianyu(LI15), Quchi(LI11), Shousanli(LI10) and Hegu(LI 4) are used to regulate the *Qi* circulation of the large intestine channel. This is done according to the principle of selecting points only from the *Yangming* channels in the treatment of a *Wei* syndrome, attempting to nourish the blood and promote its circulation. Biguan(ST31), Futu(ST32), Zusanli (ST36) are selected according to the same priniciple to enhance the function of nourishing the tendons and bones. Huantiao(GB30) is added to regulate the *Qi* circulation of the Gallbladder Channel of Foot—*Shaoyang*. Yanglingquan(GB34), the Influential point of the tendons, is added to promote the flexible movement of the tendons. Sanyinjiao(SP 6), the point at which the three *Yin* channels of the foot intersect, has the effect to nourish blood and promote its circulation. The combination of these points may reinforce *Qi*, nourish blood and marrow, and strengthen the tendons and muscles in order to cure the *Wei* syndrome.

Point Modification: Add Waiguan (SJ 5) and Zhongquan (Extra) for wrist-drop; Jiexi (ST41) for foot drop; Xuanzhong (GB39) for adduction; and Zhaohai (KI6) for abduction.

Method: Apply filiform needles with reinforcing method and retain the needles for 15-20 minutes, once daily. Moxibustion is also applicable.

4.6 Enuresis

Enuresis, also known as bed-wetting, refers to the involuntary discharge of urine during sleep in children over three years old. Such children are not aware of the bed-wetting unless they are woked up. It is usually related to fatigue or mental stress. However, bed-wetting due to excessive drinking of water on occasions is not considered as a disease condition.

Cause and Mechanism

The kidney, the origin of congenital essence, opens physiologically into both the reproductive organ and the anus, and dominates bowel movement and urination. Through its channel, the kidney forms an internal-external relationship with the urinary bladder. If an infant has kidney *Qi* deficiency, the function of the lower-*Jiao* will not be well consolidated with which the urinary bladder fails to restrain the urinary discharge, leading to enuresis when the water passage is in poor control. *Qi* deficiency of the lung and kidney may also cause enuresis because the deficiency of the upper organs may not function well in restraining the lower ones so that the urinary bladder also loses its control over urination.

Differentiation

1. Deficiency of Kidney *Yang*

Frequent discharge of profuse urine, the infant is unaware, occurs during sleep, ranging from once to several times a night. The accompanying symptoms and signs include general lassitude, pallor complexion, weakness in the lower limbs, aversion to cold with desire for warmth, clear dilute urine, pale tongue proper, and deep feeble pulse.

2. *Qi* Deficiency of the Spleen and Lung

Frequeut involuntary discharge of small amounts of urine also takes place at night during sleep. It is accompanied by lassitude, *Qi* deficiency with reluctant speech, sallow complexion, poor appetite, loose stools, pale tongue, and thready weak pulse.

Treatment

1. Deficiency of Kidney *Yang*

Principle: Warm up kidney *Yang* and consolidate urinary discharge by using points mainly from The *Ren* Channel and some Back—*Shu* points.

Prescription: Guanyuan(RN 4) Zhongji(RN 3)
             Shenshu(BL23) Pangguangshu(BL28)
             Taixi(KI 3)

Explanation: Guanyuan(RN4), Shenshu(BL23) and Taixi(KI3) are selected to reinforce the kidney *Qi* and consolidate the lower—*Jiao* function. Zhongji(RN3) and Pangguangshu (BL28), respectively the Front—*Mu* and Back—*Shu* points of the urinary bladder, known as the combination of Back—*Shu* point and Front—*Mu* point, are used to enhance the function of the urinary bladder to control urinary discharge.

Point Modification: Add Baihui(DU20) for frequent urination.

Method: Apply filiform needles with reinforcing method and retain the needles for 15—20 minutes, once daily. Moxibustion is also applicable.

2. *Qi* Deficiency of the Spleen and Lung

Prinicple: Strengthen the spleen and lung, and consolidate the urinary bladder in discharging urine by using points mainly from The *Ren* Channel, The Lung Channel of Hand—*Taiyin,* The Spleen Channel of Foot—*Taiyin* and The Stomach Channel of Foot—*Yangming*.

Prescription: Baihui(DU20) Qihai(RN 6)

Taiyuan(LU 9) Sanyinjiao(SP 6)

Zusanli(ST36)

Explanation: Baihui(DU20) and Qihai(RN 6) are used to elevate the *Yang Qi*. Taiyuan(LU 9) can reinforce the lung *Qi*. Zusanli(ST36) strengthens the *Qi* of the spleen. Sanyinjiao (SP 6), the point intersecting the three *Yin* channels of the foot, is used to regulate and tonify the spleen and kidney. The joint use of these points may help ascend the spleen *Qi*, descend the lung *Qi* so as to maintain the function of the urinary bladder in controlling the urinary discharge.

Point Modification: Add Pishu(BL20) for loose stool.

Method: Apply filiform needles with reinforcing method and retain the needles for 15—20 minutes, once daily. Moxibustion is also applicable at Baihui(DU20), Qihai(RN 6), Zusanli(ST36), Sanyinjiao(SP 6) and Pishu(BL20) for 20—30 minutes.

Alternative Treatment:

(1)Auricular Acupuncture

Prescription: Kidney   Urinary bladder   Spleen   Brain
Stem   Lung   Subcortex   Urethra   Margin
Centre

Method: Apply filiform needles at 2—3 points each time with moderate stimulation, and retain the needles for 20 minutes, once daily. Embedding of ear seeds is also applieable.

(2)Scalp Acupuncture

Prescription: Bilateral sensorimotor area of the foot

Method: Apply filiform needles with intermittent stimulation for 15 minutes. The treatment is given once daily.

4.7   Mumps

Mumps is an acute infections disease caused by invasion of exogenous pathogenic wind—heat. Clinically, it is characterized by fever, pain and swelling in the parotid region. It occurs all year around with higher incidence in children between five to nine years old, particularly in the spring time. The prognosis of this disease is often favourable. It is referred to as epidemic parotitis in modern medicine.

Cause and Mechanism

The onset of mumps is mainly due to invasion of exogenous pathogenic wind—heat into the *Shaoyang* channels. The deranged *Qi* mechanism of the *Shaoyang* channels with impaired circulation of *Qi* and blood causes pain and swelling in the parotid region, fever with aversion to cold. The *Shaoyang* channels and the *Jueyin* channels are internally—externally related channels. The Liver Channel of Foot—*Jueyin* curves around the pubic region. Extreme heat descending along this particular channel may result in swelling and pain in the testis. However, there will be high fever, convulsion and coma provided that the pathogenic heat runs into the pericardium along The Pericardium Channel of Hand—*Jueyin* to disturb the mind.

Differentiation

1. Exogenous Pathogenic Heat Invading the Exterior

Neither swelling, nor pain appears severe in the parotid region, nor the swelling feels hard by pressing. The mumps affects normal chewing. It is accompanied by slight fever with aversion to cold, general discomfort, slight yellowish tongue coating, and rapid superficial pulse.

2. Pathogenic Heat Accumulation

Both feverish sensation and pain appear in the parotid region with mass aggravated by pressing, and with difficult chewing. It is accompanied by high fever, headache, restlessness, thirst or vomiting, constipation, reduced output of straw urine, or even pain and swelling in the testis, mental confusion with syncope, red tongue proper with yellow coating, and rapid superficial pulse.

Treatment

1. Exogenous Pathogenic Heat Invading the Exterior

Principle: Relieve the exogenous pathogenic wind from the superficial portion of the body by puncturing points mainly from The *SanJiao* Channel of Hand—*Shaoyang* and The Large Intestine Channel of Hand—*Yangming*.

Prescription: Yifeng(SJ17) Jiache(ST 6)

Waiguan(SJ 5) Hegu(LI 4)

Explanation: It is imperative to eliminate the exogenous pathogenic wind—heat from The *Sanjiao* Channel of Hand—*Shaoyang* because part of its distribution passes through the parotid region. Yifeng(SJ17), the converging point of the *Shaoyang* channels of both the hand and the foot, is used to disperse the stagnant *Qi* and blood in the local area. Jiache(ST 6) and Hegu(LI 4) are also applied to eliminate the pathogenic heat since the distribution of the *Yangming* channels of both foot and hand passes through the facial area. Waiguan(SJ 5), having the effect to promote the *Qi* circulation of The *Sanjiao* channel of Hand −*Shaoyang,* is applied to assist clearing up the heat and resolving the swelling.

Point Modification: Add Dazhui(DU14)for severe fever.

Method: Apply filiform needle−reducing once daily without needle retention. Dazhui(DU14) may be pricked with a three−edged needle to cause bleeding.

2. Pathogenic Heat Accumulation

Principle: Eliminate pathogenic heat, remove channel obstruction and relieve swelling by puncturing points mainly from The *Sanjiao* Channel of Hand−*Shaoyang* and The Large Intestine Channel of Hand−*Yangming*.

Prescription: Zhigou(SJ 6) Quchi(LI11)

Hegu(LI 4) Shaoshang(LU11)

Fenglong(ST40) Guanchong(SJ 1)

Explanation: Zhigou(SJ6) and Guanchong(SJ1), having the effect of promoting the circulation of *Qi* of the *Sanjiao* are used to function in clearing away heat and relieving swelling. Quchi (LI11) and Hegu (LI4), points of the large intestine channel, are used to eliminate heat in combination with Shaoshang(LU11). Fenglong(ST40), the *Luo*−connecting point of the stomach channel, is treated to reduce the phlegm−fire, relieve swelling and pain.

Point Modification: Add Dazhui(DU14) and the twelve *Jing*—well points for high fever; Taichong(LR 3) and Ququan (LR 8) for swelling and painful testis; Fengchi(GB20) for headache; and Shuigou (DU26) for convulsion with mental confusion.

Method: Apply filiform—needle reducing once daily without needle retention.Dazhui(DU14) and the twelve *Jing*—well. points may be pricked with a three—edged needle to cause bleeding.

Alternative Treatment

1. Auricular Acupuncture

Prescription: Ear apex Ear—Shenmen Cheek Parotid region Helix 4—6

Method: Apply filiform needles once daily at 2—3 points each time with strong stimulation. Embedding of ear seeds is also applicable.

2. Rush Pith Heating

Prescription: Jiaosun (SJ20)

Method: Ignite a piece of rush pith immersed with sesame oil, and hold it closer to Jiaosun (SJ20) to heat the point area. Withdraw the burning rush pith immediately when a cracking sound is heard. Do the rush pith heating for 1—2 times each treatment. If swelling should remain, repeat the same treatment the next day.

4.8 Scarlet Fever

Scarlet fever, a term in modern medicine, is called the red rash in traditional Chinese medicine, referring to a kind of seasonal epidemic invasion into the nose and throat. Clinically, it is characterized by fever, swelling, sore throat, diffusing scarlet erythema of the general body, and subsequent casting off of the scaled skin. It usually occurs in winter and spring with high incidence in children aged from twe to eight years old.

Cause and Mechanism

The seasonal epidemic invasion affects the lung and stomach through the mouth and nose and transforms into fire steaming the fluid of the lung and stomach, and then attacking the throat. Therefore, the incipient manifestations include fever with aversion to cold and sore throat. Such a kind of pathogenic heat causes scarlet eruptions if it permeates to the superficial portion of the body. Yet, it may cause convulsions with mental confusion if it internally disturbs the heart and liver.

Differentiation

1. Seasonal Epidemics Invading the Lung and Stomach

There is a sudden onset of fever, headache, aversion to cold and sore throat, accompanied by nausea, vomiting, flushed skin, red tongue proper with thin yellow coating, and rapid superficial pulse forceful pulse.

2. Pathogenic Heat Affecting the Nutrient and Blood Systems

The strong fever remains high. The accompanying symptoms and signs include flushed face, thirst, pallor lips, sore throat with oral ulceration, dense skin rash in fresh red colour or in purplish colour with spreading spots. The skin eruption starts from the neck and chest and extends all over the body. The tongue proper is red with thorny substance like strawberries, and the pulse is rapid and forceful.

Treatment

1. Seasonal Epidemics Invading the Lung and Stomach

Principle: Promote the dispersing function of the lung, re-lieve the superficial heat and clear the throat by puncturing points mainly from The Lung Channel of Hand—*Taiyin* and The Large Intestine Channel of Hand—*Yangming*.

Prescription: Fengchi(GB20)   Quchi(LI11)
                Hegu(LI 4)   Lieque(LU 7)
                Dazhui(DU14)   Guanchong(SJ 1)

Explanation: Fengchi (GB20), Quchi (LI11), Hegu (LI 4) are selected to eliminate the wind—heat. Lieque (LU7), the *Luo*—con—necting point of the lung channel, has the effect to eliminate lung heat, clear the throat, disperse wind and activate the circulation of *Qi* and blood in the channels and collaterals. Guanchong (SJ 1) clears away the heat from the *Sanjiao* Dazhui (DU14) relieves the superficial wind—heat and promotes the func-tion of the nutrient and blood systems. The combination of these points may promote the dispersing function of the lung, relieve superficial heat, and clear the throat.

Point Modification: Add Neiguan(PC 6) for vomiting and nausea.

Method: Apply filiform—needle reducing once daily without needle retention. Dazhui(DU14) and Guanchong (SJ 1) are pricked with a three—edged needle to cause bleeding.

Alternative Treatment: Auricular Acupuncture

Prescription: Ear—Shenmen Lung Stomach Ear Apex Spleen

Method: Apply filiform needles with moderately strong stimulation, but without needling retention. Embedding of ear seeds is also applicable.

4.9 Dementia

Infantile dementia pertains to the extent of the five types of late development (late standing, late walking, late growth of hair, late growth of teeth and late speech) and the five softnesses (soft head, soft neck, soft limbs, soft muscles and soft teeth) in traditional Chinese medicine. Clinically, it is characterized by retarded growth and intellegence, similar to congenital maldevelopment of the brain in modern medicine.

Cause and Mechanism

Dementia is mainly due to either congenital deficiency or acquired malnutrition, resulting in the insufficiency of vital essence which fails to nourish the brain.

Differentiation

The growth and development of infants suffering from dementia are apparently slower than those of normal children. This may be clinically manifested by their inability to conduct speech at the age of two or three, poor intelligence, dull expression with staring vision and slow response. It is accompanied by softness of body, soft tendons and bones, weak limbs with difficulty in standing or walking.

Treatment

Principle: Reinforce liver and kidney, nourish the essence and blood and promote the intelligence by using points mainly from The *Du* Channel.

Prescription: Baihui(DU20)   Sishencong(EX−HN1)
Dazhui(DU14)   Fengchi(GB20)
Fenfu(DU16)   Shuigou(DU26)
Xinshu(BL15)   Neiguan(PC 6)

Sanyinjiao(SP 6) Zhaohai(KI 6)
Shenmai(BL62)

Explanation: Baihui(DU20) and Sishencong (Extra) are selected to replenish *Qi* to the brain, calm the mind and promte the intelligance. Dazhui(DU14), Fengfu(DU16). Fengchi(GB20) and Shuigou(DU26)promote the *Qi* circulation of all the *Yang* channels so as to activate the development of the intelligence. Xinshu (BL15), Neiguan (PC 6) and Sanyinjiao (SP 6) clear away the obstruction from the upper–*Jiao* and moisten the lower–*Jiao* invigorate heart *Yang,* reinforce heart *Yin* and clam the heart and mind. Shenmai (BL62) and Zhaohai (KI 6) reinforce the liver and kidney, replenish marrow and refill the vital essence.

Method: Apply filiform needles with reinforcing method and retain the needles for 20–30 minutes, once daily. Moxibustion is also applicable to Xinshu(BL15), Shenmai(BL62) and Zhaohai(KI6) for 30 minutes, once daily or once every other day.

Alternative Treatment: Embedding of Ear Seeds

Prescription: Ear–Shenmen Hear Kidney Brain
Stem Liver Spleen

Method: Embed two to three ear points each time alternately on both ears. Change the embedded seeds every three days.

5 Diseases of Eyes, Ears, Nose and Throat

5.1 Myopia

Myopia, an ametropic condition in ophthalmology, is mainly characterized by the fact that the eyes can see near objects but not distant ones although there is no obvious abnormality with the outer eyes. Such a condition often bothers youngsters.

Cause and Mechanism

Myopia is mostly due to continuous reading or writing for hours at close distance, dim light, incorrect posture in reading or writing, congenital deficiency or inherent factors. The liver has its opening into the eyes and human eyes can see when they are nourished by the blood. *Yin* deficiency of liver and kidney, deficiency of both *Qi* and blood, or impaired blood circulation caused by protracted fatigue of vision may all result in a near–sighted condition.

Differentiation

Clear vision for near objects but blurred vision for distant ones which may be accompanied by dizziness, tinnitus, insomnia with dream–disturbed sleep, soreness and weakness of knees and lumbus, pallor complexion, palpitation, lassitude, pale tongue proper, and weak thready pulse.

Treatment

Principle: Nourish liver and kidney, reinforce *Qi* and promote vision.

Prescription: Chengqi(ST 1) Jingming(GB1)

Fengchi(GB20) Guangming(GB37)

Ganshu(BL18) Shenshu(BL23)

Explanation: Chengqi(ST1) and Jingming(BL1), commonly used points for eye disorders, have the effect to quench liver fire and brighten the eyes. Fengchi(GB20), a coalescent point of The Gall Bladder Channel of Foot-*Shaoyang* and The *Yangwei* Channel, has the function to nourish blood and brighten the eyes. Guangming(GB37), the *Luo*-connecting point of The Gall Bladder Channel of Foot-*Shaoyang*, helps to remove obstruction from the affected channel and to brighten the eyes. Ganshu(BL18) and Shenshu(BL23) nourish the liver and kidney, promote *Qi* circulation and brighten the eyes.

Point Modifications: Add Sanyinjiao(SP6) and Zusanli (ST36) if deficiency of spleen and stomach is also involved.

Method: Apply filiform needles with even method. For points proximal to the eyes, needles should be gently inserted and thrusted. A rapid withdrawl of needle is performed when it is lifted to the subcutaneous layer, which is then followed by pressing of the point with a piece of cotton ball for about a minute. Fengchi(GB20), Guangming(GB37), Ganshu(BL18) and Shenshu(BL23) may be manipulated by intermittent thrusting and rotating of the needles. Treatment is given once a day and needles are retained for 15–20 minutes.

Alternative Treatment: Auricular Acupuncture

Prescription: Ear-shenmen Sympathetic Eye Eye1

Eye2 Liver Kidney

Method: Apply filiform needles to two to three auricular points with moderate stimulation. Treatment is given once every other day. Needles are retained for 30 minutes. Embedding of ear seeds is also applicable to the above points alternately on the two ears. The embedded seeds are renewed every three to five days.

5.2 Conjunctivitis

Conjunctivitis by Chinese convention is referred to as "wind—heat eye" or "pink—eye disease". It is characterized by redness and swelling in the palpebral, hyperemia of bulbar conjunctiva and profuse lacrimation. It is also marked by a rapid onset and epidemical nature. TCM concept of conjunctivitis may broadly include acute conjunctivitis and acute contagious corneo—conjunctivitis in modern medicine.

Cause and Mechanism

Conjunctivitis is mostly caused by invasion of wind—heat into the eye, giving rise to local wind—heat affection, or by upward disturbance of excessive fire in the liver and gallbladder along the respected channels to create a combinational affection with the exogenous wind—heat.

Differentiation

The main manifestations are swelling and pain in the eyelids, hyperemia of bulbar conjunctiva, photophobia and lacrimation with sticky discharge. The condition is mostly caused by wind—heat invasion if the patient also develops fever, aversion to wind together with a rapid pulse. It is mostly caused by excessive fire in the liver and gallbladder if the accompanying symptoms also include a bitter taste in the mouth, dysphoria, dizziness, red tongue proper with yellow coating, and a rapid wiry pulse.

Treatment

Principle: Eliminate wind—heat, relieve swelling and ease

pain by selecting points mainly from The Large Intestine Channel of Hand—*Yangming* and The Liver Channel of Foot—*Jueyin*.

Precription: Xingjian(LR 2) Hegu(LI 4)
Quchi(LI11) Taiyang(EX—HN5)
Shaoshang(LU11) Shangxing(DU23)
Fengchi(GB20) Xiaxi(GB43)

Explanation: The Liver opens into the eye. The *Yangming*, *Taiyang* and *Shaoyang* channels of the foot and hand have part of their course distributions around the eye region. Xingjian (LR 2), the *Xing*—spring point of the channel, has the function relieve blood stasis, promote *Qi* circulation and reduce swelling. It may also clear up the excessive heat from the liver and gallbladder. Hegu(LI4), the *Yuan*—source point of the channel, posesses the function of opening and dispersing. In combination with Quchi(LI11) it eliminates heat, being highly effective in clearing up the heat from the upper—*Jiao* This point is generally suggested for treating such conditions involving the sense organs. Taiyang(EX—HN5) is pricked to cause bleeding in order to eliminate heat, relieve swelling and alleviate pain. Shaoshang(LU11) and Shangxing(DU23) are used to eliminate exogenous wind—heat in the case that the condition is caused by invasion of exogenous wind—heat. Fengchi(GB20) and Xiaxi(GB43) are used to reduce excessive heat in the liver and gallbladder, particularly in guiding the heat to descend.

Point Modifications: Add Yintang(EX—HN3) for headache.

Method: Use filiform needles with reducing method. Needles may be retained for 15—20 minutes or removed simply without retention. If needling retention is intended, manipulate the needles every five minutes. Taiyang (Extra) and Shaoshang (LU11) are pricked to cause a little bit of bleeding.

Alternative Treatment: Auricular Acupuncture

Prescription: Eye   Eye 1   Eye 2 and Liver

Method: Use filiform needles with strong stimulation and manipulate the needles intermittently. Pricking may also applied to Erjian or the small veins on the dorsum of the ear.

5.3   Colour Blindness

Colour blindness is a condition of colour anomalopia. Patients who suffer from it can only identify the brightness and shape of the objects seen, but fail to tell the actual colour traits. Those who distinguish colours poorly are identified as colour weakness. Colour blindness, mostly complained of by males, is mainly related to congenital factors.

Cause and Mechanism

Factors such as congenital defect, *Yin* deficiency of liver and kidney, decline of vital energy, or derangement of *Qi* and blood in the channel portions around the eye chiefly ascribe to colour blindness, resulting in an inability to read colours.

Differentiation

There is no abnormal sign in the physical eye, but normal vision in most cases. The victims are unable to differentiate certain colour upon the objects they see, e.g. mistaking red for white, or yellow for green. Some of them may even only identify black and white. Colour blindness as a kind of physical defect that the sufferer is not aware of but is detected by examinations.

Treatment

Principle: Tonify the liver and kidney by selecting points mainly from The Urinary Bladder Channel of Foot–*Taiyang*,

The Liver Channel of Foot—*Jueyin* and The Kidney Channel of Foot—*Shaoyin*.

Prescription: Jingming(BL 1) Zanzhu(BL 2)

Fengchi(GB20) Ganshu(BL18)

Shenshu(BL23) Xingjian(LR 2)

Taixi(KI 3)

Explanation: Jingming (BL 1) and Zanzhu (BL 2), having the function of removing obstruction from the channels and collaterals, are the main points for treating eye diseases. Fengchi (GB20) clears the head and brightens the eye. This point also promotes the function of the five sense organs. Ganshu (BL18) soothes the liver and improves the eye sight. Shenshu (BL23) replenishes the vital energy of the kidney to nourish the eye. Xingjian (LR2) and Taixi (KI3) tonify the liver and kidney and nourish the eye.

Method: Use filiform needles with reinforcing method. A small amplitude of needle twisting, and slow inserting is strictly observed when puncturing the points around the eye region. Needles are retained for 15—20 minutes while the treatment is given once daily or once every other day.

Alternative Treatment: Auricular Acupuncture

Prescription: Eye 1 Eye 2 Eye Liver and Kidney

Method: Use filiform needles with mild stimulation. Retain the needles for 15—20 minutes, and treatment is given once a day. The embedding of ear seeds is also applicable.

5.4 Strabismus

Strabismus, also known as wind—deviated vision, is characterized by squinting, limited movement of the eyeball, inability for both eyes to see simultaneously the objects directly in front. The main cause of this condition is pathogenic wind atacking the channels and collaterals, similar to paralytic strabismus in modern medicine.

Cause and Mechanism

Strabismus may be due to disharmony between spleen and stomach, and collateral deficiency so that pathogenic wind invades into the eye region, resulting in local muscular spasm; or due to *Yin* deficiency of liver and kidney and subsequent insufficiency of essence and blood resulting in malnutrition of the ocular connectors.

Differentiation

One pupil or both turn abruptly towards either the inner or outer canthus with limited eye movement, double vision, ptosis, or deviation of the eye and mouth. It is considered as wind disturbing the channels if fever, headache, nausea and vomiting, white tongue coating and floating pulse also present. However, those accompanying symptoms such as dizziness, tinnitus, blurred vision, pale tongue proper and thready pulse account for *Yin* deficiency of liver and kidney.

Treatment

Principle: Eliminate wind from the affected channels and collaterals, and tonify liver and kidney by selecting points mainly from The Liver Channel of Foot—*Jueyin,* The Large Intestine Channel of Hand—*Yangming* and The Stomach Channel of Foot—*Yangming* plus some of the Back—*Shu* points.

Prescription: Sibai(ST 2) Hegu(LI 4)
                  Fengchi(GB20) Ganshu(BL18)
                  Shenshu(BL23) Zusanli(ST36)

Explanation: Sibai (ST2) is used to activate the channels and collaterals, regulate *Qi* and blood in circulation and balance *Yin* and *Yang*. Hegu (LI 4) and Fengchi (GB20) are good for clearing up pathogenic wind in the head and facial region, especially in the treatment of disorders of the five sense organs. Ganshu (BL18), Shenshu (BL23) and Zusanli (ST36) reinforce *Qi* and blood, and tonify the liver and kidney.

Point Modifications: Add Taiyang (Extra) and Tongziliao (GB1) for medial strabismus; and Jingming (BL1) and Zanzhu (BL2) for lateral strabismus.

Method: Apply filiform needles with reinforcing method. Treatment is given once a day and needles are retained for 15–20 minutes.

Alternative Treatment: Auricular Acupuncture

Prescription: Liver   Kidney   Eye 1   Eye 2

Ear seeds are implanted alternately every three days.

5.5   Stye

Stye is the inflammatory furuncle of the sebaceous gland of the eyelid. It is susceptible to becoming diabrotic, yet, an instant cure can be brought about by pricking. Since stye takes after wheat seed, it is also known as hordeolum. Such a kind of inflammation, mostly among youngsters, more often occurs in the upper eyelid.

Cause and Mechanism

Stye in many cases is the consequence of upward attack of dampheat from spleen and stomach resulted from a hot spicy diet, or due to stagnation of *Qi* and blood in the eye region caused by exogenous invasion of pathogenic wind—heat in which accumulate.

Differentiation

The onset of stye is characterized by a mild itching and subsequent local induration, redness, swelling and increasing pain. Purulent absess of a whitish yellow colour will appear in a few days. The symptoms of stye will subside promptly when the abscess is broken or relieved. The accompanying symptoms may include a bad odour in the mouth, restlessness, constipation, yellow greasy tongue coating, and soft rapid pulse if it is caused by damp—heat from the spleen and stomach. Such accompanying symptoms as aversion to cold, fever, headache, thin tongue coating and superficial rapid pulse indicate an invasion of exogenous pathogenic wind—heat.

Treatment

Principle: Eliminate pathogenic wind—heat by selecting points mainly from The Large Intestine Channel of Hand—*Yangming,* The Stomach Channel of Foot—*Yangming* and The Urinary Bladder Channel of Foot—*Taiyang.*

Prescription: Hegu(LI 4) Quchi(LI11)

Zhongchong(PC 9) Taiyang(EX—HN5)

Chize(LU 5) optional for damp—heat

in spleen and stomach;

Dazhui(DU14) and Xingjian(LR 2) optional

for exogenous wind—heat invasion.

Explanation: Hegu (LI 4) has a lifting and dispersing function. Quchi (LI11) functions in dispe ling blood—heat. Hegu (LI 4) in combination with Quchi (LI11) eliminates the wind—heat from facial area. Zhongchong (PC 9), *Jing*—river point of The Pericardium Channel of Hand—*Jueyin,* sedates the heart–fire since it is generally believed that the numerous types of furuncles and ulcerations are related to heart in TCM perception. Taiyang (EX–HN5) subdues the swelling and alleviate pain. Chize (LU 5) clears up blood heat. Dazhui (DU14) eliminates pathogenic wind–heat. Xingjian helps to dispel pathogenic heat and relieve stagnation of blood from channels and collaterals.

Point Modifications:

Add Fengchi (GB20) for head, and Zhaohai (KI6) for conjunctival congestion, swelling and pain.

Method: Use filiform needles with reducing method and retain the needles for 15–20 minutes. Treatment is given once daily.

Alternative Treatment: Auricular Acupuncture

Prescription: Eye Liver Spleen and Ear apex

Method: Use filiform needles with strong stimulation once daily. Retain the needles for 20 minutes. Pricking at Erjian is applicable. Embedding of ear seeds may also be used alternately every three days on either ear.

5.6   Ptosis

Ptosis, characterized by a disabled or incomplete elevating of the upper eyelid, can be ascribed to a number of factors. Normal vision is affected as part of or the whole pupil is covered.

Cause and Mechanism

Congenital deficiency and decline of the vital gate fire losens the eyelid and weakens its normal lifting. Stagnant Qi circulation in the channels and collaterals and malnourished tendons and vessels due to exogenous pathogenic wind invasion accounts for another factor of ptosis. Nevertheless, malnourshed Qi, blood, tendons and muscles due to deficient heat in the spleen and stomach may also result in ptosis.

Differentiation

Ptosis related to congenital deficiency is characterized by the drop of upper eyelids from childhood, a difficulty in lifting the eyelids, and tilting the head when watching objects. Frowning or wrinkling is often accompanied by some other abnormal signs in the eye region or a more extended facial area. Ptosis that occurred abruptly with limited movement of the eyeball or with double vision is caused by invasion of exogenous pathogenic wind. Ptosis as a result of weakened *Qi* of the middle–*Jiao* and malnourished *Qi* and blood due to deficient spleen and stomach is often better in the morning and worse in the afternoon. Such a kind of ptosis, often accompanied by general lassitude and poor energy, is also better with due repose but worse with stress.

Treatment

Principle: Eliminate wind from channels and collaterals and elevate *Yang Qi* by selecting points mainly from The Stomach Channel of Foot–*Yangming*, The Spleen Channel of Foot–*Jueyin* and The Kidney Channel of Foot–*Shaoyin*.

Prescription: Yangbai(GB14) Zanzhu(BL 2)
      Sizhukong(SJ23) Shenmai(BL62)
      Zhaohai(KI 6) Hegu(LI 4)

Fengchi (GB20) and Waiguan (SJ5) optional for impairment of channels and collaterals by exogenous pathogenic wind; and Zusanli (ST36) and Sanyinjiao (SP6) optional for deficiency of *Qi* of the middle–*Jiao* and malnourished *Qi* and blood.

Explanation: Yangbai (GB14), Zanzhu (BL2) and Sizhukong (SJ23) are local points for regulating *Qi* and blood in the eye region. Shenmai (BL62) promotes *Yang Qi* of the general body. Zhaohai (KI6) nourishes blood and *Yin* of the body. The use of these two points has the function of regulating nutrient and defensive systems so abundant *Qi* and blood will be infused into the eye region to perform the forceful movements of the eyelids. Hegu (LI4), lifting and dispersing, is often indicated for facial disorders. Fengchi (GB20) and Waiguan (SJ5) are selected for expelling the wind invasion of the channels and collaterals and also for eliminating the superficial syndrome caused by wind invasion. Zusanli (ST36) is used to strengthen the *Qi* of the middle—*Jiao* and Sanyinjiao (SP6) to reinforce the spleen and stomach and tonify *Qi* and blood.

Point Modifications: Add Baihui (DU20) for dizziness.

Method: Use filiform needles with even method. Penetrate Yangbai (GB14) towards Yuyao (EX—HN4), or Yuyao (EX—HN4) towards Sizukong (SJ23). Retain the needles for 20—30 minutes each time. 20—30minutes of moxa heating is applicable at Zusanli (ST36) and Baihui (DU20) after the withdrawal of needles. Treatment is given once a day.

Alternative Treatment: Embedding of ear seeds

Prescription: Liver Spleen Eye Sympathetic nerve and Ear—Shenmen.

Treat these points on either ear alternately every three days.

5.7　Sudden Blindness

Sudden blindness refers to a kind of internal oculopathy marked by abrupt diminution or loss of visual acuity in one or both eyes. It is similar to the central vessel obstruction of retina, acute optic neuritis and detatchment of retina in modern medicine.

Cause and Mechanism

Sudden blindness is mainly caused by the following factors: Violent anger, fear, fright or yin deficiency of the liver and kidney which results in the hyperactivity of liver *Yang*, and a disorderly *Qi* mechanism; or emotional depression and the poor function of the liver in maintaining the free flow of *Qi* giving rise to stagnation of *Qi* and stasis of blood obstructing the channels so that the *Qi* of the *Zangf u* fails to ascend to nourish the eye, thus leading to the sudden decline of vision because of the poor nourishment.

Differentiation

The eyes of the most patients appear asymptomatic prior to the attack until subjective awearness of loss of visual acuity in one or both eyes. A small number of patients may experience visual sparkling before the attack, distending pain, or tenderness of the eyeball, or drawing pain during the movement of the eyeball. Accompanying symptoms such as dizziness, tinnitus, fullness sensation in the chest and hypochondrium, flushed face, dark red tongue proper, and wiry rapid pulse will be present if sudden loss of visual acuity is due to hyperactivity of liver *Yang*. However, distending pain in the eyes and head, restlessness, thirst, purplish tongue proper, and uneven or wiry pulse will take place if it is due to stagnation of *Qi* and stasis of blood.

Treatment

Principle: Activiate blood circulation, soothe the liver and promote the visual acuity by selecting points mainly from the local area.

Prescription: Jingming(BL1) Zanzhu(BL2) Chengqi(ST1)
　　　　　　　　Taiyang(Extra) Fengchi(GB20)

Guangming(GB37)   Hegu(LI4)

Taixi(KI3)   Taichong(LR3)

Xingjian (LR2) optional for hyperactivity of liver *Yang*, and Geshu (BL17) optional for stagnation of *Qi* and stasis of blood.

Explanation: Jingming (BL1), Zanzhu (BL2), Chengqi (ST1), Fengchi(GB20) and Taiyang (Extra) are used to reinforce the *Qi* circulation of the related channels in order to improve the visual acuity. Guangming (GB37), the *Luo*—connecting point of The Gallbladder Channel of Foot—*Shaoyang*, regulates *Qi* and blood of the liver and gallbladder, and is therefore the principal points for treating eye diseases. Hegu (LI4), clearing up the upper—*Jiao* because of its ascending and dispersing function, is the principal point for treating disorders of the five sense organs. Taixi (KI3) and Taichong (LR3) replenish the liver and kidney, nourish the blood and brighten the eye. Xingjian (LR2), the *Xing*—spring point of The Liver Channel of Foot—*Jueyin*, sedates and quenches the wind. And Geshu (BL17), the Influential point of blood, has the function to activate blood circulation and re-solve blood stasis.

Point Modifications: Add Guanchong (SJ1) for distention of the eye.

Method: Apply filiform needles with reducing method, but without retention of needles. Pricking at Guanchong (SJ1) with a three—edged needles to cause bleeding is applicable.

Alternative Treatment: Point Injection

Prescription: Guangming(GB37)   Fengchi(GB20)

Method: Mix 100 mg of Vit B1 with 250 mg of Vit B12,then inject the mixture by equal proportions at Guangming (GB37) and Fengchi (GB20)on one side only for each treatment. Treatment is given once daily.

5.8 Lacrimation

Lacrimation in traditional Chinese medicine refers to a constant running of tears, especially when exposed to wind, even though there is no redness nor pain in the eyes. It is a common eye disorder, mostly bother the elderly, similar to dystopy of lacumal punctum, dacrycystitis, canaliculitis, trachoma and chronic conjunctivitis in modern medicine.

Cause and Mechanism

Lacrimation is often caused by malnutrition of the eye due to deficiency of *Qi* and blood, deficiency of the liver and kidney. Tears often run down because of the loseness of eye control. Or, by dysfunction of puncta lacrimalis due to wind−heat invasion which makes tears flow spontaneously.

Differentiation

There is no marginal blepharitis, swelling or pain, but lacrimation especially by expose against the wind. Lacrimation stops when the wind is avoided,but aggravates with cold. Or, lacrimation occurs from time to time and worsens with wind exposure.

Treatment

1. Deficiency of Liver and Kidney

Principle: Replenish the liver and kidney, and eliminate pathogenic wind by selecting points mainly from The Urinary Bladder Channel of Foot−*Taiyang*.

Prescription: Jingming(BL 1) Zanzhu(BL 2)
　　　　　　　Fengchi(GB20) Ganshu(BL18)
　　　　　　　Shenshu(BL23) Taixi(KI 3)

Sanyinjiao(SP 6)

Explanation: Jingming (BL1) and Zanzhu (BL2) are local points to dredge the channel and to regulate *Qi,* blood, nutrient and defensive systems so as to regain the functioning control over the eyes. Fengchi (GB20), coalescent point of The *Sanjiao* Channel of Hand−*Shaoyang* and The *Yangwei* Channel, serves as the key point for eliminating wind. It also promotes the functions of the five sense organs. Taixi (KI 3), Ganshu (BL18) and Shenshu (BL23) tonify the liver and kidney. Sanyinjiao (SP6) reinforces the spleen, liver and kidney.

Point Modifications:Add Guangming (GB37) for blurred vision.

Method: Use filiform needles with reinforcing method and retain the needles for 15−20 minutes. 20−30 minutes of moxa treatment is applicable at Ganshu (BL18) and Shenshu (BL23) when acupuncture treatment is over. Treatment is given once a day.

2. Wind−heat Invasion

Principle: Eliminate wind and heat, soothe the liver and brighten the eyes by selecting points mainly from The Urinary Bladder Channel of Foot−*Taiyang* and The Liver Channel of Foot−*Jueyin.*

Prescription: Jingming(BL 1) Zanzhu(BL 2)
　　　　　　　Hegu(LI 4) Fengchi(GB20)
　　　　　　　Xingjian(LR 2)

Explanation: Jingming (BL1) and Zanzhu (BL2) remove obstruction from channels and collaterals and activate the circulation of *Qi* and blood. Hegu (LI4) and Fengchi (GB20) clear up wind and heat. Xingjian (LR2), the *Ying*−spring point of The

Liver Channel of Foot—*Jueyin,* has the effect to disperse heat from the liver.

Point Modification: Add Shangxing (DU23) for headache and excessive lacrimation.

Method: Use filiform needles with reducing method and retain the needles for 15—20 minutes. Treatment is given once a day.

Alternative Treatment: Auricular Acupuncture

Prescription: Eye Liver Eye 1 and Eye 2

Method: Use filiform needles with strong stimulation and retain the needles for 30 minutes. Embedding of ear seeds alternately on both ears is applicable. The embedded seeds are replaced every three days.

5.9　Tinnitus and Deafness

Tinnitus and deafness are auditory disturbances caused by numerous factors. Tinnitus, mainly characterized by a ringing in the ear, disturbs normal hearing or even sleeping of the patient. Deafness refers to different degrees of poor hearing or loss of hearing. The above two often occur simultaneously. These two conditions are always mentioned together in traditional Chinese medicine because they bear similar etiology and require similar treatment as well.

Cause and Mechanism

Tinnitus and deafness are mostly caused by violent rage and fright with subsequent flaring up of fire of the liver and gallbladder disturbing the lucid organ. Obstruction of *Qi* passage due to accumulation of dampness forming into phlegm and phlegm—heat stagnation, or deficiency of kidney essence failing to ascend to the ears, on the other hand, may also lead to tinnitus and deafness.

Differentiation

1. Flaring Fire of the Liver and Gallbladder

The onset of tinnitus or deafness is abrupt with a ringing in the ear as if some wind blows in. Pressing with the hand over the ear orifice relieves neither deafness nor tinnitus, and hearing is affected. The accompanying manifestations include headache, flushed face, bitter taste with dry throat, restlessness with irritability, or disturbed sleep, discomfort sensation in the hypochondriac region, constipation, red tongue proper with yellow coating, and rapid wiry pulse.

2. Phlegm—heat Stagnation

Tinnitus in this case is like the ringing of cicada with hypoacusis, or deafness as if the ear is heavily blocked. The accompanying symptoms and signs include dizziness with a heavy sensation, fullness in the chest, bitter mouth, excessive phlegm, unsmooth urinary and stool discharge, greasy tongue coating and wiry slippery pulse.

3. Deficiency of Kidney Essence

Tinnitus bothering both ears intermittently is better in the daytime but worse at night. Hand pressing over the ear alleviates the condition. Most patients also suffer from some loss of hearing, dizziness, fatigue, soreness and weakness of the lumbar region and knee joints, fidgets of the deficient type and insomnia. The tongue proper is red with little coating, and the pulse is weak thready or rapid thready.

Treatment

1. Flaring of the Liver and Gallbladder

Principle: Clear up the gallbladder fire by selecting points mainly from The Gallbladder Channel of Foot—*Shaoyang* and The Liver Channel of Foot—*Jueyin*.

Prescription: Yifeng(SJ17) Tinghui(GB 2)
　　　　　　　Xiaxi(GB43) Zhongzhu(SJ 3)
　　　　　　　Xingjian(LR 2)

Explanation: The *Sanjiao* Channel of Hand—*Shaoyang* and The Gallbladder Channel of Foot—*Shaoyang* both curve around the ear. Therefore, Zhongzhu (SJ 3), Yifeng (SJ17) and Tinghui (GB 2) are used to promote the *Qi* circulation of the *Shaoyang* channels. Xingjian (LR2) and Xiaxi (GB43), the *Ying*—spring points of their pertaining channels, are used to clear away the fire from the liver and gallbladder. Points formed in this prescription can also be explained in light of the principles "select the lower points of the body for treating upper disorders," and "apply reducing technique for excess conditions".

Method: Use filiform needles with reducing method and retain the needles for 15—20 minutes. Treatment is given once a day.

2. Phlegm—heat Stagnation

Principle: Eliminate heat, resolve phlegm and disperse pathogenic accumulation by selecting points mainly from The *Sanjiao* Channel of Hand—*Shaoyang*, The Gallbladder Channel of Foot—*Shaoyang* and The Stomach Channel of Foot—*Yangming*.

Prescription: Yifeng(SJ17) Tinghui(GB 2) Xiaxi(GB43)
　　　　　　　Zhongzhu(SJ 3) Shangwan(RN13)
　　　　　　　Fenglong(ST40) Zusanli(ST36)

Yanglingquan(GB34)

Explanation: Yifeng (SJ17), Tinghui (GB 2), Xiaxi (GB43) and Zhongzhu (SJ 3) dredge the *Shaoyang* channels. Fenglong (ST40)clears away heat and resolve phlegm. Shangwan (RN13) in combination with Zusanli (ST36) and Yanglingquan (GB34) soothes the wood, reinforces the earth, disperses pathogenic accumulation,clears away heat from the stomach and heart, and eliminates phlegm—damp from the upper and middle—*Jiao*.

Point Modification: Add Pianli (LI 6) for deafness due to febrile disease.

Method: Use filiform needles with reducing method and retain the needles for 15—20 minutes. Treatment is given once a day.

3. Deficiency of Kidney Essence

Principle: Reinforce the kidney essence by selecting points mainly from The *Sanjiao* Channel of Hand—*Shaoyang*, The Gallbladder Channel of Foot—*Shaoyang* and The Kidney Channel of Foot—*Shaoyin*.

Prescription: Yifeng(SJ17)　Tinghui(GB 2)
　　　　　　　Zhongzhu(SJ 3)　Shenshu(BL23)
　　　　　　　Mingmen(DU 4)　Guanyuan(RN 4)
　　　　　　　Taixi(KI 3)

Explanation: Yifeng (SJ17) and Tinghui (GB 2) are local points, in combination with Zhongzhu (SJ3), promote the *Qi* circulation of the shaoyang channels. The kidney opens into the ear. The vital energy of the kidney can not ascend to nourish the ear if it is deficient. Therefore, Shenshu (BL23), Mingmen (DU 4), Guanyuan (RN 4) and Taixi (KI 3) are used to tonify the kidney energy in order that the vital energy may ascend to the ear with the expected effect of stopping tinnitus and restoring hearing.

Method: Use filiform needles with reinforcing method and retain needles for 15–20 minutes. Apply moxibustion at Shenshu (BL23), Mingmen (DU4) and Guanyuan (RN4) for 20–30 minutes when needling at these points is finished. Treatment is given once a day .

Alternative Treatment: Scalp Acupuncture

Prescription: Bilateral vertigo and hearing areas

Method: Use filiform needles with intermittent manipulations and retain the needles for 30 minutes. Treatment is given once a day or once every other day. This kind of treatment is especially indicated in neurotic tinnitus and hypoacusis.

5.10   Otitis Media

Otitis media, also know as otopysis or otorrhea, in the perception of traditional Chinese medicine is mainly characterized by pain in the ear and discharge of purulent substance from the ear. It is similar to acute and chronic otitis media suppurative in modern medicine, and more complained of by children.

Cause and Mechanism

The onset of otitis media is often caused by exogenous pathogenic wind–heat invasion into the ear, inducing the flaring up of gall–bladder fire and heat accumulation. Excessive heat accumulation ascends along The Gallbladder Channel of Foot–*Shaoyang* into the ear resulting in the forming of purulent substance. Deficiency of spleen due to protracted illness may also give rise to otitis media because the poor function of spleen in transforming and transporting causes water–damp retention in the interior and turbid phlegm flooding into the ear.

Differentiation

1. Invasion of Exogenous Pathogenic Wind—heat

The abrupt onset of otitis media occurs together with distension and pain in the internal ear that worsens increasingly. The accompanying manifestations include general fever, aversion to cold, headache and restlessness. In a few days, some sticky purulent substance of a foul smell will flow out from the ear, which is followed by some alleviation of ear pain and general symptoms. The tongue proper is red with yellow coating, and the pulse is rapid and wiry.

2. Dampness Retention due to Spleen Deficiency

The discharge of purulent substance from the ear which is diluted with a foul smell flows on and off for a prolonged period of time. Such a condition alleviates and aggravates from time to time. Other symptoms and signs may include dizziness, tinnitus and hard of hearing. The tongue proper is pale with white coating and the pulse is weak and thready.

Treatment

1. Invasion of Exogenous Pathogenic Wind—heat

Principle: Dispel wind and heat and promote the auditory function of the ear by selecting points mainly from The Gallbladder Channel of Foot—*Shaoyang* and The *Sanjiao* Channel of Hand—*Shaoyang*.

Prescription: Fengchi(GB20)　Wangu(GB12)

　　　　　　　Hegu(LI 4)　Xingjian(LR 2)

　　　　　　　Guanchong(SJ 1)　Ear apex

Explanation: Fengchi (GB20), Wangu (GB12) and Ear apex (ear point) may disperse wind—heat from the part of the shaoyang channel in the area of the ear. Hegu (LI 4) eliminates wind—heat from the head and facial areas, and promotes the function of the five sense organs. Xingjian (LR 2) and Guanchong (SJ 1) clears away heat from the liver, gallbladder and the *Sanjiao*.

Point Modifications: Add Dazhui (DU14) for severe heat; Taiyang (EX—HN5) and Shangxing (DU23) for headache.

Method: Use filiform needles with reducing method. Dazhui (DU14) may be pricked with a three—edged needle for bleeding.

2. Dampness Retention due to Spleen Deficiency

Principle: Strengthen the spleen and resolve dampness by selecting points mainly from The *Sanjiao* Channel of Hand—*Shaoyang*, The Spleen Channel of Foot—*Taiyin* and The Stomach Channel of Foot—*Yangming*.

Prescription: Yifeng(SJ17) Zusanli(ST36)
               Yinlingquan(SP9) Yinbai(SP1)

Explanation: Yifeng (SJ17) is a local point for removing obstruction from the local channels and promoting the function of the ear. Zusanli (ST36) and Yinlingquan (SP 9), the He—sea points of their pertaining channels, are used in combination with Yinbai (SP1) to reinforce the spleen *Qi* and activate spleen *Yang* for the purpose of strengthening spleen and resolving dampness.

Point Modification: Add Shenshu (UB23) and Taixi (KI 3) for dizziness and tinnitus.

Method: Use filiform needles with reinforcing method and retain the needles for 15—20 minutes. Moxibustion can be added at Shenshu (UB23) and Zusanli (ST36) for 20—30 minutes each time after acupuncture treatment. Treatment is given once a day.

Alternative Treatment: Auricular Acupuncture

Prescription: Ear apex Kidney Occiput outer ear

Sub—cortex inner ear

Method: Use filiform needles with moderate stimulation and retain the needles for 20—30 minutes. Treatment is given once daily or once every other day. Embedding of ear seeds is also applicable.

5.11   Deafness and Mute

Although deafness and mute are distinctly two different conditions, mute is mostly related to a complete loss of hearing. There is a common saying which goes like this, "Mute is generally the result of deafness. Priority is given to treat deafness first in order to treat patients for mute." Also, "Deafness is the cause of mute and mute is the consequence of deafness." Clinically, most patients receiving treatments for such conditions are children.

Cause and Mechanism

A congenital deficiency accounts basically for the cause of deafness and mute. However, exogenous pathogenic heat invasion with subsequent obstruction of the channels and dysfunction of the respective sense organs, or drug toxication may also be the cause of the condition.

Differentiation

Deafness and mute are characterized by severe hypoacusis or complete loss of hearing. Generally, the phonatory organ is normal.

Treatment

Principle: Remove obstruction from the channels and restore the auditory and speech functions by selecting points mainly from The *Sanjiao* Channel of Hand—*Shaoyang* and The Gallbladder Channel of Foot—*Shaoyang*.

Prescription: Shuaigu(GB 8) Xuanlu(GB 5)

                 Tianchong(GB 9) Tinggong(SI19)

                 Zhongzhu(SJ 3) Yanglingquan(GB34)

                 Tinghui(GB 2) Yamen(DU15)

Explanation: Shuaigu (GB 8), Xuanlu (GB 5), Tianchong (GB 9), Tinggong (SI19) and Tinghui (GB 2) are points from The *Sanjiao* Channel of Hand—*Shaoyang* and The Gallbladder Channel of Foot—*Shaoyang* located in the ear area. The distribution of these channels here runs from the orifice of external acoustic meatus to the front of the auricle. Therefore, the above points can promote the *Qi* circulation of these channels in the ear area. Zhongzhu (SJ 3), Yanglingquang (GB34) promote the circulation of *Qi* of their pertaining channels and assist the previous points to remove obstruction from the channels and restore normal functions of the sense organs involved. Yamen (DU15), promoting the function of the throat and speech, is an important point for treating the mute.

     Method: Use filiform needles with horizontal insertion. Penetrate from Shuaigu (GB 8), Xuanlu (GB 5) and Tianchong (GB9) towards Jiaosun (SJ20) for 1−1.5 *Cun* deep;Tinggong (SI19) towards Tinghui (GB 2) obliquely for 1−1.2 *Cun* deep. Also, Shuaigu (GB 8) and Xuanlu (GB 5) are applied with electric stimulation. Densesparse wave is maintained for 40 minutes.

5.12　Epistaxis

     Epistaxis refers to nasal bleeding caused by factors other than traumatic injuries. In traditional Chinese medicine, profuse nasal bleeding is called nasal flooding or heavy expistaxis.

Cause and Mechanism

The lung opens into the nose. Invasion of exogenous pathogenic wind, heat or dryness first attacks the lung, obstructing the nasal cavity and impairing the nasal collaterals by means of burning. Constitutional retention of heat in the stomach channel plus a hot, spicy diet causes excessive stomach heat ascending along the channel. Weak constitution in the aged with *Yin* deficiency of the liver and kidney leads to the flaring up of asthenic fire. The above factors may all result in epistaxis when the blood is forced to flow outside of the vessels.

Differentiation

1. Heat Accumulation in the Lung

Dripping of fresh blood accompanied by dry nose, general feverish sensation, dry mouth, cough with little sputum, red tongue proper with thin white coating, and rapid superficial pulse.

2. Burning of Stomach Heat

Heavy nasal bleeding of fresh red or deep red colour accompanied by dry throat, foul smell in the mouth, thirst desiring for cold drinking, constipation and scanty urine. The tongue proper is red with yellow coating and the pulse is rapid superficial.

3. *Yin* Deficiency of the Liver and Kidney

Small amount of fresh red bleeding which goes on and off, accompanied by dry mouth, dizziness, vertigo, palpitation, tinnitus, restlessness, insomnia and red tongue proper with less coating. The pulse is thready, rapid and feeble.

Treatment

1. Heat Accumulation in the Lung

Principle: Clear wind, eliminate heat and stop bleeding by selecting points mainly from The Lung Channel of Hand—*Taiyin* and The Large Intestine Channel of Hand—*Yangming*.

Prescription: Fengchi(GB20)   Yingxiang(LI20)
Hegu(LI 4)   Shaoshang(LU11)

Explanation: Pricking at Shaoshang (LU11) is to help clear away heat from lung. Hegu (LI4) and Yingxiang (LI20) have the effect of sedating fire from their pertaining channel. Fengchi (GB20) assists eliminating wind.

Point Modification: Add Dazhui (DU14) and Quchi (LI11) for severe heat; and prick Weizhong (BL40) to cause bleeding for heavy nasal bleeding.

Method: Use filiform needles with reducing method and retain the needles for 15—20 minutes. Pricking at Shaoshang (LU11) and Dazhui (DU14) to cause bleeding is applicable.

2. Burning of Stomach Heat

Principle: Eliminate stomach fire and stop bleeding by selecting points mainly from The Large Intestine Channel of Hand—*Yangming*, The Stomach Channel of Foot—*Yangming* and the *Du* Channel.

Prescription: Yingxiang(LI20)   Hegu(LI 4)
Lidui(ST45)   Shangxing(DU23)

Explanation: Yingxiang (LI20) and Hegu (LI 4), points of The Large Intestine Channel of Hand—*Yangming*, clear away heat from the *Yangming* channel. Lidui (ST45), the *Jing*—well point of The Stomach Channel of Foot—*Yangming*, clears away stomach heat and restrains the adverse flow of stomach *Qi*. The *Du* Channel is known as the sea of all *Yang* channels. Shangxing (DU23), a point of The *Du* Channel, is punctured to eliminate the pathogenic heat from all of the *Yang* channels, resulting in a normal blood circulation in the vessels and stop of nasal bleeding.

Point Modification: Add Yinbai (SP1) for massive nasal bleeding.

Method: Use filiform needles with reducing method and retain the needles for 15—20 minutes. Manipulation is maintained every 3—5 minutes.

3. *Yin* Deficiency of the Liver and Kidney

Principle: Tonify the liver and kidney, sedate fire and stop nasal bleeding by selecting points mainly from The Kidney Channel of Foot—*Shaoyin* and The Liver Channel of Foot—*Jueyin*.

Prescription: Taixi(KI 3) Taichong(LR 3)
　　　　　　　Tongtian(BL 7) Feiyang(BL58)

Explanation: Taixi (KI 3) and Taichong (LR 3), the two *Yuan*—source points of their pertaining channels, tonify kidney *Yin* and sedate liver fire. These two points in combination with Tongtian (BL 7) are indicated in epistaxis. Feiyang (BL58), the *Luo*—connecting point of The Urinary Bladder Channel of Foot—*Taiyang,* is the principal point for treating epistaxis due to *Yin* deficiency of the liver and kidney.

Point Modification: Add Yongquan (KI 1) with moxibustion for massive nasal bleeding.

Method: Use filiform needles with even method and retain the needles for 15—20 minutes. Treatment is given once daily.

Alternative Treatment: Auricular Acupuncture

Prescription: Inner nose lung stomach adrenal gland
　　　　　　　forehead

Method: Use filiform needles with moderate stimulation and retain the needles for 20—30 minutes. Treatment is given once a day. Embedding of ear seeds is also applicable at these ear points.

5.13 Rhinorrhea

Rhinorrhea in the perception of traditional Chinese medicine is mainly characterized by nasal discharge of turbid substance, nasal obstruction and poor sense of smell. Since the turbid discharge often bothers the patient over a prolonged period of time, as if the spring emerging from the bottom of a deep pond, such a condition has been traditionally called as nasal pond by practitioners of traditional Chinese medicine. The accompanying symptoms and signs include a distending pain in the forehead and dizziness. It is one of the commonly encountered nasal conditions similar to sinusitis in modern medicine.

Cause and Mechanism

The lung dominates over skin pores and opens into the nose. Invasion of exogenous pathogenic wind–cold attacks primarily the superfitial portion of the body and the lung. This invasion sometimes gives rise to wind–cold transforming into heat and the poor function of the lung in descending and dispersing, resulting in nasal obstruction. And accumulation of heat in the nasal cavity develops into rhinorrhea with turbid discharge. Excessive fire of the liver and gallbladder ascending to the orifices of the sense organs may also cause rhinorrhea.

Differentiation

1. Wind–cold Transforming into Heat

Fever with aversion to cold, productive cough, headache, distension of the forehead, stuffy nose with massive discharge, poor sense of smell, red tongue proper, thin yellow coating, and rapid floating pulse.

2. Excessive Fire of the Liver and Gallbladder

Stuffy nose with yellowish discharge of sticky quality and foul smell, tenderness in the glabella and xygomatic area. Other manifestations include fever, headache, dizziness, bitter taste, irritability, dream−disturbed sleep, red tongue proper and rapid wiry pulse.

Treatment

1. Wind−cold Transforming into Heat

Principle: Remove wind, clear away heat, and promote the function of lung in descending and dispersing by selecting points mainly from The Lung Channel of Hand−*Taiyin* and The Large Intestine Channel of Hand−*Yangming*.

Prescription: Lieque(LU 7) Hegu(LI 4)

                 Yingxiang(LI20) Yintang(EX−HN3)

Explanation: The nose the specific organ that the lung opens into. Lieque (LU7), the *Luo*−connecting point of the lung channel, helps the lung in dispersing and eliminates wind−heat. The Lung Channel of Hand−*Taiyin* and The Large Intestine Channel of Hand−*Yangming* are internally−externally related two channels. Part of the distribution of the Large Intestine Channel of Hand−*Yangming* passes along the nostrils. Therefore, Hegu (LI 4) and Yingxiang (LI20) are selected to regulate the *Qi* circulation of The Large Intestine Channel of Hand−*Yangming* for the purpose of clearing away lung heat. These two points are believed to be most effective in the treatment of nasal obstruction with poor sense of smell. Yintang (Ex−HN3) has the function of dispersing heat accumulation and removing nasal obstruction.

Point Modification: Add Yuyao (EX−HN4) and Zhaohai

(KI6) for pain in the supra—orbital bone.

Method: Use filiform needles with reducing method and retain the needles for 15—20 minutes. Treatment is given once a day.

2. Excessive Fire of the Liver and Gallbladder

Principle: Clear up the heat of the liver and gallbladder and remove the nasal obstruction by selecting points mainly from The Large Intestine Channel of Hand—*Yangming*, The Liver Channel of Foot—*Jueyin* and The Gallbladder Channel of Foot—*Shaoyang*.

Prescription: Xingjian(LR 2) Fengchi(GB20)
          Shangxing(DU23) Yingxiang(LI20)

Explanation: Xingjian (LR2) is the *Xing*—spring point of the liver channel, and Fengchi (GB20) is the coalescent point crossing The Gallbladder Channel of Foot—*Shaoyang* and The *Yangwei* Channel. These two points have the functions to expel wind and clear away heat, and remove heat from the liver and gallbladder. Shangxing (DU23) in combination with Yingxiang (LI20) promotes blood circulation and remove nasal obstruction as well.

Point Modification: Add Taiyang (EX—HN5) for headache.

Method: Use filiform needles with reducing method and retain the needles for 15—20 minutes. Treatment is given once daily.

Alternative Treatment: Auricular Acupuncture

Prescription: Inner nose Forehead Lung Adrenal gland
Add asthma—relief only for patients with allergic history.

Method: Use filiform needles with strong stimulation and intermittent manipulation. Retain the needles for 20—30 minutes. Embedding of ear seeds is also applicable.

5.14   Toothache

Toothache, a common symptom in stomatopathy, can be due to pulpitis, dental caries and periodentitis, and be aggravated by stimulation of either cold or heat. It is more complained of by children and the aged with poor body constitution.

Cause and Mechanism

Invasion of exogenous pathogenic wind—fire obstructs the *Yangming* channel resulting in subsequent stagnation of *Qi* and blood, and heat accumulation forming inflammation. Retention of heat in the gastrointestinal system due to a hot spicy diet causes fire of the *Yangming* channel ascending to develop toothache. The kidney governs bones, and the teeth are part of the bones. Kidney *Yin* deficiency leads to the emptying of the dental pulp and flaring up of asthenia fire to burn in the dental pulp and ail the teeth.

Differentiation

1. Toothache due to Exogenous Pathogenic Wind—fire

Toothache, gingival swelling and worse pain with hot drinking or food, accompanied by general fever, aversion to cold, thirst, red tongue proper with white coating, and rapid floating pulse.

2. Toothache due to Stomach Fire

Severe toothache with redness and swelling of the dental pulp, or abcess and oozing of blood, headache, foul mouth, thirst desiring drinking, constipation, yellow tongue coating and full rapid pulse.

3. Toothache due to Asthenia Fire

Dull toothache marked by an intermittent pain, loose teeth,

red tongue proper with little coating and thready pulse, but normal dental pulp without any redness or swelling, nor foul breath.

Treatment

Principle: Remove the obstruction in the channels and relieve pain with respective sub—principles to dispel wind—fire, eliminate stomach fire, and nourish *Yin* to sedate fire.

Prescription: Hegu(LI 4) Xiaguan(ST 7) Jiache(ST 6)

On the basis of the above main points, plus Yemen (SJ2) and Fengchi (GB20) for toothache due to pathogenic wind—fire, Neiting (ST44) and Laogong (PC8) for toothache due to stomach fire, and Taixi (KI3) and Xingjian (LR2) for toothache due to asthenic fire.

Explanation: Hegu (LI 4), the effective point for treating toothache, can clear away the heat from the *Yangming* channel. Xiaguan (ST 7) and Jiache (ST 6), points of the stomach channel, promote the *Qi* circulation of the channel, sedate the fire and stop pain. Yemen (SJ 2) drives away the wind—heat of the *Sanjiao* from the exterior of the body. Neiting (ST44), the *Ying*—spring point of The Stomach Channel of Foot—*Yangming*, relieves the excess heat from the channel. Laogong (PC 8), the *Ying*—spring point of The Pericardium Channel of Hand—*Jueyin*, eliminates heart fire. Taixi (KI 3) nourishes kindey *Yin* and sedates fire. Xingjian (LR 2) eliminates liver fire.

Point Modification: Add Erjian (LI 2) for pain due to dental caries, and Taiyang (EX—HN5) for headache.

Method: Use filiform needles with reducing method for most of the points, but reinforcing method for Taixi (KI3), and retain the needles for 15—20 minutes. Manipulation of needles is maintained every five minutes.

Alternative Treatment: Auricular Acupuncture

Prescription: Upper jaw Lower jaw Ear—shenmen
Toothache point

Method: Use filiform needles with strong stimulation and retain the needles for 20—30 minutes. Embedding of ear seeds is also applicable.

5.15 Sore Throat

Sore throat can be caused by many commonly encountered throat conditions. Its main manifestations are local redness, swelling, pain and discomfort sensation which may be accompanied by fever, headache and cough. It is similar to pharyngitis, laryngitis, and acute or chronic tonsillitis in modern medicine.

Cause and Mechanism

Invasion of exogenous pathogenic wind—heat attacking the lung and stomach to cause heat accumulation in the throat; constitutional heat accumulation in the lung and stomach flaring up to the throat; or deficiency of kidney *Yin* and over consumption of stomach *Yin* resulting in the ascending of asthenic fire and the lack of fluid to moisten the throat, etc., all these factors may contribute to the onset of sore throat.

Differentiation

1. Excess of Wind—heat

More severe fever than aversion to cold, headache and cough accompanied by redness, swelling and pain in the throat, red tongue proper with thin yellow coating and rapid floating pulse.

2. Excess Heat

Continuous strong fever without headache or aversion to cold, severe sore throat, flushed face with congestion of eyes, mouth ulceration, thirst desiring for drinking, constipation, scanty urine, red tongue proper with burnt yellow coating, and rapid slippery pulse.

3. Asthenic Heat

Dull pain in the throat, thirst desiring no drinking, soreness in the lumbar region and knees, dizziness, tinnitus, tidal fever, red tongue proper with less coating, and rapid thready pulse.

Treatment

1. Excess of Wind–heat

Principle: Relieve the exogenous pathogenic wind–heat from the throat by selecting points mainly from The Lung Channel of Hand–*Taiyin*, and The Large Intestine channel of Hand–*Yangming*.

Prescription: Fengchi(GB20) Shaoshang(LU11)
                Hegu(LI 4) Quchi(LI11) Lieque(LU 7)

Explanation: Fengchi (GB20) expels wind and removes heat. Quchi (LI11) and Hegu (LI 4) clear the pathogenic heat from their pertaining *Yangming* channel. Shaoshang (LU11), the *Jing*–well point of The Lung Channel of Hand–*Taiyin*, may clear away the heat from the lung and promote the throat. Lieque (LU 7), having the effect to resolvephlegm and stop cough, helps to expel wind, remove heat and promote the throat.

Point Modification: Add Taiyang (EX–HN5) and Dazhui (DU14) for headache.

Method: Use filiform needles with reducing method and retain the needles for 15–20 minutes, or puncture these points with a three–edged needle to cause bleeding. Treatment is given once daily.

2. Excess Heat

Principle: Eliminate heat from lung and stomach and promote throat by selecting points mainly from The Lung Channel of Hand—*Taiyin*, The Large Intestine Channel of Hand—*Yangming* and The Stomach Channel of Foot—*Yangming*.

Prescription: Shaoshang(LU11) Hegu(LI 4) Chize(LU 5)
Xiangu(ST43)   Guanchong(SJ1)

Explanation: Shaoshang (LU11), the *Jing*—well point of The Lung Channel of Hand—*Taiyin,* is the principal point to treat sore throat because it can eliminate lung heat. Chize (LU 5), the *He*—sea point of the same channel, can clear away the excess heat from its pertaining channel. It is used according to the principle of reducing the son in case of excess syndrome. Hegu (LI4) and Xiangu (ST43), respectively belonging to the *Yangming* channels of both hand and foot, are used in combination to disperse the accumulated heat of their pertaining channels. Guanchong (SJ1), the *Jing*—well point of the *Sanjiao* Channel of Hand—*Shaoyang,* here helps to clear away the pathogenic heat from the lung and stomach for the purpose of relieving the sore throat.

Point Modification: Add Zhigou (SJ 6) for constipation.

Method: Use Filiform needles with reducing method and retain the needles for 15—20 minutes. Shaoshnag (LU11) and Guanchong (SJ1) are pricked with a three—edged needle to cause bleeding.

3. Deficient Heat

Principle: Nourish yin, sedate fire and relieve sore throat by selecting points mainly from The Lung Channel of Hand—*Taiyin,* and The Kidney Channel of Foot—*Shaoyin*.

Prescription: Taixi(KI 3)   Zhaohai(KI 6)
Yuji(LU10)   Jinjin(EX—HN12)

Yuye(EX-HN13)

Explanation: Taixi (KI3) is the *Yuan*-source point of its pertaining channel, and Zhaohai (KI6) the coalescent point of the same channel crossing The *Yinqiao* Channel, which both travel to the throat. Therefore, these two points have the function to nourish *Yin* and sedate the fire, particularly to guide the asthenic fire to run downward. Yuji (LU10), the *Ying*-spring point of its pertaining channel, eliminates the asthenic heat from the Lung Channel of Hand-*Taiyin*. Jinjin(EX-HN12) and Yuye(EX-HN 13) are used to replenish body fluid and moisten the throat.

Point Modification: Add Shenshu (BL23) for soreness in the lumbar region and knees.

Method: Use filiform needles with even method and retain the needles for 15-20 minutes. Treatment is given once daily.

Alternative Treatment: Auricular Acupuncture

Prescription: Throat Lung Tonsil Helix 1-6

Method: Use filiform needles with strong stimulation. Embedding of ear seeds is also applicable. Helix 1-6 are pricked with a three-edged needle to cause bleeding.

5.16 Plum Throat

Plum throat refers to the subjective feeling of a foreign body sensation in the throat, as if the throat were stuck by a piece of plum pit, thus acquiring the term plum throat. The main characteristic is that the patient suffers from constant dry cough and repeated empty swallowing, which may accompanied by fullness sensation in the chest and hypochondriac region, and depression. It is often complained of by adult females. Referring to modern medicine, it is included in the extent of neurosis.

Cause and Mechanism

The onset of plum throat is mostly caused by mental irritation, emotional depression resulted from liver *Qi* stagnation. The liver condition overacts the spleen, leading to the dysfunction of the spleen in transporting the fluid so that dampness retention transforms into phlegm mixing with the abnormal ascending of *Qi* obstructing the throat.

Differentiation

Patients have the subjective feeling of some foreign substance in the throat which can neither be expectorated out nor swallowed in. Such a sensation often goes with an underlying course of emotional disturbance, mental depression and over suspicion, accompanied by hypochondriac pain, anorexia, or irregular menstruation in women. it fluctuates from time to time, often in accordance with dramatic emotional changes. There is no pain in the throat, nor difficulty in food intake. Physical examination appears normal. The tongue proper is pale with white sticky coating, and the pulse is wiry.

Treatment

Principle: Relieve the abnormal *Qi* mechanism in the chest, promote the circulation of *Qi* and resolve the phlegm by selecting points mainly from The *Ren* Channel, The Pericardium Channel of Hand—*Jueyin* and The Liver Channel of Foot—*Jueyin*.

Prescription: Tiantu(RN22)   Danzhong(RN17)

Xingjian(LR2)   Fenglong(ST40)

Neiguan(PC6)

Explanation: Tiantu (RN22) may clear the throat and relieve the discomfort in the diaphragm. Danzhong (RN17), the Influential point of *Qi*, is used to promote the circulation of *Qi*. Neiguan

(PC6), the *Luo*—connecting of The Pericardium Channel of Hand—*Jueyin,* can regulate the *Qi* circulation in the chest. Xingjian (LR2) soothes the depressed liver *Qi.* Fenglong (ST40), the *Luo*—connecting point of The Stomach Channel of Foot—*Yangming,* resolves phlegm, promotes bowel movement and relieves the abnormal *Qi* circulation.

Point Modification: Add Sanyinjiao (SP6), Taixi (KI3) and Zhaohai (KI 6) for *Yin* deficiency, and Guanyuan (RN 4), Zusanli (ST36) and Geshu (BL17) for deficiency of *Qi* and blood.

Method: Use filiform needles with even method and retain the needles for 15—20 minutes. Treatment is given once daily.

Alternative Treatment: Embedding of Ear Seeds

Prescription: Ear—Shenmen Sympthetic Throat Liver

Embed ear seeds on these points on a alternative basis, changing the points every three days.

6　Emergency Cases

6.1　High Fever

High fever refers to a sudden rise of body temperature over 39℃ with general hot sensation, restlessness, thirst and rapid pulse. The causative factors of high fever can commonly be either exogenous or endogenous. This section mainly deals with the high fever due to exogenous pathogenic factors, similar to that as a main symptom in acute epidemic or infectious diseases and chronic diseases complicated by acute infection in modern medicine.

Cause and Mechanism

Factors that can lead to onset of high fever are various. Wind-heat invasion into the body through the mouth, nose or the skin pores can impair the function of the lung in descending and dispersing. The inability of the lung to disperse energy to protect the defensive system results in high fever. Stagnant warm ractor in the body surface transmitting into *Qi* system, or retaining in the nutrient and blood systems can cause the struggle between the pathogenic warmth and the *Qi* as well as blood to produce high fever. Summer heat invasion disturbing the heart and mind, because of the extreme hot property of summer heat as a pathogenic factor, may also cause high fever and coma. Lastly, invasion of seasonal epidemics remaining in the body surface or sinking into the internal *Zangfu* organs cause the struggle between the anti-pathogenic *Qi* and pathogenic *Qi*, resulting in high fever as well.

Differentiation

1. Wind—heat Affecting the Lung

The chief manifestations include high fever, slight aversion to wind and cold, sore throat, cough, yellow sticky sputum, thirst, red tongue proper with thin yellow coating, and rapid superficial pulse.

2. Retention of Pathogenic Warmth in the Interior

If the pathogenic warmth stays in the *Qi* system, the chief manifestations include high fever without aversion to cold, red face, congestion in the eyes, thirst in the mouth with desire to drink, cough with pain in the chest, distending pain over the abdominal region which does not respond to hand pressing, or constipated stools, red tongue proper with dry yellow coating, and full rapid pulse. If the pathogenic warmth affects the nutrient and blood systems, the chief manifestations include high fever, worse at night, restlessness, dry mouth without desire for drinking, skin eruptions, or mental confusion with delirium, convulsion of the four limbs, dark red tongue proper with lack of fluid, and rapid thready pulse.

3. Summer Heat Disturbing the Heart

The chief manifestations include high fever, sweating, restlessness, feverish sensation over the skin, dry mouth and tongue, thirst with desire for drinking, and deep feeble pulse. In the severe case, it is also accompanied by headache, shortness of breath and coma with loss of consciousness.

4. Seasonal Epidemic Steaming

The seasonal epidemics affect the body in a very rapid process. Therefore, the chief manifestations include high fever, swollen eyes with congestion, headache, sore throat, restlessness, or dense skin eruptions of the body surface, ulceration in throat, red tongue proper with yellow coating, and rapid pulse.

Treatment

1. Wind—heat Affecting the Lung

Principle: Eliminate wind—heat, promote the lung in dispersing and stop cough by using points mainly from The *Du* Channel, The Lung Channel of Hand—*Taiyin*, and The Large Intestine Channel of Hand—*Yangming*.

Prescription: Dazhui (DU14) Fengchi(GB20)

Shaoshang(Lu11) Yuji(LU10) Hegu(LI14)

Quchi(LI11)

Explanation: Dazhui (DU14), a point from The *Du* Channel and converging the *Yang* of the body, can eliminate heat from the super ficial portion of the body. Fengchi (GB 20) is good for eliminating wind and clearing away heat. The joint use of these two points may disperse wind and clear away heat. Shaoshang (LU11) and Yuji (LU·10)are respectively the *Jing*—well and *Ying*—spring points of The Lung Channel of Hand—*Taiyin*. The combination of *Jing*—well and *Xing*—spring points can eliminate heat from the lung and clear the throat. Both Hegu (LI 4) and Quchi (LI11) are points from The Large Intestine Channel of Hand—*Yangming*. The former has a ascending and dispersing effect while the latter has the property of removing pathogenic factors. The joint use of these two points can regulate the harmony between *Qi* and blood, disperse pathogenic factors from the superficial portion of the body, promote the lung in dispersing, and eliminate heat.

Point Modification: Add Taiyang (EX—HN5) for headache; Lieque (LU 7) and Feishu (BL13) for severe cough.

Method: Apply filiform needles with reducing method and retain the needles for 10−15 minutes, manipulating them two to three times. Shaoshang (LU11) can be applied with a three−edged needle to cause bleeding.

2. Retention of Pathogenic Warmth in the Interior

(1) Retention of Warmth in the *Qi* System

Principle: Eliminate pathogenic heat from the *Qi* system by using points mainly from The *Du* Channel, The Large Intestine Channel of Hand−*Yangming* and The Stomach Channel of Foot−*Yangming*.

Prescription: Dazhui(DU14) Chize(LU 5) Hegu(LI 4)
Guanchong(SJ 1) Neiting(ST44)

Explanation: Dazhui (DU14) is used to clear away heat from the superficial portion of the body. Chize (LU 5) and Hegu (LI 4) are also combined to eliminate retention of pathogenic heat in the superficial portion of the body. These two points assist Dazhui (DU 14) to repel pathogenic heat from the nutrient and defensive systems to the very body surface. Guanchong (SJ 1), the *Jing*−well point of the *Sanjiao* channel, may disperse heat from the *Qi* system, and promote the *Qi* mechanism of the *Sanjiao*. Neiting (ST44), the *Ying*−spring point of the stomach channel, may eliminate heat from the stomach. The joint use of these five points may eliminate heat not only from the body surface but also from the interior of the body.

(2) Retention of Warmth in the Nutrient and Blood Systems

Principle: Clear away heat from the blood, cool the blood and eliminate toxic materias.

Prescription: Quze (PC 3) Weizhong(BL40)
Zhongchong(PC 9) Shaochong(HT 9)

Quchi(LI11)   Taichong(LR   3)

Explanation:In this case, the mechanism of the high fever is that the pathogenic dampess invades into the nutrient and blood systems. Therefore, Quze (PC 3) and Weizhong (BL 40), also known as the *Xi*–cleft point for the blood, are used to eliminate the pathogenic heat from the blood system. Heart dominates blood and vessels. Zhongchong (PC 9) and Shaochong(HT 9), respectively the *Jing*–well points of the pericardium and heart channels, are used to sedate heart fire and eliminate heat from the blood. Quchi(LI 11), the *He*–sea point of the large intestine channel, may regulate the *Qi* and blood. Taichong (LR 3), the *Yuan*–source point of the liver channel, is good for clearing up heat and cooling blood. The joint use of these points eliminate heat from the nutrient system and cool the blood.

Point Modification: Add Shixuan (EX–UE 11) and Shuigou (DU26) for mental confusion and delirium; Shangxing (DU23) for epistaxis; Kongzui (LU 6) for hemoptysis; Erbai (EX–UE 2) for bloody stools; and Jinsuo (DU 8) and Yanglingquan (GB 34) for convulsions of the four limbs.

Method: Apply filiform needles with reducing method and retain the needles for 15–20 minutes, manipulating them two to three times, Quze (PC 3), Weizhong (BL40), Zhongchong (PC 9) and Shaochong (HT 9) can be pricked with a three–edged needle to cause bleeding.

3. Summer Heat Disturbing the Heart

Principle: Eliminate summer heat and resuscitate the patient by using points mainly from The *Du* Channel and The Pericardium Channel of Hand–*Jueyin*.

Prescription: Dazhui (DU14)   Shangxing (DU23)

Quze (PC 3)   Shuigou (DU26)

Shixuan(EX-UE 11)   Hegu(LI   4)

Laogong (PC   8)   Neiguan (PC 6)

Juque (RN14)   Danzhong (RN17)

Explanation: Dazhui (DU 14), the converging point of *Yang*, is used in combination with Shangxing(DU23) to eliminate summer heat from the superficial portion of the body. Quze (PC 3), the *He*-sea point of the pericardium channel, is pricked to cause bleeding in order to disperse the summer heat from the heart. Shuigou (DU26), Shixuan (EX-UE 11) and Hegu(LI 4) which is penetrated towrad Laogong (PC 8) may clear up heat and resusciate the patient with a clear mind. Neiguan(PC 6), Juque (RN14) and Danzhong (RN17) relieve fullness sensation in the chest, regulate *Qi* circulation and calm the heart and mind.

Method: Apply filiform needles with reducing method and retain the needles for 20-30 minutes, manipulating them intermittent for five to six times. Quze (PC 3) and Shixuan (Extra) are pricked to cause bleeding.

4. Seasonal Epidemic Steaming

Principle: Eliminate heat from the body by using points mainly from The Large Intestine Channel of Hand-*Yangming*.

Prescription: Quchi (LI11)   Shaoshang (LU11)

Shangyang (LI   1)   Shaoze(SI 1)

Zhongchong(PC 9)   Hegu(LI 4)

Fengchi(GB20)   Waiguan (SJ 5)

Weizhong (BL 40)

Explanation: Shaoshang (LU 11), Shaoze (SI 1), Shangyang (LI 1) and Zhongchong (PC 9) are respectively the *Jing*-well points of the lung, small intestine, large intestine and pericardium channels. The joint use of these four points may relieve the pathogenic factors both from the interior and exterior of the body, viz, the nutrient and defensive systems. Quchi (LI 11) and Hegu (LI 4) eliminate wind and heat, particularly the wind and heat from the head and facial areas. Fengchi(GB20) and Waiguan(SJ 5) disperse the *Qi* of the *Sanjiao*, eliminate wind-heat, swelling and stop pain. Weizhong (BL 40), the *Xi*-cleft point of blood, can eliminate heat and cool the blood if it is pricked with a three-edged needle.

Point Modification: Add Lieque(LU 7) for sore throat; Tianzhu (BL 10) for headache.

Method: Apply filiform needles with reducing method and retain the needles for 15-20 minutes, manipulating them three to four times. Weizhong (UB40) is pricked with a three-edged needle to cause bleeding.

Alternative Treatment: Auricular Acupuncture

Prescription: Ear Apex   Adrenal gland   Subcortex

Sunjiao Lung   Stomach

Method: Apply filiform needles with strong stimulation and retain the needles for 15-20 minutes, manipulating them one to two times.

6.2 Syncope

The syndrome of syncope, characterized by sudden fainting with loss of consciousness and cold limbs, can be seen in many kinds of diseases. A mild case of syncope only makes the patient faint for a short period of time, then recover spontanously without leaving any sequela, while the severe one can make the patient lose consciousness for a long time, or even cause death. For syncope appearing in shock, sunstroke, hypoglycemia coma and mental diseases in modern medicine, the differentiation and treatment in this section can be referrred to.

Cause and Mechanism

The onset of syncope in most cases is due to a sudden disorder of *Qi* mechanism which leads to abnormal ascending and descending of *Qi* and incoordination between *Yin* and *Yang*. However, the disorderly *Qi* mechanism can be excessive and deficient in nature. The excess type of syncope is characterized by ascending of excessive *Qi* that also causes an excessive upward blood flow. Or the ascending *Qi* brings up food or phlegm to have upward obstruction or lucid *Yang* disturbing. The deficient type of syncope is characterized by poor ascending of lucid *Yang*, sinking of *Qi* and difficult ascending flow of blood to nourish the brain in consequence of syncope. Besides, in the progression of febrile diseases, factors such as excess of *Yin*, deficiency of *Yang*, heat retention in the interior, stagnant *Qi* that can not be dispersed, or stasis of blood can all lead to the incoordination of *Qi* between the *Yin* and *Yang*, leading to onset of syncope.

1. *Qi* Type Syncope

The disorderly *Qi* mechanism due to over emotional upset such as anger, fear or frightening can disturb the *Qi* mechanism in the chest and blocking of lucid *Yang* to end in syncope. Constitutional deficiency of *Yuan*—source *Qi* occasionally aggravated by over strain or stress, or sudden sorrow or fear, can lead to massive dispersing of *Yang* energy and sinking of *Qi* so that the lucid *Yang* can not ascend in consequence of sudden onset of syncope.

2. Blood Type Syncope

Constitutional excess of liver *Yang* plus emotional upset of anger cause the abnormal mechanism of Qi as well as blood in circulation. Excessive upward flowing of Qi and blood disturb the lucid $Yang$ to end in loss of consciousness. Also, collapse of Qi followed by excessive loss of blood may result in sudden syncope.

3. Phlegm Type Syncope

Impaired function of the spleen and stomach in adipose patient with deficient Qi due to diet of greasy or sweat food causes poor spleen in transforming and transporting, retention of dampness to form phlegm and internal retention of turbid phlegm, leading to poor Qi mechanism. Such a poor Qi mechanism encountered by emotional upset will bring the phlegm upward together with the abnormal ascending of Qi to disturb the lucid $Yang$, resulting in sudden onset of syncope.

4. Food Type Syncope

Food retention and dysfunction of transforming and transporting due to improper intake of food causes obstructed Qi mechanism so that suffocating sensation leads to the onset of syncope which is more common in children. However, over—eating enountered by emotional upset can cause abnormal ascending of Qi together with the food. The obstructed Qi mechanism with fullness in the stomach and abdomen can also disturb the lucid $Yang$ to develop syncope.

5. Cold Type Syncope

Constitutional deficiency of kidney yang can cause direct invasion of cold into the interior of the body, leading to onset of syncope because kidney $Yang$ deficiency fails to warm up the channels and collaterals.

6. Heat Type Syncope

The excessive heat retained in the interior of the body that can not be dispersed out causes the heat type of syncope.

Differentiation

Clinically, syncope is manifested by some critical symptoms and signs such as sudden fainting with loss of consciousness, cold limbs and pallor complexion. However, there are apparently some inducing factors for the onset of syncope. Therefore, it is very crucial to know the past history of the condition in order to differentiate if the present attack of syncope is due to any of the following factors such as deficiency, excess, cold, heat, Qi, blood, phlegm or food intake.

1. Qi Type Syncope

(1) Excess Type of Qi Syncope

The main manifestations include sudden fainting due to emotional upset, loss of consciousness, cold limbs, locked jaws and tight fists, rough breathing , thin tongue coating ,and deep wiry pulse.

(2) Deficient Type of Qi Syncope

The patient has deficient body constitution. The onset of syncope follows dizziness after overstrain or sudden fear of frightening. The accopmanying symptoms and signs include pallor complexion, weak breathing, profuse sweating with cold limbs, pale tongue, and deep fainting pulse.

2. Blood Type Syncope

(1) Excess Type of Blood Syncope

The chief manifestations include sudden fainting after violent anger, loss of consciousness, lacked jaws, purplish facial expression and lips, red tongue proper, and deep wiry pulse in most cases.

(2) Deficient Type of Blood Syncope

The chief manifestations include sudden fainting due to excessive loss of blood, pallor complexion, pale lips, tremor of the limbs, sinking eyes and opening mouth, spontaneous sweating, cold skin, weak breathing, pale tongue proper, and rapid thready but forceless pulse.

3. Phlegm Type Syncope

The chief manifestations include sudden fainting, rattling sound in the throat or vomiting of saliva, rough breathing, white greasy tongue coating, and deep slippery pulse.

4. Food Type Syncope

The syncope occuring after food intake together with severe emotional upset, is manifested by sudden fainting, suffocating breathing, distention in the abdominal and epigastric regions, thick greasy tongue coating, and forceful slippery pulse.

5. Cold Type Syncope

The chief manifestations include greenish facial complexion, severe cold limbs, lying with knees drawn up, stools with undigested food but no thirst, pale tongue proper with white coating, and deep thready pulse.

6. Heat Type Syncope

The chief manifestations include fever in the body, headache, thirst, restlessness, feverish sensation in the abdomen and chest, scanty urine and constipation in the first stage, and subsequent mental confusion, cold limbs, red tongue proper with dry yellow tongue coating, and deep forceful rapid pulse.

Treatment

1. Excess Type of Syncope

Principle: Bring back resuscitation by using points mainly from The *Du* Channel and The Pericardium Channel of Hand—*Jueyin*.

Prescription: Shuigou (DU26)   Zhongchong (PC 9)

Neiguan(PC 6)   Zusanli(ST36) Yongquan(KI 1)

Explanation: Shuigou (DU26), a point from The *Du* Channel that communicates with the brain and governs the *Yang*, is used to bring back resuscitation. Zhongchong(PC 9) and Neiguan (PC 6), respectively the *Jing*—well points and Luo—connecting points, also have the effect of resuscitating the patients. Zusanli (ST36) and Yongquan (KI 1) are respectively the *He*—sea point of the stomach channel and the *Jing*—well point of the kidney channel. These two points applied together with moxibustion may restore *Yang Qi* from collapse.

Point Modification: Add Taichong(LR 3) for *Qi* type syncope; Xingjian (LR 2) for blood type syncope; Shenque (RN 8) and Mingmen (DU 4) for cold type syncope; the 12 *Jing*—well points for heat type syncope; Tiantu (RN 22), Juque (RN 14) and Fenglong (ST 40) for phlegm type syncope; and Zhongwan (RN 12) for food type syncope.

Method: Apply filifomr needles with reducing method and retain the needles for 20—30 minutes, manipulating them four to six times. Zusanli (ST36) and Yongquan (KI 1) are applied with moxibustion for 20—30 minutes; and Zhongchong (PC 9) with three—edged needle to cause bleeding.

2. Deficient Type Syncope

Principle: Restore *Yang Qi* from collapse by using points using points mainly from The *Du* Channel and The *Ren* Channel.

Prescription: Shuigou (DU26)   Neiguan (PC 6)

Baihui (DU 20) Qihai (RN 6)

Hegu (LI 4)   Zusanli (ST 36)

Explanation: Renzhong (DU 26) may resuscitate the patient

and clear up the mind. Neiguan (PC 6) can relieve fullness sensation in the chest, strengthen the heart and restore the collapsed *Yang Qi*. Baihui (DU 20) is a point from The *Du* Channel that governs the *Yang* of the general body. Qihai(RN 6) is a point of The *Ren* Channel that governs *Yin* of the body. Baihui(DU 20) may lift yang and restore patients from collapse. Qihai (RN 6) may also restore *Yang Qi* from collapse. The joint use of these two points may regulate *Yin* and *Yang*. Hegu (LI 4) and Zusanli (ST 36) are points from the *Yangming* channels that are richer with *Qi* and blood. These two points in combination may reinforce *Qi* of the middle—*Jiao* regulate *Qi* and blood, and reinforce the anti—pathogenic *Qi*.

Point Modification: Add Shanzhong(RN17) for *Qi* type syncope; Taichong(LR 3) and Sanyinjiao (SP 6) for blood type syncope; Shenque(RN 8) for cold type syncope; and Shixuan (EX—UE 11) for heat type syncope.

Method: Apply filiform needles with reinforcing method and retain the needles for 20—30 minutes, manipulating them four to six times. Baihui(DU20) and Qihai (RN 6) can be applied with moxibustion. Shenque (RN 8) is applied with moxibustion with salt in between.

Alternative Treatment: Auricular Acupuncture

Prescription: Heart Brain Ear—Shenmen

Subcortex Adrenal gland Sympathetic

Method: Apply filiform needles with strong stimulation for 15—20 minutes.

6.3 Collapse Syndrome

Collapse syndrome refers to a critical internal condition

mainly due to exhaustion of *Yang* and *Yin*. It is characterized by pale complexion, cold limbs, shortness of breath with sweating, dull expression, drop of blood pressure with fainting pulse, and even loss of consciousness in the severe cases. It may cover infectious shock, hemorrhagic shock, cardiogenic shock, allergic shock, and drug or food toxic shock in modern medicine.

Cause and Mechanism

Collapse syndrome is often the consequence of exhaustion of Yuan—source energy due to severe constitutional deficiency with lingering diseases, or sudden profuse sweating, heavy vomiting, severe diarrhea, or massive loss of blood. Exhaustion of *Yin* ends the source of nouirshing for the *Yang* that subsequently collapses too. Exhaustion of *Yang* ends the energy to produce more *Yin* which subsequently disappears. Therefore, collapse is the final consequence when *Yin* and *Yang* do not promote, but separate from each other.

Differentiation

1. *Yin* Type Collapse

This type of collapse is mostly seen in many febrile diseases. The chief manifestations include pale complexion and lips, feverish sensation, restlessness, palpitation, profuse sweating that hot and sticky, thirst with desire for drinks, short scanty urine, loss of consciousness in the severe case, and rpaid thready, deep fainting pulse.

2. *Yang* Type Collapse

This type of collapse is mostly due to the aggravation of *Yin* collapsing. The chief manifestations include dark complexion, profuse sweating that is dilute and cool, ice—cold body with no thirst, discharge of stools with undigested food, short urine or enuresis, dull expression, mental confusion in the severe cases, pale tongue with white coating, and weak fainting pulse.

3. Collapse of Both *Yin* and *Yang*

The chief manifestations include loss of consciousness, dull eye expression, opened mouth, platycoria, laryngeal rales, shortness of breath, thick sweating, curled tongue proper, general cold sensation, in continence of urine and stools, and weak fainting pulse.

Treatment

Principle: Restore *Yang* from collapse, regulate *Yin* and *Yang* by using points mainly from The *Ren* Channel, and The *Du* Channel.

Prescription: Shuigou(DU26)　Suliao(DU25)
　　　　　　　Guanyuan (RN 4)　Shenque(RN 8)
　　　　　　　Yongquan(KI 1)　Zusanli (ST 36)
　　　　　　　Neiguan (PC 6)

Explanation: Shuigou (DU 26) and Suliao (DU 25) may resusciatate the patient, invigorate *Yang* and increase the blood pressure. Shenque (RN 8) and Guanyuan (RN 4) restore *Yang* as well as *Yin* from collapsing. Yongquan (KI 1) the *Jing*—well point of the kidney channel moistens *Yin*, recuperating *Yang* and resuscitate the patient. Zusanli (ST 36) strengthens *Yang Qi* and consolidate the superficial to stop sweating. Neiguan(PC 6) strengthens the heart and increases the blood pressure.

Point Modification: Add Hegu (LI 4) and Fuliu (KI 7) for profuse sweating; Fenglong (ST 40) for profuse sputum; and Taiyuan (LU 9) for weak fainting pulse.

Method: Apply filiform needles with reinforcing method and retain the needles for 30–40 minutes, manipulating them five to eight times.

Note: Collapse syndrome is a kind of critical condition due to various factors. Such a condition is often very perplexing with rapid changes. Therefore, it is imperative to closely observe the patient, seize the time and take comprehensive measures to save the patients. It is better to combine traditional Chinese medicine and modern medicine together such as acupuncture with drugs for treating the patient. The combination of acupuncture and drugs in the treatment of collapse not only produces a rapid effect, but also saves the patients who can not be saved by using drugs only.

6.4   Sunstroke

Sunstroke is a kind summer heat attack in dry hot summer days. It is the invasion of summer mixed with dampness into the body for those who stay too long or work under hot sun. Clinically, it is characterized by over consumption of *Yin* by forceful sweating, sudden onset of high fever, profuse sweating, sleepiness, mental confusion, restlessness and convulsions. It is also called sunstroke in modern medicine.

Cause and Mechanism

The invasion of summer heat or summer heat with dampness due to deficiency of body constitution causes heat steaming in the body. The over consumption of body energy, disturbance of summer heat to lucid *Yang* and exhaustion of *Qi* in the channesl and collaterals develop sunstroke.

Differentiation

Clinically, sunstroke is mainly divided into mild and severe types in accordance with the varied severity of the condition. The mild type is manifested by headache, dizziness, suffocating sensation in the chest, nausea, thirst, sweating, high fever, restlessness, soreness and lassitude of the general body. The severe type may repeat all the above manifestations plus profuse sweating, cold limbs, pale complexion, palpitation, shortness of breath, and mental confusion, sudden fainting and convulsion of the four limbs in the severe case.

Treatment

1. Mild Type of Sunstroke

Principle: Eliminate heat and pacify the stomach by using points mainly from The *Du* Channel and The Stomach Channel of Foot−*Yangming*.

Prescription: Dazhui(DU14)   Quze(PC 3)   Hegu(LI 4)
                Taiyang(EX−HN5)   Zusanli(ST 36)
                Neiguan (PC 6)

Explanation: Dazhui (DU 14), the converging of all *Yang,* may eliminate summer heat from the general body. Quze (PC 3) clears away heat from the heart, relieve restlessness sensation and restore the function of the heart in housing the mind. Hegu (LI 4) is combined with Taiyang (EX−HN5) to clears away heat from facial and head areas in order to relieve headache and dizziness. Zusanli (ST 36) is combined with Neiguan (PC 6) to pacify the stomach and stop vomiting, strengthen the heart and calm the mind.

Method: Apply filiform needles with reducing method and retain the needles for 5−10 minutes manipulating them one to two times. Dazhui (DU14), Quze (PC 3) and Taiyang (Extra)may be pricked to cause bleeding.

2. Severe Type of Sunstroke

Principle: Eliminate heat, restore *Yang Qi* from collapse and resuscitate the patient by using points mainly from The *Du* Channel and The Bladder Channel of Foot−Taiyang.

Prescription: Shuigou (DU26)   Dazhui (DU14)

Quze (PC 3)   Weizhong(BL40)

Chegnshan (BL57)   Neiguan(PC6)

Guanyuan(RN 4)   Shenque (RN 8)

12 *Jing*—well points

Explanation: Shuigou (DU26) resuscitates the patient, calms and clears the mind. Dazhui (DU14) eliminates summer heat of the general body. Quze (PC 3) is combined with Weizhong (BL40) to elimnate heat from the heart, relieve retlessness sensation, restore the function of heart in housing the mind and relieve spasm. The 12 *Jing*—well points may eliminate summer heat and clear the mind. Chengshan (BL57) relieves spasm and stop convulsion. Neiguan (PC 6) pacifies the stomach, strengthens the heart and increases the blood pressure . Guanyuan (RN 4) and Shenque (RN 8) strengthen the *Yuan*—source *Qi* and restore patients from sunstroke.

Method: Apply filiform needles with reducing method and retain the needles for 10—15 minutes, manipulating them one to two times. Dazhui (DU 14), Quze (PC 3), Weizhong (BL 40) and the 12 *Jing*—well points may be pricked to cause bleeding.

Alternative Treatment: Scrapping Method

Prescription: Quze(PC 3)   Weizhong(BL40)   Dashu(BL19)
to Sanjiaoshu (BL 22) on both sides of medial line of The urinary Bladder Channel of Foot—*Taiyang*.

Method: Wash and moisten the skin to be scrapped before scrapping is done. Scrap the skin with moisture until local redness of the skin with red purplish spots appear.

7   Miscellaneous Conditions

7.1   Sciatica

Sciatica is a kind of radiating and continuous pain in the course of sciatic nerve distribution, i.e. pain in the hip region, the posterior lasteral aspect of the thigh and leg, and lateral aspect of the foot. According to its etiology, sciatca can be divided into the primary and secondary types. Sciatic neuritis, the primary type, is caused mainly by pathological stimulation, pressing or injuring of the adjacent nerves affecting the sciatic nerve. This is also clinically known as symptomatic sciatica. The secondary sciatica is more common than the primary.

Clinical Manifestations

Primary sciatica is characterized by a sudden onset of continuous sharp pain that aggravates in paroxysmal attacks. The paroxysmal pain, burning and sharp in nature, worsens with cold, but alleviates with warmth. There may appear some points of tenderness along the sciatic nerve. Stretching and raising of leg tests are positive. An increase of ankle flexing is seen in the early stage, but decreases in the later stage without apparent muscular atrophy.

Secondary sciatica is marked by a slow onset of pain which may sometimes involve primary lesions. It is mainly a kind of radiating pain due to lumbar disc degeneration. The pain is often worse with cough, sneezing or halting of the breath. Disc and spinal tenderness are involved. Fewer points of tenderness are found along the course of the sciatic nerve. Stretching and raising of legs tests also appear positive. Chin—chest and Queckenstedt's test appear positive but ankle flexing is mostly decreasing, or disappearing in the severe case. There will be muscular atrophy in the severe case.

Treatment

1. Primary Sciatica

Prescription: Huantiao(GB30)　Fengshi(GB31)
　　　　　　　Yanglingquan(GB34)　Kunlun(BL60)
　　　　　　　Chengshan (BL 57)

Method: Apply filiform needles with reducing method and retain the needles for 15—20 minutes, manipulating them once or twice.

2. Secondary Sciatica

Prescription: Dachangshu(BL25)　Guanyuanshu(BL26)
　　　　　　　Zhibian(BL54)　Weizhong(BL40)
　　　　　　　Yanglingquan(BL40)　Xuanzhong(GB39)
　　　　　　　Kunlun(BL 60)　Huatuojiaji points from L4 to
　　　　　　　L5 on both sides.

Method: Apply filiform needles with even method and retain the needles for 15—20 minutes, manipulating them once or twice.

Alternative Treatment

1. Auricular Acupuncture

Prescription: Sciatic nerve　Buttock　Ear—Shenmen
　　　　　　　Sub—cortex　Sympathetic
　　　　　　　Lumbosacral　vertebrae

Method: Apply filiform needles with moderate stimulation and retain the needles for 20 minutes. Embedding of ear seeds is also applicable.

2. Electric Stimulation

Prescription: Zhibian(BL54)　Yanglingquan(GB34)
　　　　　　　Huantiao(GB30)　Huatuojiaji from L4 to L5

Method: Select two points each time to use electric stimulation in dense–disperse wave form. Electric stimulation is applied for 20minutes each time.

7.2 Occipital Neuralgia

Occipital neuralgia refers to pain in the occipital and upper cervical areas, often caused by some infectious conditions, neck sprain or changes in the cervical vertebrae from C1 to C4.

Clinical Manifestations

Pain in the occipital area and upper cervical area is often induced by awkward movement of the neck, sneezing or cough. During the attack, the patient feels rigid in the neck, and pain that is mostly continuous or aggravated in paroxysmal attacks. There may also some sharping pain even when the attack is over. Tenderness can be detected in the examination. The tender point of the greater occipital nerve is located between the mastoid process and the posterior part of the cervical vertebrae, proximal to Fengchi(GB 20) . The tender point for the minor occipital nerve is near the posterior–superior aspect of them. sternocleidomastoideus, proximal to Yiming (Extra). Patient feel severe pain when these tendernesses are pressed. The pain may also disperse according to the distribution of nerves. Skin allergy or dystrophy may often accompany the condition.

Treatment

Prescription: Fengchi (GB20)   Tianzhu(BL10)

Naokong (GB19)   Head–Wangu (GB12)

Houxi(SI 3)   Kunlun (BL 60)

Method: Apply filiform needles with reducing method and retain the needles for 15–20 minutes, manipulating them two or

three times.

Alternative Treatment: Auricular Acupuncture

Prescription: Ear—Shenmen   Sub cortex   Occipital Neck.

Method: Apply filiform needles with moderate stimulation and retain the needles for 15—20 minutes. Embedding of ear seeds is also applicable.

7.3   Facial Spasm

Facial spasm, more common in women over middle age, refers to spasm on one side of the face in irregular attacks.

Clinical Manifestations

At the beginning, there are only intermittent spasms of the orbicular muscles. Gradually, the spasm involves other muscle of the face. There will be convulsions of the mouth corner in the severe case. The severity of the convulsions or spasm may be aggravated by fatigue, mental stress or physical movement. Convulsions spontaneously stop during the sleep. Some patients may also have headache, and tinnitus. Neurological system examinations show positive signs.

Treatment

Prescription: Taiyang(EX—HN5)   Sibai(ST2)   Dicang(ST 4)

Taichong(LR 3)   Yingxiang(LI20)

Xiaguan(ST 7)   Hegu(LI 4)

Method: Apply filiform needles with reducing method and retain the needles for 15—30 minutes. Electric stimulation with dense—disperse wave for 15—20 minutes is also applicable.

Alternative Treatment: Auricular Acupuncture

Prescription: Sympathetic   Ear—Shenmen   Liver   Taiyang

Cheeks   Subcortex

Method: Apply filiform needles at three to four points with strong stimulation each time and retain the needles for 20 minutes. Embedding of ear seeds or ear subcutaneous needles is also applicable.

7.4 Multiple Neuritis

Multiple neuritis, also known as peripheral neuritis, is a condition chiefly manifested by symmetrical disturbances of the motor, sensory and autonomic nerves in the distal regions of the four extremities. It is mainly caused by infections, toxication, metabolic disorders and allergies among which infections and toxication are considered as the leading causative factors.

Clinical Manifestations

In the early stage of multiple neuritis, numbness and prickly pain may appear in the fingers and toes as if ants are running around in these areas. The condition progressively worsens with typical sensory disturbance like glove–wearing or sock–wearing sensations. In the meanwhile, there will be poor physical movement of the four limbs, muscular atrophy, wrist–drop, foot–drop, and decrease or disappearance of tendon flexing. Besides, there is also cold sensation in the distal ends of the limbs with profuse sweating or without sweating. The clinical manifestations indicating the disturbance of the motor, sensory and autonomic nerves vary due to the fact that there can be different causative factors.

Treatment

Prescription: Jianyu(LI15) Quchi(LI11) Waiguan(SJ 5)
                        Hegu(LI 4) Baxie(EX–UE9) Dazhui(DU14)
                        Taodao(DU13) Zusanli(ST36)
                        Yanglingquan(GB34) Sanyinjiao(SP 6)

Jiexi(ST41)   Bafeng(EX−LE10)

Method: Apply filiform needles with reducing method in the early stage, but reinforcing or even method in the later stage, and retain the needles for 20−40 minutes, manipulating them two to four times. Acupuncture can be combined with moxibustion.

7.5   Radial Nerve Paralysis

Radial nerve paralysis refers to the declined or disappeared motor function of the skeletal muscles controlled by the radial nerve after injury. It is mainly manifested by wristdrop, difficulty in palm extension and wrist lifting. There are many causative factors that can lead to radial nerve paralysis, such as wrist or elbow sprain, fracture of the humerus, or arm pressing due to using the arm as pillow during the sleep, prolonged abduction of the arm during surgical operation, pressure of crutches or tourniquet in incorrect position, as well as lead or alcoholic poisoning.

Clinical Manifestations

The chief manifestations of radial nerve paralysis include wristdrop, dysfunctions of extensor digitorum muscles and thumb in abduction. Sensory function associated with the lesions of the radial nerve is light or confined in most cases to a small area on the posterior radial surface of the hand and the first and second metacarpals of the thumb, index and middle fingers.

Treatment

Prescription: Quchi(LI11)   Zusanli(ST36)   Waiguan(SJ 5)
Yangxi(LI 5)   Yangchi(SJ 4)   Hegu(LI 4)

Method: Apply filiform needles with even method and retain the needles for 20−30 minutes, manipulating them two to three times. Acupuncture and moxibustion may be combined in the treatment. Electric stimulation is also applicable to Quchi (LI 11) and Waiguan (SJ 5) for 20 minutes.

7.6 Paralysis of Ulnar Nerve

Ulnar nerve paralysis refers to the declined or disappeared motor function of skeleton and muscles controlled by the ulnar nerve after injury. The deformity of the fingers is accompanied by sensory disturbance in the affected area. This condition is often caused by injury of the ulnar nerve due to prolonged period of supporting the body with the elbow during work or traumatic injury.

Clinical Manifestations

The chief manifestations include deviation of the hand towards the ulnar side, abducted thumbs, flat thenar eminence minor, flexion of the ring and little fingers, atrophy of hypothenar muscles, lost motor function of the little finger, loss of fine movements of the fingers which appear like claws, and about fifty percent sensory loss on the ulnar aspect of the dorsum of the hand, thenar eminence minor, and the ulnar side of the ring and little finger.

Treatment

Prescription: Xiaohai (SI 8)   Zhizheng (SI 7)

Waiguan (SJ 5)   Yanggu (SI 5)

Hand−Zhongzhu (SJ 3)   Baxie (EX−UE9)

Method: Apply filiform needles with even method and retain the needles for 20−30 minutes, manipulating them two to three times. Electric stimulation may also be applied at Xiaohai (SI 8) and Zhizheng (SI 7) for 20 minutes.

7.7 Paralysis of Common Peroneal Nerve

Paralysis of common peroneal nerve refers to the motor

dysfunction of the skeleton or muscles controlled by the nerve after injury. It is characterized by foot—drop and sensory loss in the
area distributed by the nerve. This condition is caused mainly by
injury, fracture of the head of the fibula, compression in crossing
the knees while the patient is under a plaster splintage or stretching by prolonged squatting.

Clinical Manifestations

The manifestations include foot—drop and inversion of the
foot, difficulty for dorsiflexing of the ankle, extending the toes, or
everting the foot. The gait is characterized by overflexion of the
hip and knee, and slapping of the foot on the floor—step—page
gait. Hypoesthesia or anesthesia in the lateral aspects of the leg or
foot dorsum, and atrophy of anterior tibial muscle.

Treatment

Prescription: Zusanli(ST36)   Yanglingquan(GB34)

                  Tiaokou(ST 38)   Xuanzhong(GB 39)

                  Jiexi(ST41)   Shenmai(BL 62)   Zhaohai(KI 6)

Method: Apply filiform needles with even method and retain
the needles for 20—30 minutes, manipulating them two to three
times. Electric stimulation may be applied to Yanglingquan (GB
34) and Xuanzhong (GB 39) for 20 minutes.

7.8   Neuritis of Lateral Cutaneous Nerve of Thigh

Neuritis of the lateral cutaneous nerve of thigh, also
known   as   meralgia   paresthetica,   is   characterized   by
formication, numbness, pins and needles sensation of the lower
two thirds of the lateral aspect of the thigh. It is more common
inmiddle—aged men who have obese body shape, or pregnant
women.

Clinical Manifestations

The chief manifestations include abnormal formication, prickling or numbness limited to the lower 2 / 3 cutaneous distribution of the anterior lateral aspect of the thigh, and pain which is aggravated by walking or standing. Areas of dysesthesia or anesthesia in different sizes as well as tender points can be detected in the lateral aspect of the thigh.

Treatment

Prescription: Fengshi (GB 31)   Yanglingquan (GB 34)

Sanyinjiao (SP 6)   local areas

Method: Apply filiform needles with even method and retain the needles for 15−30 minutes, manipulating them two to three times. Surrounding needles are applied at hypoesthesia areas. Moxibustion can also be applied for 20−30 minutes.

Alternative Treatment: Plum−blossom Needles

Prescription: Affected areas

Method: Tap the affected areas with the plum−blossom needles mildly until local redness appears, once daily or once every other day.

7.9 Cervical Spondylopathy

Cervical spondylopathy, also called retrograded cervical spondylosis, includes hyperplastic cervical spondylosis and herniation of cervical disc. It is very common in the clinic characterized by numbness and pain in the neck, head, arm and hand accompanied by progressive functional disturbance of sensation and movement caused by opressing of the nerve root or spinal cord. It is more common in adult men than women ranging from 40−60 years of age.

Clinical Manifestation

Pain in the neck and nape often radiates to the shoulder, forearm, finger and frontal chest. The pain is worse by movement of the head or tapping of the vertex. The neck is rigid with movement limitation. There may be sensory disturbance in the corresponding areas together with poor leg flexion. If the condition also affectes the spine, there will be numbness of the lower limbs, heavy sensation, hypermyotonia, muscular weakness and pathological flexes of the lower limbs. There can be incomplete colic paralysis in the severe case. Some patients may be accompanied by headache, head distention, dizziness, vertigo or even fainting when they extend or turn the neck.

Treatment

Prescription: Fengchi(GB20) Bingfeng(SI12) Jianyu (LI15)
Quchi(LI11) Waiguan(SJ 5) Hegu(LI 4)
Houxi(SI 3) Cervical Huatuo Jiaji points

Also, add Huatuo Jiaji points in the lumbar region, Zusanli (St 36) and Yanglingquan (GB 34) for paralysis of the lower limb.

Method: Apply filiform needles with even method and retain the needles for 20—30 minutes, manipulating them two to three times.

Alternative Treatment: Plum—blossom Needles

Prescription: Cervical Huatuo Jiaji points

Method: Tap with mild stimulation once every other day until local redness appears.

7.10 Raynaud's Disease

Raynaud's disease, more often complained by young

women, refers to apasmodic or functional occlusion in the vessels of the distal extremities. Intermittent paleness or cyanosis of the skin may occur due to sudden exposure to cold or abrupt emotional upset. It is accompanied by pain in the toes and fingers.

Clinical Manifestations

The fingers, toes, tip of the nose, and external ears suddenly turn white when there is an abrupt drop of temperature or emotional disturbances. It is accompanied by cold sensation, cold sweating, cyanosis or waxy appearance of the skin with numbness and pain. Before long, the skin turns red, warm and returns normal. In the advanced stage, there will apear continuous pain in the fingers and toes, malnutrition of the fingers and toes, crevices of the fingers and toes and small areas of ulceration but not necrosis. The necrosis only involves the skin provicled that it does happen.

Treatment

Prescription: Points on the upper limb:

        Quchi (LI 11)   Taiyuan (LU 9)

        Neiguan(PC 6) Hegu(LI 4) Houxi(SI 3)

        Points on the lower limb:

        Zusanli (ST 36)   Sanyinjiao (SP 6)

        Taixi (KI 3)   Chongyang (ST 42)

        Taichong (LR 3)

Method: Apply filiform needles with reinforcing method and retain the needles for 15−20 minutes, manipulating them two to three times. Moxibustion is also applicable.

Alternative Treatment: Auricul ar Acupuncture

Prescription· Ear−Shenmen Sympathetic Heart Lung

        Endocrine Adrenal gland

Subcortex Toes Fingers

Method: Apply filiform needles at three to four points with mild stimulation and retain the needles for 15−20 minutes. Embedding of ear seeds is also applicable.

7.11 Erythromelalgia

Erythromelalgia, a kind of vascular disease, is characterized by paroxysmal increase of the temperature at the end of limbs, flushed skin, swelling and severe pain of a burning nature, especially in the soles of the feet or toes. The pain is aggravated by the increase of natural temperature. This condition mosrly affects youngsters although its cause still remains unknown.

Clinical Manifestations

The onset of erythromelalgia is usually slow, but sometimes out of a sudden. In the beginning, the paroxysmal burning pain only involves the distal ends of the limbs such as soles or palms. There can be flushed skin, fever, swelling and perspiration, and increased vascular pulsation in the affected areas. Then the pain further involves the whole limbs. Most attacks occur at night, and the seizure lasts only a few minutes or even a few hours. There still remains local numbnes and pain in between the attacks. The various factors of vasodilation or vascular congestion such as local heat, warming temperature, physical exercices, standing, or even natural lowering of the limbs may lead to the aggravation of the pain. Yet, the pain can relieved by resting, cooling, raising or exposing the affected limbs. Profuse sweating and hypoesthesia in the affected areas makes the patient feel reluctant to wear socks or gloves. The affected nails or terminal skin in the body limbs in repeated attacks may become thickened or suffer from diabrosis, or even occasional necrosis. Generally, there is no sensory or motor disturbance.

Treatment

Prescription:

Upper Extremities: Quchi(LI11)   Waiguan(SJ 5) Hegu(LI 4)
Laogong(PC 8)   Renying (ST 9)

Lower Extremities: Zusanli(ST 36)   Sanyinjiao(SP 6)
Xingjian(LR 2)   Neiting(ST 44)
Yongquan(KI 1)

Method: Apply filiform needles with reducing method and retain the needles for 15–30 minutes, manipulating them three to five times.

Alternative Treatment: Auricular Acupuncture

Prescription: Sympathetic   Ear–Shenmen   Subcortex
Endocrine   Finger   Toe   Adrenal gland

Method: Use filiform needles at three to five points each time with moderate stimulation and retain the needles for 15–20 minutes. Embedding of ear seeds is also applicable.

7.12   Simple Goiter

Simple goiter is a compensatory enlargement of the thyroid gland due to iodine deficiency. The lack of iodine in the body reduces the synthesis of thyroxin and lowers the thyroxin concentration in the blood, resulting in increased secretion of pituitary thyropic hormone, hyperplasia and hypertrophy of the thyroid cells to lead to the enlarge ment of the t yroid glands. Simple goiters, more common in women, can be endemic as well as sporadic.

Clinical Manifestations

Most goiters appear to have diffuse or nodular enlargement without pain nor abnormal change of skin colour. The enlargement is soft by palpating without general symptoms. The endemic goiters have more severe enlargement of thyroid glands surrounding the neck. The enlargement may also press over nearby body organs causing dyspnsea, cough, dysphagia and hoarseness of voice. Sporadic goiters, often symmetrical and lustrous, have less severe enlargement of the thyroid glands in comparason to the endemic type. The thyroid moves upward and downward with swallowing. Over a prolonged period, the goiters may turn hard or become nodular. Laboratory examinations show that the basal metabolic rate and determination of plasma protein—bound iodine appear normal.

Treatment

Prescription: Renying(ST 9)   Shuitu(ST10)

                    Hegu(LI 4)   Quchi(LI 11)   Fengchi (GB 20)

                    Huatuo Jiaji from C3 to C5.

Method: Apply filiform needles with reducing or even method and retain the needles for 15—30 minutes, mani pulating them two to three times.

Alternative Treatment: Auricular Acupunctnre

Prescription: Endocrine   Ear—Shenmen   Thyroid

                    gland   Neck

Method: Apply filiform needles with moderate stimulation and retain the needles for 20 minutes. Embedding of ear seeds is also applicable.

7.13   Hyperthyroidism

Hyperthyroidism is one of the common endocrinal diseases due to excessive secretion of the thyroid gland. Clinically, the accompanying symptoms and signs also include palpitation, profuse sweating, hand tremor, increased intake of food emaciation and restlessness in addition to enlargement of the thyroid glands. Its incidence is high in women at any age, but higher among the young and middle−aged women. The onset of hyperthyroidism is related to many factors such as severe emotional disturbance, menstruation, pregnancy or infectious diseases, for they result in the cerebral cortex dysfunction and produce pathological excitement, leading to hyperthyroidism, hyperplasia and hypertrophy of thyroid gland.

Clinical Manifestations

Mild or medium type of diffuse and symmetric enlargement appears in the anterior neck. Some patients may have simple leaf or nodular enlargement with local tremor or murmuring. The accompanying symptoms and signs include irritability, mental stress with easy emotional disturbances, insomnia, tachycardia, aversion to heat, profuse sweating, slight tremor of the fingers when the hands are horizontally extended, lower grade fever, hyperorexia, emaciation and hypermenorrhea. Some patients also suffer from exophthalmos. Laboratory tests can prove high metabolic rates and higher serum protein−bound iodine synthesis than normal.

Treatment

Prescription: Renying (ST 9)   Jianshi (PC 5)

Sanyinjiao (SP 6)   Taichong (LR 3)

Hegu (LI 4)   Huatuo Jiaji from C3 to C5

Method: Apply filiform needles with both reinforcing and reducing method and retain the needles for 15−20 minutes, manipulating them two to three times.

Point Modification: Add Yinxi (HT 6) and Fuliu (KI 7) for

profuse sweating: Shenmen (HT 7) and Anmian (Extra) for insomnia; and Neiguan (PC 6) and Tongli (HT 5) for tachycardia.

Alternative Treatment: Auricular Acupuncture

Prescription: Ear—Shenmen　Subcortex　Endocrine

Thyroid gland　Dingchuan　Heart　Lung

Method: Apply filiform needles at three to four points each time and retain the needles for 15 minutes. Embedding of ear seeds is also applicable.

7.14　Paralysis Agitans

Paralysis agitans, also known as Parkinson's disease, is a degenerative disease of the central nerve system, usually complained of by patients over middle age. Its main clinical features include tremor, muscular rigidity and hypokinesia.

Clinical Manifestations

The onset of paralysis agitans is slow, but aggravates gradually as time passes by. The incipient tremor occurs at the distal end of the extremities, usually starting from the distal end of the arm such as fingers, which then extends gradually to the lower limb of the same side, and then to the opposite arm and leg. The fingers tremble rhythmically as if to roll balls in the palm, which is also called ball—rolling tremor. This kind of tremor takes place when the patient is quiet, but lessens when he exercises at random; it is aggravated by emotional excitement but disappears completelyduring the sleep. The accompanying symptoms and signs include muscular rigidity and hypermyotonia. Cog—wheel rigidity, the movements interpreted by a series of jerks, may occur with passive flexing or extending of the muscles of the extremities. Patients often show a special body pos-ture typical of forward bending, stooping of shoulders and body trunk and arching of the spine. The gait is slow and shuf-fling without any arm swinging. Some patients may have diffi-culty to start walking, which is then followed by brisk walk to be broken into short—step running with difficulty in stopping or turning directions. Such a gait is called facinating walk. All movements are apparently slow and reduced with indifferent facial expression as if masked face. The hands are unable to perform meticulous actions. Writing is difficult with a tendency of micrographia. Letters in the first part of the sentence may be of normal size, but become progressively smaller in each succes-sive word or phrase. In the advanced stage, patients may suffer from slow and monotonous speech and difficulty in swallowing.

Treatment

Prescription: Renying(ST 9)　Neck—Futu(LI18)

　　　　　　Hegu(LI　4)　Taichong (LR 3)

　　　　　　Yinlingquan (SP 9)

Method: Apply filiform needles with even method and retain the needles for 15—20 minutes, manipulating them two to three times.

Alternative Treatment: Scalp Acupuncture

Prescription: Motor area　Chorea—tremor control area

Method: Apply filiform needles for 30—40 minutes, manip-ulating them three to four times. Electric stimulation with dense—disperse wave for 60 minutes is also applicable.

7.15　Minor Chorea

Minor chorea, also known as rheumatic chorea, is charac-terized by involuntary movements, accompanied by disturbance of voluntary movement, weakness of myodynamia and emotional change. It is mostly seen in children, youngsters, but more often in women. It is mainly caused by rheumatism. However, factors like scarlet fever, diphtheria, encephalitis, hypothyroidism, etc. may also give rise to minor chorea.

Clinical Manifestations

Early symptoms of minor chorea are not always remarkable. It is just manifested by daily restlessness, distractibility, poor progress in studies, clumsy body movements, deviated writings, and frequent losing of objects holding in hand. In certain period of time, patients may have involuntary, rapid and irregular choreiform movements which start on one side and gradually extend to the opposite side. The face often shows unintended frownings, winklings, mouth taping, tongue projecting and nose contracting. These actions can be aggravated by emotional stress. Speech, chewing and sleep can be affected in the severe case, accompanied by weak muscular force, lower muscle tone, poor or even disappeared tendon flexing.

Treatment

Prescription: Dazhui(DU14)　Fengchi(GB20)　Ganshu(BL18)
　　　　　　　Neiguan(PC 6)　Hegu(LI 4)
　　　　　　　Yanglingquan(GB34)　Zusanli(ST 36)
　　　　　　　Taichong(LR 3)　Sanyinjiao (SP 6)

Method: Aplly filiform needles with even method and retain the needles for 20—40 minutes, manipulating them three to four times.

Alternative Treatment:

1. Auricular Acupuncture

Prescription: Heart　Liver　Kidney　Ear—Shenmen

Subcortex   Sympathetic   Occipital bone
Brain stem Tender points in the coresponding
areas

Method: Apply filiform needles at four to five points with moderate stimulation and retain the needles for 15—20 minutes. Embedding of ear seeds or subcutaneous needles is also applicable.

2. Scalp Acupuncture

Prescription: Chorea control area   Motor area

Method: Apply filiform needles for 30—40 minutes, manipulating them three to five times. Electric stimulation with dense—disperse wave can also be applied for 60 minutes.

7.16 Leukopenia

Leukopenia refers to a continual lower index of leukocytes below $4\ 000 / mm^3$. This condition is mainly caused by neutropenia. Clinically, it is divided into primary and acquired types of leuko—penia, but the former is more common.

Clinical Manifestations

Patients with primary leukopenia may appear asymptomatic, or become easily tired with general weakness, lower grade fever, night sweating and insomnia following a chronically benign course. Most patients do not show obvious deteriorative manifestations despite prolonged history of the condition. The absolute leukocyte index may remain between $3\ 000$ to $4\ 000 / mm^3$. The index of granulocyte is normal or slightly lower with occasional marked fluctuation. The hemoglobin concentration and platelet indexes are mostly normal or slightly lower. The clinical manifestations of acquired leukopenia depend on the primary one.

Treatment

Prescription: Dazhui(DU14) Ganshu(BL18) Pishu(BL20)
Gaohuangshu(BL43) Geshu(BL17)
Quchi(LI 11) Zusanli(ST36) Sanyinjiao(SP 6)
Shenshu(BL 23)

Method: Apply filiform needles with even method and retain the needles for 15−20 minutes, manipulating them two to three times. Dazhui(DU14), Gaohuangshu(BL43), Pishu(BL20) and Zusanli(ST 36) may also be applied with moxibustion for 10−15 minutes in addition to acupuncture treatment.

Note: The primary diseases of secondary leukopenia should be mainly treated, and acupuncture can be also applied.

7.17 Obesity

Obesity refers to excessive accumulation of fat in the subcutaneous or other body tissues by at least 15−20% over the normal weight. Clinically, obesity can be divided into simple and secondary types. The former is mainly due to over eating of greasy or sweet food that exceeds the normal consumption of body heat, resulting in the accumulation of fat in the body. Such patients do not present endocrinal dysfunctions despite their obesity. Secondary obesity is caused by hypothalamic pituitary lesions and over secretion of hydrocortisone. I n the meantime, such patients do present some neurological and endocrinal dysfunctions.

Clinical Manifestations

Patients are at certain level of obese condition, especially fat accumulations in the neck, lower abdomen and buttock. Mild obese patients do not present other symptoms and signs. However, severe obese patients do have some metabolic disturbances such as aversion to heat, profuse sweating, fatigue, dizziness and headache palpitation, and abdominal distention..

Treatment

Prescription: Renying(ST 9)   Yishu(EX)   Zusanli(ST36)
            Shuifen (RN 9)   Fuliu (KI 7)

Method: Apply filiform needles with even method and retain the needles for 15–30 minutes, mamipulating them two to three times.

Alternative Treatment

1. Auri cular Acupuncture

Prescription: Sympathetic   Ear–Shenmen   Stomach
            Mouth   Endocrine   Subcortex
            Hunger point   Sunjiao

Method: Apply filiform needles at three to four points with mild stimulation and retain the needles for 15–20 minutes. Embedding of ear seeds or subcutaneous needles is also applicable..

2. Plum–blossom Needle Therapy

Prescription: Huatu Jiaji points from T7 to T12.

Method: At the time when the body points are used, tap the above points until local redness appears. Treatment is given once every other day.

Note: 1. Acupuncture is more effective for the treatment of simple obesity. It is imperative to combine acupuncture with other comprehensive treatments for secondary obesity according to the exact cause.

2. Auxillary treatment is necessary when acupuncture treatment is being given. It is highly significant to advise patients to go on a diet and take part in physical exercises. Patients are encouraged to have food of low salt, low protein, low fat and low sugar, and to eat plenty of vegetables.

7.18 Motion Sickness

Carsickness or seasickness refers to the dizziness and vomiting during travelling by bus, train, plane or ship. Irregular movement, over stimulation of vestibulum of the inner ear cause neurological dysfunctions. In the meantime, mental stress, visual effects or unpleasant smells may also cause the problem.

Clinical Manifestations

In the mild case, there may appear nausea, vomiting, dizziness and blurring of vision. In severe case, there can be fainting, pallor complexion, cold limbs, and profuse cold sweat.

Treatment

Prescription: Neiguan (PC 6)   Zusanli (ST 36)
　　　　　　　Baihui (DU 20)   Fengchi (GB 20)

Method: Apply filiform needles with even method and retain the needles for 20—30 minutes, 40—60 minutes, manipulating them three to four times.

Alternative Treatment: Auricular Acupuncture

Prescription: Ear—Shenmen   Sympathetic   Occipitus
　　　　　　　Stomach   Adrenal gland   Subcortex

Method: Apply embedding of ear seeds or subcutaneous needles and press the embedded points every 10 to 20 minutes for 10—20 times for the pressing of each point.

Note: For people who have habitual sickness by travel, Neiguan (PC 6) and Zusanli (ST 36) before the proposed trip in order to prevent sickness. Embedding of ear seeds or subcutaneous needles can also be applied for preventive purposes. But for very severe case of trainsick or shipsick passengers, firstaid is necessary.

7.19 Acupuncture for Quitting Smoking

This is an approach through acupuncture treatment to cause smokers to dislike the smell from cigarette smoking in order to achieve the purpose of stopping smoking.

Clinical Manifestations

Chain smokers may have lassitude, restlessness, frequent yawning and slow responses when they suddenly stop smoking.

Treatment

Prescription: Renying(ST 9) Zusanli(ST36)

Taichong(LR 3) Hegu(LI 4)

Method: Apply filiform needles with reducing method and retain the needles for 20—30 minutes, manipulating them two to three time. Zhusanli(ST36) and Taichong(LR 3) can be needled with electric stimulation in densedisperse wave form. Electric stimulalion is applied for 15~20 minutes.

Aternative Treatment: Auricular Acupuncture

Prescription: Sympathetic Shenmen Lung Bronchea

Stomach Mouth Endocrine

Method: Apply filiform needle at three to four points with strong stimulation and retain the needles for 15—20 minutes. Subcutaneous needles are also applicable.

Note: Patients receiving acupuncture treatment will have apparently less desire for smoking in two to three days. Some of them may even stop smoking. They also taste change in the mouth which drives the patients to smoke less and less. It is advisable to ask the patient to increase nutritional food in his diet, and take some herbal pills that have the effect to calm the heart and mind as well as some vitamin pills.

6

针 灸 治 疗 学

序

　　《英汉实用中医药大全》即将问世,吾为之高兴。

　　歧黄之道,历经沧桑,永盛不衰。吾中华民族之强盛,由之。世界医学之丰富和发展,亦由之。然而,世界民族之差异,国别之不同,语言之障碍,使中医中药的传播和交流受到了严重束缚。当前,世界各国人民学习、研究、运用中医药的热潮方兴未艾。为使吾中华民族优秀文化遗产之一的歧黄之道走向世界,光大其业,为世界人民造福,徐象才君集省内外精英于一堂,主持编译了《英汉实用中医药大全》。是书之问世将使海内外同道欢呼雀跃。

　　世界医学发展之日,当是歧黄之道光大之时。

　　吾欣然序之。

中华人民共和国卫生部副部长

兼国家中医药管理局局长

世界针灸学会联合会主席

中国科学技术协会委员

中华全国中医学会副会长

中国针灸学会会长

胡熙明

1989 年 12 月

序

　　中华民族有同疾病长期作斗争的光辉历程，故而有自己的传统医学——中国医药学。中国医药学有一套完整的从理论到实践的独特科学体系。几千年来，它不但被完好地保存下来，而且得到了发扬光大。它具有疗效显著、副作用小等优点，是人们防病治病，强身健体的有效工具。

　　任何一个国家在医学进步中所取得的成就，都是人类共同的财富，是没有国界的。医学成果的交流比任何其他科学成果的交流都应进行得更及时，更准确。我从事中医工作30多年来，一直盼望着有朝一日中国医药学能全面走向世界，为全人类解除病痛疾苦作出其应有的贡献。但由于用外语表达中医难度较大，中国医药学对外传播的速度一直不能令人满意。

　　山东中医学院的徐象才老师发起并主持了大型系列丛书《英汉实用中医药大全》的编译工作。这个工作是一项巨大工程，是一种大型科研活动，是一个大胆的尝试，是一件新事物。对徐象才老师及与其合作的全体编译者夜以继日地长期工作所付出的艰苦劳动，克服重重困难所表现出的坚韧不拔的毅力，以及因此而取得的重大成绩，我甚为敬佩。作为一个中医界的领导者，对他们的工作给予全力支持是我应尽的责任。

　　我相信《英汉实用中医药大全》无疑会在中国医学史和世界科学技术史上找到它应有的位置。

中华全国中医学会常务理事
山东省卫生厅副厅长

张奇文

1990年3月

出 版 前 言

中国医药学是我中华民族优秀文化遗产之一，建国以来由于党和国家对待中医药采取了正确的政策，使中医药理论宝库不断得到了发掘整理，取得了巨大的成绩。当前，世界各国人民对中国医药学的学习和研究热潮日益高涨。为促进这一热潮更加蓬勃的发展，为使中国医药学能更好地为全人类解除病痛服务，就必须促进中医中药在世界范围内的传播和交流，而要使这一传播和交流进行得更及时、更准确，就必须首先排除语言障碍。因此，编译一套英汉对照的中医药基本知识的书籍，供国内外学习、研究中医药时使用，已成为国内外医药学界和医药学教育界许多人士的迫切需要。

多年来，在卫生部门的号召下，在"中医英语表达研究"方面，已经作出了一些可喜的成绩。本书《英汉实用中医药大全》的编辑出版就是在调查上述研究工作的历史和现状的基础上，继续对中医药英语表达作较系统、较全面的研究，以适应中国医药学对外传播交流的需要。

这部"大全"的版本为英汉对照，共有 21 个分册，一个分册介绍论述中国医药学的一个分科。在编著上注意了中医药汉文稿的编写特色，在内容上注意了科学性、实用性、全面性和简明易读。汉文稿的执笔撰写者主要是有 20 年以上实践经验的教授、副教授、主任医师和副主任医师。各分册汉文稿撰写成后，均经各学科专家逐一审订。各分册英文主译、主审主要是国内既懂中医又懂英语的权威人士，还有许多中医院校的英语教师及医药卫生部门的专业翻译人员。英译稿脱稿后，经过了复审、终审，有些译稿还召开全国 22 所院校和单位人员参加的英译稿统稿定稿研讨会，对英译稿进行细致的研讨和推敲，对如何较全面、较系统、较准确地用英语表达中国医药学进行了探讨，从而推动整个译文达到较高水平，因此，这部"大全"可供中医院校高年级学生作为泛读教材使用。

这部"大全"的编纂得到了国家教育委员会、国家中医药管理局、山东省教育委员会、山东省卫生厅等各部门有关领导的支持。在国家教委高等教育司的指导下，成立了《英汉实用中医药大全》编译领导委员会。还得到了全国许多中医院校和中药生产厂家领导的支持。

希望这部"大全"的出版，对中医院校加强中医英语教学，对国内卫生界培养外向型中医药人才，以及在推动世界各国人民对中医药的学习和研究方面，都将产生良好的影响。

高等教育出版社

1990 年 3 月

前　言

　　《英汉实用中医药大全》是一部以中医基本理论为基础，以中医临床为重点，较为全面系统、简明扼要、易读实用的中级英汉学术性著作。它的主要读者是：中医药院校高年级学生和中青年教师，中医院的中青年医生和中医药科研单位的科研人员，从事中医对外函授工作的人员和出国讲学或行医的中医人员，西学中人员，来华学习中医的外国留学生和各类进修人员。

　　由于中国医药学为我中华民族之独有，因此，英译便成了本《大全》编译工作的重点。为确保译文能准确表达中医的确切含义，我们邀集熟悉中医的英语人员、医学专业翻译人员、懂英语的中医药人员乃至医古文人员于一堂，共同翻译、共同对译文进行研讨推敲的集体翻译法，这样，就把众人之长融进了译文质量之中。然而，即使这样，也难确保译文都能尽如人意。汉文稿虽反映了中国医药学的精髓和概貌，但也难能十全十美。我衷心地盼望读者能提出批评和建议，以便《大全》再版时修改。

　　参加本《大全》编、译、审工作的人员达 200 余名，他们来自全国 28 个单位，其中有山东、北京、上海、天津、南京、浙江、安徽、河南、湖北、广西、贵阳、甘肃、成都、山西、长春等 15 所中医学院，还有中国中医研究院，山东省中医药研究所等中医药科研单位。

　　山东省教育委员会把本《大全》的编译列入了科研计划并拨发了科研经费，山东省卫生厅和一些中药生产厂家也给了很大支持，济南中药厂的资助为编译工作的开端提供了条件。

　　本《大全》的编译成功是全体编译审者集体劳动的结晶，是各有关单位主管领导支持的结果。在《大全》各分册即将陆续出版之际，我诚挚地感谢全体编译审者的真诚合作，感谢许多专家、教授、各级领导和生产厂家的热情支持。

愿本《大全》的出版能在培养通晓英语的中医人才和使中医早日全面走向世界方面起到我所期望的作用。

主编　徐象才

于山东中医学院

一九九〇年三月

目　录

说　明

　　《针灸治疗学》是大型系列丛书《英汉实用中医药大全》的第 6 分册。

　　本分册有内科病证、外科病证、妇科病证、儿科病证、五官科病证、急证和其他病证共七章。按病证特点，病因病机，辨证分型，分型治疗，其他疗法等项详细介绍了 135 个临床常见病证的针灸治疗方法。分型治疗包括治则、处方、方义、随证取穴和针刺法，其他疗法包括灸法、耳针、耳穴压豆、头针、火针、皮肤（即梅花）针、电针、刺络拔罐、挑治、激光治疗等疗法的取穴和操作。因此，本分册可供国内外广大读者作为针灸临床的参考。

　　中国针灸学会副会长、北京国际针灸培训中心副主任程莘农教授审定了汉文稿。南京国际针灸培训中心的尤本林先生，新西兰朋友约翰·布莱克审校了英文稿。北京中医学院的方廷钰教授审校了部分英文稿。

　　本分册采用了中华人民共和国国家技术监督局 1990 年发布，1991 年 1 月 1 日实施的标准经穴部位。

编　者

1 内科病证

1.1 感冒

感冒，俗称伤风，是以鼻塞，流涕，咳嗽，头痛，发热，恶寒，脉浮为主证的临床常见外感病。一年四季均可发生，但以秋冬发病率为高。

本病包括由病毒或细菌感染引起的上呼吸道炎症，流行性感冒等。

病因病机

本病多因感受风邪所致。但风邪多与寒热暑湿之邪夹杂为患，秋冬多感风寒，春夏多感风热，长夏多夹暑湿。感受风寒则寒邪束表，毛窍闭塞，肺气不宣；感受风热则热邪犯肺，肺失清肃，皮毛疏泄失常；挟有暑湿则阻遏清阳，留连难解。

辨证

1. 风寒　恶寒重，发热轻，无汗，头痛，鼻塞流涕，咽痒咳嗽，痰白清稀，肢体酸痛，舌苔薄白，脉浮紧。

2. 风热　发热重，恶寒轻，恶风汗出，头痛，鼻塞流浊涕，咽喉肿痛，口干欲饮，咳嗽，咯痰黄稠，舌苔薄黄，脉浮数。

3. 暑湿　高热无汗，头胀痛如裹，身重困倦，胸闷泛恶，食欲不振，腹胀便溏，咳嗽不甚，痰白而粘，舌苔厚腻或黄腻，脉濡数。

治疗

1. 风寒

治则：祛风散寒，解表宣肺。取手太阴、阳明和足太阳经穴为主。

处方：列缺　风门　风池　合谷

方义：列缺为手太阴之络穴，取之以宣肺止咳；太阳主一身之表，取风门以疏调太阳经气，祛风散寒解表；风池为足少阳与阳维之会，阳维主阳主表，故取之以疏解表邪；太阴阳明互为表里，取阳明原穴合谷以增祛邪解表之功力，助上穴功效更捷。

随证选穴：头痛加印堂、太阳；鼻塞配迎香。

刺灸法；毫针刺，用泻法。体虚者亦可用平补平泻手法。留针15～20分钟，间歇行针2～3次。风池、风门亦可针后加灸。

2. 风热

治则：疏散风热，清利肺气。取督脉，手太阴、阳明经穴为主。

处方：大椎　曲池　合谷　鱼际　尺泽

方义：大椎为诸阳之会，取之以表散阳邪，疏散高热；合谷、曲池分别为手阳明原穴和合穴，阳明与太阴相表里，泻之能清肺气而退热；手太阴荥穴鱼际配合穴尺泽能清泄肺热，通利咽喉，化痰止咳。五穴相配可达宣散风热，清肃肺气之目的。

随证选穴：咽喉肿痛加少商；高热、痉厥加十宣。

刺灸法：毫针刺，用泻法。留针15～20分钟，间歇行针2～3次。大椎、少商、十宣用三棱针点刺放血。

3. 暑湿

治则：清暑，解表，化湿。取太阴、阳明、三焦经穴为主。

处方：孔最　合谷　中脘　足三里　外关

方义：取孔最、合谷宣肺解表，清暑化湿；中脘、足三里化痰降浊，和胃止呕；外关为手少阳之络穴，可通调三焦气化。配合诸穴共收祛暑化湿之效。

随证选穴：热重加大椎，委中；湿重加阴陵泉；腹胀便溏加天枢。

刺灸法：毫针刺，用泻法。留针15～20分钟，间歇行针2～3次。大椎、委中可用三棱针点刺出血。

其他疗法

1. 耳针

取穴：肺 气管 内鼻 咽喉 耳尖 胃 脾 三焦 肾上腺 皮质下

操作方法：毫针刺，每次选 3～4 穴，用强刺激。留针 10～20 分钟。亦可用耳针埋藏或耳穴压豆法。

2. 艾灸

感冒流行期间，早晚灸大椎、风门、足三里，每次每穴灸 15～20 分钟，有益气固表，健运脾胃，增强人体自身免疫功能，是预防感冒有效之法。

1.2 咳嗽

凡因感受外邪或脏腑功能失调，而影响肺的正常肃降功能，造成肺气上逆作咳，咳吐痰涎的即称咳嗽。中医认为有声无痰叫咳，有痰无声叫嗽，有痰有声谓之咳嗽。因为临床二者并见，所以总称咳嗽。根据发病原因不同，可分为外感和内伤咳嗽两大类型。

咳嗽常见于现代医学的上呼吸道感染，急慢性支气管炎，支气管扩张、肺炎、肺结核等。

病因病机

外感咳嗽，多因风寒，风热之邪侵袭肺卫，肺气失宣，清肃失常引起。

内伤咳嗽，多由咳嗽反复发作，肺气久伤，肺虚及脾，脾虚生湿，湿盛生痰，痰湿上渍于肺，肺气不降而致。或因肝气郁结，气郁化火，灼肺伤津导致咳嗽。

辨证

1. 外感咳嗽

（1）风寒　咳嗽喉痒、痰稀色白，咯吐不畅，伴有恶寒，发热，无汗，头痛，鼻塞流涕，肢体酸楚，舌苔薄白，脉浮紧。

（2）风热 咳嗽频剧，气粗，咽痛口干，咯痰不爽，痰黄质粘，兼有头痛，身热恶风，有汗不畅，鼻流黄涕等，舌苔薄黄，脉浮数。

2. 内伤咳嗽

（1）痰浊阻肺 咳嗽多痰，痰白而粘，胸脘痞闷，神倦纳呆，舌苔白腻，脉滑。

（2）肺燥阴虚 干咳无痰或痰少，不易咳出，咳引胸胁而痛，口渴咽干，手足心热或午后潮热，舌红，苔薄黄少津，脉弦数或细数。

治疗

1. 外感咳嗽

（1）风寒

治则：疏风散寒、宣肺止咳。取手太阴、阳明经穴为主。

处方：列缺 肺俞 合谷 外关

方义：列缺为手太阴之络穴，配肺俞以宣肺止咳；合谷配外关以发汗解表。四穴同用共奏疏风散寒、宁肺止咳之功效。

随证选穴：头痛加风池、上星；痰多加丰隆；肢体酸楚加昆仑、温溜。

刺灸法：毫针刺，用泻法。留针15～20分钟，间歇行针3～4次。肺俞可针后加灸，每次灸15～20分钟。

（2）风热

治则：疏风清热，止咳化痰、取手太阴、阳明、督脉经穴为主。

处方：尺泽 肺俞 大椎 曲池

方义：尺泽是手太阴肺经之合穴，五行输中的水穴，配肺俞以泻肺化痰止咳，大椎为诸阳之会，督脉要穴，取之通阳解表；配曲池疏风清热。诸穴相配可使风热外解，痰火得降，肺气平顺而咳嗽可止。

随证选穴：咽痛加少商；汗出不畅加合谷；咳嗽痰多加天

突、丰隆。

刺灸法：毫针刺，用泻法。留针 15～20 分钟，间歇行针 2～3 次。大椎、少商多用三棱针点刺出血。

2. 内伤咳嗽

(1) 痰浊阻肺

治则：调补肺气，健脾化痰。取背俞、手足太阴、阳明经穴为主。

处方：肺俞　脾俞　太渊　太白　丰隆

方义：脾为生痰之源，肺为贮痰之器。取肺之原穴太渊和脾之原穴太白，配其肺俞、脾俞为标本同治，是医痰浊阻肺之大法；丰隆为足阳明络穴，能健运中焦脾胃之气，使气行津布，痰浊得化，而肺脏自安。

随证选穴：咳嗽兼喘加定喘穴；胸脘痞闷加足三里、内关。

刺灸法：毫针刺，用补法或平补平泻法。留针 15～20 分钟，间歇行针 2～3 次。脾俞、肺俞可用灸法，灸 10～15 分钟。

(2) 肺燥阴虚

治则：益阴润燥，清肺止咳。取手太阴、足厥阴经穴为主。

处方：肺俞　中府　列缺　照海　太冲

方义：中府为肺之募穴，与肺俞合用为俞募配穴，以宣调肺道，清肃肺气；列缺、照海二穴合用为八脉交会配穴，以益阴润燥，清利咽喉，肃降肺气；太冲为肝之原穴，可平肝降火。诸穴相配共奏益阴润燥降火，清肺化痰止咳之效。

随证选穴：咯血加孔最、膈俞。

刺灸法：毫针刺，用平补平泻法，太冲用泻法。留针 15～20 分钟，间歇行针 2～3 次。

其他疗法：耳针

取穴：肺　支气管　神门　枕点　肾上腺　交感　脾　肾

操作方法：毫针刺。每次选 3～4 穴，用中等刺激，留针 10～20 分钟，亦可用耳穴压豆法。

1.3 哮喘

哮喘是一种发作性的以哮鸣气促，呼气延长，发作时不能平卧为主要临床特征的疾患。哮喘本属两症："哮以声响言"，即以呼吸急促，喉中有哮鸣声为主证；"喘以气息言"，即以呼吸急促，甚至张口抬肩为特征。但两者在临床上每同时举发，难以分开，而且病因病机，治则也大致相似，故作一症名为"哮喘"。

本病具有反复发作的特点，一年四季都可发作，尤以寒冷季节气候急剧变化时发病较多。

哮喘包括现代医学的支气管哮喘，喘息性支气管炎等。

病因病机

导致哮喘的病因甚多，但总不外外感和内伤两种因素引起。故凡因外感风寒，侵袭于肺，肺气不得宣畅；或饮食不节，脾失健运，积湿生痰，久郁化热，痰热内结，阻塞气道；或久病肺弱，咳伤肺气；或劳欲伤肾，正气亏损，精气内伤，肾不纳气等均可致哮喘。

辨证

1. 发作期

(1) 寒邪伏肺　　呼吸困难，咳嗽气促，喉中有哮鸣音，咯痰清稀色白，形寒无汗，面色晦暗带青，四肢不温，口不渴，或兼头痛身痛等证，舌苔白或白腻，脉浮紧或浮滑。

(2) 痰热伏肺　　呼吸急促，声高气粗，发热面红，痰稠色黄，咯痰不爽，胸膈满闷，渴喜冷饮，小便黄赤，大便秘结，舌苔黄腻，脉滑数。

2. 缓解期

(1) 脾肺气虚　　喘促气短，语言无力，咳声低沉，动则汗出，面色㿠白，食少纳呆，颜面、四肢浮肿，舌质淡，苔白，脉濡弱。

(2) 脾肾两虚　　咳嗽气短，动则气促，张口抬肩，气短不续，形疲神惫，腰膝酸软，脑转耳鸣，盗汗遗精，形寒肢冷，面色黧黑，舌质淡，脉沉细。

治疗

1. 发作期

(1) 寒邪伏肺

治则：宣肺散寒，豁痰平喘。取手太阴、足太阳经穴为主。

处方：列缺　肺俞　风门　人迎　定喘

方义：列缺为手太阴络穴，能宣肺解表散寒；肺俞、风门为足太阳经穴而位近肺脏，有宣肺散寒之效；人迎为足阳明经穴，位于结喉旁，配经外奇穴定喘可豁痰平喘。诸穴合用以达解表散寒，宣肺豁痰，平喘之目的。

刺灸法：毫针刺，用泻法或平补平泻法。留针 15～20 分钟，间歇行针 2～3 次。肺俞、风门多用灸法或针灸并用，每穴灸 10～15 分钟，或针后拔火罐。

(2) 痰热伏肺

治则：宣肺清热，涤痰利气。取手太阴、阳明经穴为主。

处方：尺泽　孔最　大椎　丰隆　膻中　合谷

方义：尺泽为手太阴合穴，五行输中之水穴，配手太阴肺经之郄穴，孔最能宣肺清热；合谷，大椎疏表散热；足阳明络穴丰隆配气之会穴膻中，有涤痰利气之功。诸穴配伍可达清热肃肺、涤痰平喘之功效。

随证选穴：喘甚者加肺俞、中府。

刺灸法：毫针刺，用泻法。留针 15～20 分钟，间歇行针 2～3 次。

2. 缓解期

(1) 脾肺气虚

治则：健脾益气、补土生金。取太阴、阳明、背俞穴为主。

处方：太渊　肺俞　足三里　太白　膏肓俞

方义：肺之原穴太渊，为手太阴经之土穴，配肺俞以补益肺气；足三里为足阳明经之土穴，太白为脾之原穴，肺属金，脾胃属土，土能生金，虚则补其母，故取之以培土生金；膏肓俞善治虚劳咳嗽气喘。诸穴相配共收扶正培本，化痰平喘之功效。

刺灸法：毫针刺，用补法。留针 20～30 分钟，间歇行针 2～3 次。肺俞、膏肓俞可用灸法，每穴灸 10～15 分钟。

(2) 肺肾两虚

治则：肺肾双补，益气定喘。取足少阴，任脉经穴为主。

处方：太溪　肾俞　肺俞　膻中　关元

方义：太溪为肾之原穴，配肾俞可补肾中真元之气；膻中为气之会穴，配肺俞以益气定喘；关元亦名丹田，可通调三焦，补益一身之气。五穴配伍应用有补肾纳气，益气定喘的作用。

随证选穴：兼见心气虚弱，心慌气喘不得息者加内关，以强心定喘。

刺灸法：毫针刺，用补法。留针 20～30 分钟，间歇行针 2～3 次。肾俞、肺俞、关元可用灸法，每穴灸 10～15 分钟。

其他疗法

1. 耳针

取穴：肺　平喘　气管　肾　肾上腺　皮质下　交感　神门　内分泌

操作方法：毫针刺。每次选 3～4 穴，用强刺激，留针 10～15 分钟。亦可用耳穴压豆或耳针埋藏。

2. 伏灸

取穴：肺俞　膏肓俞　脾俞　肾俞

操作方法：用艾炷如枣核大，隔姜灸，每穴 3～5 壮，不发泡，皮肤微红为度，每日一次，在夏季三伏天施灸。

1.4 咳血

咳血是肺络受伤所引起的病证，其血由肺而来。以咳嗽痰中带血丝或痰血相兼或纯血鲜红，间夹泡沫为主症。

咳血常见于现代医学的支气管扩张，肺脓肿，肺结核，肺癌等。

病因病机

咳血常因肺阴素虚，复感风热燥邪，上犯肺系，清肃失司，肺络受伤而致；或因情志内伤，肝火偏旺，火邪上乘迫肺，灼伤肺络引起；亦有因久病肺肾阴亏，阴虚火旺，虚火上炎，扰及脉络而致咳血。

辨证

1. 风热伤肺　　喉痒咳嗽，痰中带血，血色鲜红，口渴，咽痛，或有恶寒发热，头痛，舌苔薄黄，脉浮数。

2. 肝火犯肺　　咳嗽，痰中带血或见纯血鲜红，烦躁易怒，胸胁牵痛，口苦而干，大便干燥，小便短赤，舌质红，苔薄黄，脉弦数。

3. 阴虚火旺　　干咳痰少，痰中带血或反复咳血，血色鲜红，潮热盗汗，颧部红艳，口干咽燥，形体消瘦，眩晕耳鸣，舌质红，少苔、脉细数。

治疗

1. 风热伤肺

治则：清热润肺，宁络止血。取手太阴，阳明经穴为主。

处方：列缺　鱼际　孔最　合谷

方义：列缺为手太阴之络穴，配荥穴鱼际及大肠之原穴合谷的清泄风热，润肺凉血；孔最为手太阴之郄穴，可益肺止血，是治咳血之要穴。诸穴合用，共奏清热润肺，宁络止血之功效。

随证选穴：发热恶寒加大椎、曲池。

刺灸法：毫针刺，用泻法。留针15～20分钟，间歇行针2～3次。

2. 肝火犯肺

治则：泻肝清肺，和络止血。取厥阴，手太阴经穴为主。

处方：肺俞　鱼际　孔最　行间　劳宫

方义：肺俞配鱼际、孔最可泻肺热以和络止血；行间泻肝火，降逆气，使血有所藏；劳宫可清血热以止血妄行。四穴相合共达泻肝清热，和络止血之目的。

随证选穴：烦躁易怒加神门、太冲；便秘加支沟。

刺灸法：毫针刺，用泻法。留针 15～20 分钟，间歇行针 2～3 次。

3. 阴虚火旺

治则：益阴养肺，清热止血。取手太阴，足少阴经穴为主。

处方：尺泽 鱼际 孔最 太溪 然谷

方义：尺泽为手太阴之合穴，五行输中属水，鱼际为手太阴之荥穴属火，补尺泽、泻鱼际，可益肺阴、清肺热以止血；肺经郄穴孔最益肺止血；肾之原穴太溪与肾经荥穴然谷，可益阴清热。诸穴共奏滋阴降火，清热止血之功。

随证选穴：潮热盗汗加阴郄、大椎。

刺灸法：毫针刺，补泻兼施，尺泽、太溪、然谷多用补法，鱼际、孔最多用泻法。留针 15～20 分钟，间歇行针 2～3 次。

其他疗法：耳针

取穴：肺 气管 心 肾 肾上腺 皮质下 内分泌 神门

操作方法：毫针刺。每次选 3～4 穴，用中等刺激，留针 10～15 分钟。或用耳穴压豆法。

1.5 失音

失音亦称喉瘖。以讲话声音嘶哑，甚至不能发音为主证。发病有急有缓，急者猝然而起，缓者逐渐形成，故根据病情缓急又有"暴瘖"、"久瘖"之分。

本病属于喉咙、声道的局部疾患，应与中风舌强不语，语言塞涩之"舌瘖"和妊娠的"子瘖"作鉴别。

现代医学的急慢性喉炎，喉头结核，声带劳损，声带小结以及癔病性失音等，均可参考本节辨证施治。

病因病机

导致失音的原因甚多，但概括起来可分为外感、内伤两大类。凡因风寒外袭，邪郁于肺，肺气失宣，气机不利，或因风热犯肺，蒸热成痰，壅塞肺气，或因情志郁结，气郁化火，声门不利而致猝然声哑者为外感。外感属实，中医称为"金实不鸣"；凡因久病体虚，肺燥津伤或肺肾阳虚，精气耗损，声道失于润泽而致失音由轻渐重者多为内伤，内伤属虚。中医称为"金破不鸣"。

辨证

1. 实证

（1）风寒　　猝然声音嘶哑，兼有咳嗽不爽，胸闷，鼻塞，头痛，寒热等症，舌苔薄白，脉浮。

（2）痰热　　猝然声音重浊不扬或嘶哑，兼有咳嗽，痰黄，咽痛，鼻干，发热，口渴，舌苔薄黄，脉浮数。

（3）气郁　　突然声哑不出，或呈发作性，常因情志悲忧郁怒引发，心烦易怒，胸闷气窒，或觉咽喉梗塞不舒，舌苔薄黄，脉弦。

2. 虚证　　声音嘶哑由轻渐重，咽干口燥，潮热盗汗、干咳，心悸，头晕耳鸣，舌红苔少，脉细数。

治疗

1. 实证

（1）风寒

治则：疏风散寒，宣通肺气。以取手太阴，阳明经穴为主。

处方：列缺　合谷　人迎　天鼎

方义：列缺为手太阴之络穴，又为八脉交会穴之一，通于任脉，与大肠之原穴合谷同用可疏风散寒，宣通肺气，清利咽喉；人迎、天鼎为阳明经穴，可直接疏通患部气血，通利气机。诸穴配用可使风寒得散，肺气宣通，气机通利，音哑得复。

刺灸法：毫针刺，用泻法。留针 15～20 分钟，间歇行针 2～3 次。人迎、天鼎穴应避开动脉进针，针刺时不可大幅度提插捻转。

(2) 痰热

治则：泄热化痰，清利肺窍。取手太阴、足阳明经穴为主。

处方：鱼际　丰隆　人迎　天鼎　天突

方义：鱼际为手太阴之荥穴，刺之有清热、润肺、利喉之功效；丰隆为足阳明之络穴，可清热化痰；人迎、天鼎、天突以通调局部经气、清利咽喉。诸穴配用可使痰热得化，咽喉清利而音自开。

随证选穴：发热加合谷；咽痛加二间、少商。

刺灸法：毫针刺，用泻法。留针15～20分钟，间歇行针2～3次。

(3) 气郁

治则：疏肝理气，开郁利咽。取厥阴、少阳、阳明经穴为主。

处方：太冲　支沟　关冲　合谷　人迎

方义：太冲为肝之原穴，刺之以疏肝理气；支沟为手少阳三焦之经穴，可理气散郁，配关冲清泄少阳之热邪以启闭；取合谷、人迎清利咽喉。诸穴共用可达疏肝理气散郁，通利声门之目的。

刺灸法：毫针刺，用泻法。留针15～20分钟，间歇行针2～3次。

2. 虚证

治则：滋阴降火、清肺润燥。取手太阴、足少阴经穴为主。

处方：鱼际　列缺　照海　太溪　人迎

方义：鱼际为手太阴之荥穴，配手太阴之络穴列缺可清肺降火；肾之原太溪与八脉交会穴之一照海可滋补肾阴；人迎以疏通局部经气。五穴同用可奏滋阴降火，清肺润燥，利喉增音之功效。

刺灸法：毫针刺，用补法。留针15～20分钟，间歇行针2

～3次。

其他疗法：耳针

取穴：肺　咽喉　气管　大肠　肾

操作方法：毫针刺，每次选3～4穴，轻刺激，留针10～15分钟。可用耳穴压豆法。

1.6　呃逆

呃逆俗称打嗝，古称"哕"。是指气逆上冲，喉间呃呃连声，声短而频，令人不能自止的病证。呃逆可偶然单独发生，亦可见于其他病之兼证，呈连续或间歇性发作。

呃逆包括现代医学的膈肌痉挛。如在其他急慢性疾病过程中或腹部手术后出现呃逆者，亦可参考本节辨证治疗。

病因病机

本病多因素体虚弱，过食生冷，损伤胃阳，胃阳被遏，气不顺行而上逆为呃；或暴饮暴食，过食辛辣，伤及中焦，中焦阻滞不通，燥热内盛，气不顺行，气逆动膈；或情志不畅，郁怒伤肝，气机不利，肝气犯胃，胃失和降；或因久病脾肾阳虚，胃气衰败，清气不升，浊气不降，气逆动膈而致呃声连作。

辨证

1. 胃中寒冷　　呃声沉缓有力，得热则减，遇寒愈甚，胸膈及胃脘不舒，纳少，小便清长，大便溏薄，舌苔白润，脉迟缓。

2. 胃火上逆　　呃声洪亮有力，冲逆而出，脘满纳少，呃逆酸臭、小便黄赤，大便秘结，舌苔黄，脉滑数。

3. 肝气横逆　　呃声连连，脘胁胀满，烦闷不舒，嗳气，胸闷，舌苔薄白，脉弦。

4. 脾肾阳虚　　呃声低长，气不接续，面白少华，食少困倦，气怯神疲，腰膝酸软，手足不温，舌质淡，苔薄白，脉细弱。

治疗

治则：和胃降逆平呃。取阳明、厥阴经穴为主

处方：膈俞　膻中　内关　足三里　中脘

方义：血会膈俞，气会膻中，二穴均为八会穴，同用有理气宽胸，利膈镇逆之功；内关为手厥阴心包之络穴，又为八脉交会之一，通于阴维，可和中降逆；足三里为足阳明之合穴，与胃之募中脘合用以和胃降逆。诸穴配伍共达通利气机，和胃降逆，利膈平呃之目的。

随证选穴：胃寒加灸梁门；胃热加陷谷；肝气横逆加太冲、期门；脾肾阳虚加脾俞、肾俞、气海。

刺灸法：毫针刺，用泻法，脾肾阳虚型用补法。留针15～30分钟，间歇行针2～3次。

其他疗法：耳针

取穴：膈　交感　胃　肝　脾　神门

操作方法：毫针刺，强刺激，留针30分钟。

1.7　反胃

反胃，又称胃反。是以食后脘腹痞满，宿食不化，朝食暮吐，暮食朝吐为主症。本病男女老幼皆有之，但以年高者多见。

反胃多见于现代医学的幽门痉挛，幽门梗阻，胃神经官能症等。

病因病机

本证多因饮食不当，嗜食寒凉，或情志失调，损及脾阳，以致脾胃虚寒，不能消化谷食，终至尽吐而出；或酒食不节，劳倦伤脾，脾失健运，积湿生痰，痰浊阻胃，胃失通降，宿食不化而致反胃。

辨证

1. 脾胃虚寒　　食后脘腹胀满，朝食暮吐，暮食朝吐，吐出宿食不化及清稀水液，吐尽始觉舒适，神疲乏力，面色青白，

大便溏少，舌淡苔白，脉细弱。

2. 痰浊阻胃　　脘腹胀满，食后尤甚，上腹或有积块，朝食暮吐，暮食朝吐，吐出宿食不化兼有痰涎水饮，或吐白沫，或有眩晕，心下悸，舌苔白滑，脉弦滑。

治疗

1. 脾胃虚寒

治则：温中散寒、和胃降逆。取背俞、任脉、足阳明经穴为主。

处方：脾俞　胃俞　章门　中脘　足三里　内关

方义：脾俞、胃俞与脾之募章门，胃之募中脘合用为俞募配穴，可健脾和胃，升清降浊；足三里、内关理气宽中，降逆止呕。诸穴相配共达健补脾胃，温中散寒，和胃降逆止呕之目的。

刺灸法：毫针刺，用补法。留针 20～30 分钟，间歇行针 2～3 次。脾俞、胃俞多用灸法，每穴灸 10～15 分钟。亦可用温针灸。

2. 痰浊阻胃

治则：涤痰化浊，和胃降逆。取足阳明、任脉经穴为主。

处方：中脘　丰隆　建里　足三里　内关

方义：中脘为胃之募，配丰隆以调中健胃，祛痰化浊；建里以健胃消食；足三里、内关可调理胃气，宽中降逆。诸穴共奏涤痰化浊，和胃降逆之功。

刺灸法：毫针刺，用泻法或平补平泻法。留针 20～30 分钟，间歇行针 2～3 次。

其他疗法：耳针

取穴：胃　脾　神门　枕　皮质下

操作方法：毫针刺，每次选 3～4 穴，中等刺激，留针 20 分钟。亦可用耳穴压豆或耳针埋藏。

1.8 噎膈

噎膈，是指饮食吞咽受阻，或食入即吐的一种病证。噎即噎塞，是吞咽时梗塞不顺；膈为胸膈梗阻，饮食格拒不下，或食入即吐。噎证既可单独出现，又可为膈证的前兆，故以噎膈并称。

噎膈相当于现代医学的幽门梗阻、食道憩室，食道神经官能症，食道炎等。亦可见于现代医学的食道癌，胃癌，贲门癌，贲门痉挛。

病因病机

本病多因情志不畅，气机郁结，津液不得输布，凝集成痰；或嗜酒辛辣，积热伤阴，食道干枯，痰瘀胶固，气血郁结，阻碍饮食而成噎膈。或由于饮食日渐减少，导致气血生化之源亏乏，津液枯涸，元气亏耗，出现严重衰竭证候。

辨证

1. 痰气交阻　　吞咽梗阻，胸膈痞满隐痛，嗳气呃逆，或呕吐痰涎及食物，大便艰涩，口干咽燥，体质逐渐消瘦，舌质红，脉弦细而滑。

2. 痰瘀内结　　吞咽困难，胸膈疼痛，食不能下，甚则滴水难进，进食即吐，泛吐粘痰，大便坚如羊屎，或吐下如赤豆汁，或便血，形体消瘦，肌肤枯燥，舌红少津，脉细涩。

3. 气虚阳微　　吞咽受阻、饮食难下，面色㿠白，形寒气短，泛吐涎沫，面浮足肿，腹胀，舌胖，苔淡白，脉细弱。

治疗

1. 痰气交阻

治则：开胸膈，调胃气，降痰浊。取任脉、足阳明经穴为主。

处方：天突　膻中　巨阙　内关　上脘　丰隆

方义：膻中为气之会穴，配天突以开胸理气，散结利咽；巨阙为心之募，内关为手厥阴心包之络，取二穴宽胸利气，通调三焦气机；上脘、丰隆祛痰湿，降痰浊。诸穴合用共达开胸利膈，清降痰浊，调气止痛之目的。

随证选穴：胸膈痞满加膈关；大便艰涩加天枢。

刺灸法：毫针刺，用泻法。留针 20~30 分钟，间歇行针 2~3 次。

2. 痰瘀内结

治则：滋阴祛瘀开结、除痰降逆利膈。取背俞，任脉经穴为主。

处方：膈俞　膈关　膻中　中脘　照海　关冲

方义：膈俞为血之会穴与膈关均位近胸膈，取之可调气行血，祛瘀开膈；膻中为气之会穴与中脘同用可祛痰宽肠降逆；照海以滋阴润燥；关冲能清相火，益津液。诸穴同用共奏滋阴涤痰，化瘀开结，降逆利膈之功。

刺灸法：毫针刺，用泻法，照海穴用补法。留针 15~20 分钟，间歇行针 2~3 次。

3. 气虚阳微

治则：温补脾肾，益气回阳。取背俞，任脉经穴为主。

处方：脾俞　肾俞　胃俞　气海　膈俞　足三里

方义：脾俞、胃俞、肾俞以健脾胃，益肾阳；膈俞宽胸开膈；气海、足三里以补中气，升清阳。诸穴配伍以健脾胃，温肾阳，益气宽胸利膈，扶正祛邪。

刺灸法：毫针刺，用补法。留针 15~30 分钟，间歇行针 1~2 次。背俞穴可用灸法，每穴可灸 10~15 分钟，亦可针后加灸。

其他疗法：耳针

取穴：神门　胃　食道　膈

操作方法：毫针刺，用中等刺激，留针 30 分钟。或用耳穴压豆，亦可用耳针埋藏。

按语

针刺治疗食道炎，贲门痉挛等食道功能性疾患，疗效较好。对食道癌，贲门癌能改善胸闷、胸痛和咽下困难等症状。

临床对于噎膈患者，应注意排除癌症，以防延误手术时机。

1.9　胃脘痛

胃脘痛又称胃痛。以胃脘部近心窝处经常发生疼痛为主要症状。由于痛近心窝部，故又有心痛、心腹痛之称，但与真心痛不同（应有所区别）。

现代医学的急、慢性胃炎，胃、十二指肠溃疡，胃神经官能症，胃癌等均属胃脘痛范畴。

病因病机

本病多因忧思恼怒，气郁伤肝，肝失疏泄，横逆犯胃，气机阻滞，胃失和降；或饮食不节，嗜食生冷，损伤脾胃，脾不健运，食滞中焦；或脾胃素虚，感受寒邪，凝滞于胃脘，以致胃气不降而发生胃脘部疼痛。

辨证

1. 肝气犯胃　　在本型中按其临床症状之不同又可分为气滞、火郁、血瘀三种类别。

（1）气滞　胃脘胀满，攻痛两胁，走窜不定，嗳气频作，呕逆酸苦，苔薄白，脉弦。

（2）火郁　胃脘部疼痛，痛势急迫，心烦易怒，泛酸嘈杂，口干口苦，胃脘部有灼热感，舌红苔黄，脉弦数。

（3）血瘀　痛有定处而拒按，食后较甚，或见吐血，大便发黑，甚者舌质紫暗，脉涩。

2. 饮食停滞　　胃脘胀满作痛，嗳腐吞酸，不思饮食，食则痛甚，或呕吐不消化食物，吐后痛减，舌苔厚腻，脉沉实或滑。

3. 脾胃虚寒　　胃脘隐痛，泛吐清水，喜暖欲得按，神疲乏力，四肢欠温，纳食减少，大便溏薄，舌质淡，脉虚弱。

治疗

1. 肝气犯胃

(1) 气滞

治则：疏肝理气，和胃止痛。取足厥阴、足阳明经穴为主。

处方：中脘　内关　期门　足三里　太冲

方义：取胃之募中脘配胃经之合穴足三里以和胃止痛；内关为八脉交会穴之一，通于阴维，刺之可宽胸解郁、降逆止呕；期门为肝之募穴，太冲为肝之原穴，二穴可疏肝理气、消胀定痛。诸穴配伍共奏疏肝理气，和胃止痛之功效。

刺灸法：毫针刺，用泻法。留针 15～20 分钟，间歇行针 2～3 次。

(2) 火郁

治则：清肝泄热，和胃止痛。取足厥阴，足阳明经穴为主。

处方：行间　中脘　内关　足三里　太溪

方义：行间为肝经之荥穴，刺之有清热泄火之功，配肾之原穴太溪以滋水养肝，清热泄火；中脘、内关、足三里理气和胃止痛。诸穴合用可达疏肝郁泻肝火，理气和胃止痛之目的。

刺灸法：毫针刺，用泻法。留针 15～20 分钟，间歇行针 2～3 次。

(3) 血瘀

治则：活血通络，和胃止痛。取足阳明、足太阴经穴为主。

处方：中脘　内关　足三里　公孙　血海　膈俞

方义：脾与胃相表里，取脾经络穴公孙，与内关、中脘、足三里配用以理气、和胃、止痛；取血之会穴膈俞及脾经血海可活血散瘀通络。诸穴相配共奏理气活血通络，和胃止痛之效。

刺灸法：毫针刺，用泻法。留针 15～20 分钟，间歇行针 2～3 次。

2. 饮食停滞

治则：消食导滞，和胃止痛。取足阳明经穴为主。

处方：中脘　足三里　梁门　天枢

方义：中脘、足三里疏通阳明腑气，和胃止痛；梁门调中和胃，消积化滞；天枢为大肠募穴，可通大肠腑气，以消食除滞。四穴配用共达消食导滞止痛之目的。

刺灸法：毫针刺，用泻法。留针 20～30 分钟，间歇行针 3～4 次。

3. 脾胃虚寒

治则：温中健脾，散寒止痛。取背俞、任脉经穴为主。

处方：脾俞　胃俞　章门　中脘　足三里　内关

方义：胃俞与中脘，脾俞与章门皆为俞募配穴，用以健脾和胃；足三里，内关以调和胃气。诸穴并用共奏温中散寒、健脾和胃止痛之功。

随证选穴：久病加灸气海。

刺灸法：毫针刺，用补法。留针 20～30 分钟，间歇行针 2～3 次。背俞穴与足三里多针灸并用，每穴灸 15～20 分钟，或用温针灸。

其他疗法：耳针

取穴：脾　胃　肝　交感　神门　十二指肠　皮质下　内分泌

操作方法：毫针刺，每次选 3～4 穴，疼痛剧时用强刺激，疼痛轻时用轻刺激，留针 15～30 分钟。或用耳穴压豆法。

1.10　胃下垂

胃下垂又称胃缓，是以食后脘腹痞满，嗳气不舒，胃脘坠痛或漉漉有声为主症的一种病证。其特点是平卧时坠痛减轻或消失，站立或活动时坠痛加剧。

病因病机

本病多因饮食不节，七情内伤，劳倦过度以致脾胃虚弱，中气下陷，升降失常而致。

辨证

食后脘腹胀闷，嗳气不舒，胃脘坠痛，平卧时减轻，兼见形体消瘦，面色萎黄，精神倦怠，不思饮食，或见恶心呕吐，大便时溏时秘，舌苔薄腻，脉濡软无力或沉细。

治疗

治则：健脾和胃，升举中气。取任脉、阳明经穴为主。

处方：中脘　胃上　提胃　气海　足三里　百会

方义：中脘为胃之募穴配足三里以健脾和胃，益气升阳，配百会，气海以增升提中气之功；胃上、提胃均属经外奇穴，为治疗胃缓之经验穴。诸穴配用共奏补气升陷、健脾和胃之功用。

随证选穴：恶心呕吐加内关；消瘦面黄加脾俞、胃俞。

刺灸法：毫针刺，用补法。留针20～30分钟，间歇行针2～3次。亦可用电针，疏密波刺激30分钟。百会穴可针灸并用，中脘、胃上、提胃均呈45度向下斜刺，深1.5～2寸，取针后卧床15分钟。

其他疗法：耳针

取穴：胃　交感　神门　脾　皮质下

操作方法：毫针刺，每次选3～4穴，轻刺激。留针15～20分钟。或用耳穴压豆法。

按语

1. 治疗期间应鼓励病人参加体育锻炼，增加腹部肌力。

2. 注意饮食营养，避免暴饮暴食。

3. 进食后最好平卧一段时间，有助胃下垂的恢复。

1.11　呕吐

呕吐又名吐逆，是指食物或痰涎等由胃中上逆而出的病证。古人谓：有声有物谓之呕，有物无声谓之吐，有声无物谓之哕（干呕），只吐涎沫谓之吐涎。由于临床呕与吐常兼见，难以截然分开，故合称呕吐。

呕吐可见于现代医学的急、慢性胃炎，幽门痉挛或梗阻，神经性呕吐，胆囊炎 胰腺炎等。

病因病机

凡外感风寒暑湿之邪，循阳明内犯胃腑，胃失和降，水谷随气逆而上；或恣食生冷甘肥以及误食腐败食物，食积不化，胃气不得下降；或抑郁暴怒，肝气横逆犯胃，饮食随气上逆；或脾胃素弱及病后脾胃受损，中阳不振，运化无力，水谷停滞，胃气上逆；或胃阴不足，失其润降等均可导致呕吐。

辨证

1. **外邪犯胃** 突然呕吐，起病较急，胸闷不舒，兼见恶寒发热，头痛身痛等证 舌苔白，脉浮。

2. **饮食停滞** 呕吐腐酸，脘腹胀满，嗳气厌食，腹痛，吐后则舒，大便或溏或结，舌苔腻，脉滑实。

3. **肝气犯胃** 呕吐吞酸，嗳气频作，胸胁满痛，烦闷不舒，常因精神刺激而使病情加重，舌苔薄腻脉弦。

4. **脾胃虚弱** 面色㿠白，饮食稍多即吐，时作时止，倦怠乏力，纳少，大便溏薄，舌质淡，脉濡弱。

5. **胃阴不足** 呕吐反复发作，或时作干呕，口燥咽干，似饥而不欲食，舌红少津，脉细数。

治疗

1. 外邪犯胃

治则：解表、调中、止呕。取阳明、任脉经穴为主。

处方：大椎 合谷 内庭 中脘 内关

方义：大椎为诸阳之会，取之以宣通阳气，疏达表邪；合谷、内庭以清泄阳明；中脘为胃之募，腑之会穴，可通降胃气，和胃止呕；内关开胸降逆，宣通气机。诸穴配伍可使外邪得解，胃气得安，呕吐自止。

刺灸法：毫针刺，用泻法。留针 15～20 分钟，间歇行针 3～4 次。

2. 饮食停滞

治则：行气消食导滞。取任脉、足阳明经穴为主。

处方：下脘　璇玑　足三里　内关　腹结

方义：下脘、璇玑行气导滞而清宿食；足三里、内关和胃止呕；腹结除脘腹膨胀。五穴合用共达行气导滞，消食止呕之目的。

随证选穴：便秘加支沟；便溏加天枢、上巨虚；腹胀加气海。

刺灸法：毫针刺，用泻法。留针 15～20 分钟，间歇行针 2～3 次。

3. 肝气犯胃

治则：疏肝和胃止呕。取足厥阴、少阳、阳明经穴为主。

处方：上脘　阳陵泉　太冲　梁门　内关　足三里

方义：上脘宽胸膈，配梁门平胃止呕；太冲平肝降逆与阳陵泉合用以疏肝解郁；内关、足三里宽胸理气，和胃止呕。诸穴配伍共达疏肝和胃止呕之目的。

随证选穴：烦闷不舒加膻中。

刺灸法：毫针刺，用泻法。留针 15～20 分钟，间歇行针 2～3 次。

4. 脾胃虚弱

治则：健脾温中和胃。取背俞、任脉　足阳明经穴为主。

处方：脾俞　胃俞　中脘　章门　足三里　公孙　内关

方义：脾俞、胃俞配脾之募章门、胃之募中脘；俞募相合可振奋脾胃之气，疏导升降气机；足三里通降胃气；公孙配内关以调中焦、平冲逆。诸穴合用可补益脾胃，振奋中气，运化有权，水谷得以消磨，升降恢复常度，而呕吐得愈。

随证选穴：大便溏泄加天枢、上巨虚。

刺灸法：毫针刺，用泻法。留针 20～30 分钟，间歇行针 3～4 次。背俞穴可用灸法，亦可针灸并用，每穴灸 10～20 分钟。

5. 胃阴不足

治则：滋养胃阴，降逆止呕。取背俞，足太阴、足阳明经穴为主。

处方：胃俞　阴陵泉　足三里　内关　公孙　内庭

方义：胃俞配脾之合穴阴陵泉、胃之合穴足三里可滋养胃阴，健脾益胃；内关、公孙调中焦、平冲逆以宽胸和胃；内庭为足阳明胃经之荥穴以清胃经之邪热。诸穴同用共达清胃泄热，滋养胃阴，降逆止呕之功效。

随证选穴：呕吐不止加金津、玉液；口燥咽干加照海、阴郄

刺灸法：毫针刺，用补法，内庭穴用泻法。留针15～20分钟，间歇行针2～4次。金津、玉液可用三棱针点刺出血。本证禁用灸法。

其他疗法：耳针

取穴：胃　肝　交感　神门　皮质下　枕

操作方法：毫针刺，每次选3～4穴，强刺激，留针15～30分钟。或用耳针埋藏，或用耳穴压豆。

1.12　腹痛

腹痛是指胃脘以下，耻骨毛际以上部位发生疼痛的症状而言。在临床上极为常见，可伴发于多种脏腑疾病。

本节所述腹痛常见于现代医学的急、慢性肠炎，胃肠痉挛，肠神经官能症，消化不良性腹痛等。至于外科及妇科病症所出现的急性腹痛等，另详见外科及妇科疾病中的有关篇章。

病因病机

本证的发生多由于过食生冷或脐腹受寒，寒性收引以致气机痹阻，不通则痛；或暴饮暴食，过食肥甘厚味和不洁食物，食积化热，壅滞肠间，腑气通降不利，遂成腹痛；或因素体阳虚，脾阳不振，脾胃运化失职而发腹痛。

辨证

1. 寒邪内积　痛势急剧，喜温恶冷，大便溏薄，腹中雷鸣，小便清利，饮食减少，口不渴，四肢不温，舌苔薄白，脉沉紧或沉迟。

2. 饮食停滞　脘腹胀满，疼痛拒按或痛而欲泻，泻后痛减，恶食，嗳腐吞酸，恶心呕吐，舌苔腻，脉滑。

3. 脾阳不振　腹痛绵绵，时作时止，痛时喜按，喜热恶冷，大便溏泄，神疲肢倦，舌质淡，边有齿龈，苔薄白，脉沉细。

治疗

1. 寒邪内积

治则：温中散寒止痛。取任脉、足阳明、太阴经穴为主。

处方：中脘　神阙　足三里

方义：腑之会穴中脘配足阳明胃经之合穴足三里以升清降浊，通调胃肠，健中祛寒，艾灸神阙可温中散寒。诸穴配伍可使中焦得温，寒邪得化，气机得通，而腹痛自止。

随症选穴：脐腹痛剧加气海、三阴交；大便溏薄加天枢，大肠俞。

刺灸法：毫针刺，用泻法。留针20～30分钟，间歇行针2～3次。神阙隔盐灸15～30分钟。

2. 饮食停滞

治则：消食化滞止痛。取任脉、足阳明经穴为主。

处方：下脘　梁门　公孙　足三里　里内庭

方义：取下脘、梁门以健胃消食；足太阴之络穴公孙配足阳明之合穴足三里健脾理气，消食化滞，以疗胃肠之诸疾；奇穴里内庭为治疗伤食的经验效穴。诸穴合用共达通降气机、消食化滞、止痛之目的。

随证选穴：嗳腐吞酸加阳陵泉。

刺灸法：毫针刺，用泻法。留针15～30分钟，间歇行针2

～3次。

3. 脾阳不振

治则：温中散寒、益气健脾。取背俞、任脉经穴为主。

处方：脾俞　胃俞　中脘　章门　气海　足三里　关元

方义：脾俞配章门，胃俞配中脘为俞募配穴，有振奋脾胃之阳之功效；气海、关元可温下焦，固元气，以益气壮阳；配足三里健运脾胃，补益中气；脾胃不虚，中阳得振，则腹痛得愈。

随证选穴：腹痛时作者加灸神阙。

刺灸法：毫针刺，用补法。留针15～30分钟，间歇行针2～3次。背俞穴及气海穴多用灸法或针灸并用，每穴灸10～15分钟。神阙用隔姜灸10～20分钟。

其他疗法：耳针

取穴：大肠　小肠　脾　胃　腹　神门　皮质下

操作方法：毫针刺，每次选3～5穴，中等刺激，留针10～20分钟，或用耳穴压豆。

1.13　腹胀

腹胀是指以腹部胀满不舒为主证的疾患，甚则兼见腹痛，嗳气，呕吐。本病多因胃肠功能失调所致。

现代医学的胃下垂，肠麻痹，肠梗阻，胃肠神经官能症，急性胃扩张等病出现以腹胀为主症时均可参考本篇辨证治疗。

病因病机

本病多因暴饮暴食，损伤脾胃，以致胃肠运化功能失调，宿食积滞，阻塞气机；或素体脾胃虚弱及久病体虚，脾胃失于健运，胃肠气机不利而致。此外，腹部手术后，亦可导致腹胀。

辨证

1. 实证　　腹部胀满不减，腹满拒按，甚至腹痛，嗳气，口臭，小便黄赤，大便秘结，或有发热，呕吐，舌苔黄厚，脉滑数有力。

2. 虚证　　腹胀时轻时重，喜按，肠鸣便溏，食少身倦，精神不振，小便清白，舌质淡，苔白，脉弱无力。

治疗

1. 实证

治则：通调腑气。取手足阳明经穴为主。

处方：中脘　天枢　足三里　上巨虚

方义：胃募中脘，大肠募天枢与胃之合穴足三里，大肠之下合穴上巨虚同用可通调胃肠气机，消食化滞，从而使腑气通畅，腹胀消失。

刺灸法：毫针刺，用泻法。留针 15～20 分钟，间歇行针 2～3 次。

2. 虚证

治则：健脾和胃，理气消胀。取足阳明，足太阴经穴为主。

处方：建里　天枢　足三里　太白　关元

方义：建里健胃益气；天枢通调胃肠气机；足三里、太白、关元健脾和胃，以助运化。诸穴相配共达健补脾胃，调理气机，消胀除满之目的。

刺灸法：毫针刺，用补法。留针 15～30 分钟，间歇行针 2～3 次。

其他疗法：耳针

取穴：脾　胃　大肠　小肠　交感　皮质下

操作方法：毫针刺，每次选 3～4 穴，轻刺激，留针 15～20分钟。或用耳穴压豆法。

1.14　泄泻

泄泻是指大便次数增多，粪质溏薄，完谷不化，甚至泻如水样的一种病证。临床上根据发病情况及病情长短又分为急性泄泻和慢性泄泻。本病一年四季均可发生，但以夏秋两季较为多见。

泄泻与现代医学的腹泻含义相同，可见于多种疾病，如急、慢性肠炎，肠结核，肠功能紊乱，结肠过敏等。

病因病机

导致泄泻的原因很多，但以脾胃失调为主要因素。

急性泄泻多因饮食生冷、不洁食物，或暴饮暴食，或兼受寒湿暑热之邪，尤以湿邪，困阻脾阳，脾胃受损，脾失健运，水谷不化，清浊不分，并走大肠而下致成泄泻。

慢性泄泻多由思虑伤脾，脾胃素虚；或情志失调，肝失疏泄，肝气横逆，脾胃受克；或久病之后，肾阳虚亏，命门火衰，不能温暖脾胃而腐化水谷，脾胃运化失常而致。

辨证

1. 急性泄泻　　发病急骤，大便次数显著增多，小便减少。

(1) 寒湿　　泄泻清稀，甚则如水样，腹痛肠鸣，脘闷食少，身寒喜温，口不渴，舌淡苔白，脉沉迟或濡缓。

(2) 湿热　　泄泻腹痛，泻下急迫或泻而不爽，粪色黄褐，气味臭秽，肛门灼热，烦热口渴，小便短赤，舌苔黄腻，脉滑数或濡数。

(3) 伤食　　腹痛肠鸣，泻下粪便臭如败卵，泻后痛减，脘腹胀满，嗳腐酸臭，不思饮食，矢气频作，舌苔垢浊或腻，脉滑。

2. 慢性泄泻　　多由急性泄泻演变而来，发病势缓，便泄次数较急性泄泻为少，病程较长，迁延日久。

(1) 脾虚　　大便时溏时泻，迁延反复，完谷不化，饮食减少，食后脘闷不舒，稍进油腻食物，则大便次数明显增加，面色萎黄，神疲倦怠，舌苔白腻，脉濡缓。

(2) 肝脾不和　　腹痛即泻，泻后而痛不减，每当精神刺激，情绪紧张之时，即发生腹痛泄泻，泻时常有脘胁痞闷，嗳气，苔薄，脉弦。

(3) 肾虚　　多在黎明之前脐腹作痛，肠鸣即泻，泻后则安，形寒肢冷，腰膝酸软，舌苔白，脉沉细。

治疗

1. 急性泄泻。

(1) 寒湿

治则：温中利湿。取足阳明、任脉经穴为主。

处方：天枢　建里　气海　上巨虚　阴陵泉

方义：天枢为大肠募穴，可疏调大肠气机，驱腹中寒湿；建里、气海针灸并用以理气温中，散寒祛湿；大肠之下合穴上巨虚配脾之合穴阴陵泉以理肠胃，分清浊，利水湿。诸穴合用其达温中利湿止泻之目的。

刺灸法：毫针刺，用泻法。留针 15～20 分钟，间歇行针 2～3 次。建里、气海、天枢可用灸法，每穴灸 10～15 分钟，亦可用隔姜灸，每穴灸 5～7 壮。

(2) 湿热

治则：清热利湿。取足阳明，足太阴经穴为主。

处方：中脘　天枢　阴陵泉　内庭　曲池

方义：中脘、天枢调理胃肠气机；阴陵泉健脾利湿；内庭为足阳明荥穴，曲池为手阳明之合穴，取之以清泄胃肠之湿热。诸穴共用以奏调理肠胃气机，清热利湿止泻之功效。

刺灸法：毫针刺，用泻法。留针 15～20 分钟，间歇行针 2～3 次。

(3) 伤食

治则：消食导滞止泻。取任脉、足阳明经穴为主。

处方：天枢　中脘　璇玑　里内庭　足三里

方义：天枢、中脘、足三里三穴合用可疏导通降肠胃气机；配璇玑、里内庭以消食化滞。诸穴配伍可使食滞消散，积热得解，脾胃调和，而泄泻自止。

随证选穴：嗳腐酸臭加内关、内庭。

刺灸法：毫针刺，用泻法。留针 15～20 分钟，间歇行针 2

～3次。

2. 慢性泄泻

(1) 脾虚

治则：健脾止泻。取脾经及有关腧穴为主。

处方：脾俞　章门　太白　中脘　足三里　天枢

方义：脾俞、章门俞募相配有健脾益气之功；中脘、足三里、天枢调理肠胃气机；太白为脾之原穴，以补益脾气。诸穴同用具有振奋脾阳，健运止泻的作用。

刺灸法：毫针刺，用补法。留针15～30分钟，间歇行针1～2次。脾俞、天枢、足三里可用灸法，每穴灸10～15分钟。

(2) 肝脾不和

治则：疏肝理气、健脾和胃止泻。取足厥阴、足阳明、背俞穴为主。

处方：肝俞　太冲　脾俞　章门　天枢　足三里

方义：肝俞、太冲疏泄肝气；脾俞、章门健脾益气；天枢、足三里调理胃肠气机。诸穴合用，可使肝气条达，脏腑之气机和调，而痛泻自止。

随证选穴：脘胁痞闷加阳陵泉、内关。

刺灸法：毫针刺，用平补平泻法。留针15～20分钟，间歇行针2～3次。

(3) 肾虚

治则：温补脾肾。取背俞、任脉经穴为主。

处方：肾俞　命门　关元　脾俞　天枢　上巨虚

方义：肾俞、命门、关元温肾壮阳，疗腹中寒冷；脾俞以补益脾气；天枢，上巨虚调理大肠气机。诸穴合用共达温补脾肾，腐熟水谷，散寒止泻之效。

随证选穴；虚泻日久，中气下陷者加灸百会。

刺灸法：毫针刺，用补法。留针15～30分钟，间歇行针1～2次。每次可选2～3穴加灸，每穴灸10～20分钟。

其他疗法: 耳针

取穴: 大肠 小肠 脾 胃 肝 肾 交感 神门

操作方法: 毫针刺, 每次选 3～5 穴, 中等刺激, 留针 10～20 分钟。亦可用耳穴压豆或耳针埋藏。

1.15 痢疾

痢疾是夏秋季节常见的肠道传染病。以大便次数增多, 腹痛里急后重, 痢下赤白脓血为特征。临床分为湿热痢, 寒湿痢, 噤口痢, 休息痢等。

现代医学的细菌性痢疾、中毒性菌痢, 阿米巴痢疾, 慢性非特异性溃疡性结肠炎等, 均可参照本节辨证治疗。

病因病机

本病多因饮食不洁, 过食生冷或感受暑湿疫毒之邪, 损伤肠胃而致。若湿热偏盛则化火伤血, 肠络受伤遂致大便脓血, 赤多白少成为湿热痢; 若寒湿偏盛, 其邪搏结于肠间, 滞积于肠腑, 下痢夹杂粘液白冻; 或白多赤少而为寒湿痢; 如邪热犯胃以致呕恶不能食而发为噤口痢; 痢疾迁延日久, 中气虚弱, 正虚邪恋则成休息痢。

辨证

1. 湿热痢　　腹痛, 里急后重, 下痢赤白相杂, 赤多白少, 日数次或十余次, 肛门灼热, 小便短赤, 甚者身发高热, 心烦口渴, 舌苔黄腻, 脉滑数。

2. 寒湿痢　　腹痛拘急, 痢下赤白粘冻, 白多赤少或为纯白冻, 里急后重, 喜暖畏寒, 兼有胸脘痞闷, 口淡不渴, 舌苔白腻, 脉沉迟。

3. 噤口痢　　痢下赤白, 饮食不进, 恶心呕吐, 腹痛或胸腹胀满, 舌苔黄腻, 脉濡数。

4 休息痢　　下痢时作时止, 或轻或重, 缠绵难愈, 常因饮食不慎, 过于劳累, 或感受外邪而使其痢下加重, 兼有倦怠乏力，怯冷嗜卧，腹胀纳差，舌淡苔腻，脉濡软或虚大。

治疗

1. 湿热痢

治则：清热导滞，调气行血。取手足阳明经穴为主。

处方：天枢　上巨虚　曲池　内庭　合谷

方义：天枢为大肠募穴，配大肠之下合穴上巨虚，原穴合谷以通调大肠腑气；手阳明经合穴曲池，足阳明经荥穴内庭上下相配，共同清泄肠胃湿热之气。诸穴合用可达清热导滞，调气行血之功，气调而湿化滞行，下痢得止。

随证选穴：发热加大椎；里急后重甚者加气海。

刺灸法：毫针刺，用泻法。留针 15～20 分钟，间歇行针 2～3 次。

2. 寒湿痢

治则：温化寒湿，行气和血。取任脉，足阳明经穴为主。

处方：中脘　天枢　气海　上巨虚　阴陵泉

方义：中脘为胃之募配大肠之下合穴上巨虚以通调肠胃气机，和胃气化湿浊；天枢、气海可温中散寒，调气行滞；足太阴之合穴阴陵泉可健脾利湿；诸穴配伍共奏温中散寒，健脾化湿，行气和血之目的。

刺灸法：毫针刺，用平补平泻法。留针 15～20 分钟，间歇行针 1～2 次。气海、天枢可用灸法，每穴灸 10～15 分钟。

3. 噤口痢

治则：和胃开噤。取手足阳明、任脉经穴为主。

处方：中脘　合谷　内关　内庭　天枢

方义：取胃之募中脘以和胃气，分清降浊；合谷、内庭以清泄胃肠积滞湿热；内关通降三焦，降逆气，止呕吐；天枢为大肠之募穴，可通调大肠气机。诸穴共奏升清降浊，清热化湿，降逆和中，开噤止呕之功能。

刺灸法：毫针刺，用泻法。留针 15～20 分钟，间歇行针 2

～3 次。

4. 休息痢

治则：健脾益气，消积化滞。取背俞、任脉经穴为主。

处方：脾俞　胃俞　大肠俞　关元　天枢　足三里

方义：脾俞、胃俞、足三里健脾益胃，补后天之本，资生化之源；大肠俞配天枢，一俞一募以通调肠腑之气，消积化滞；关元为小肠之募温下焦，固元气，以助分利清浊之功。诸穴合用共达扶正祛邪，补中益气，通调肠腑之目的。

随证选穴：脱肛加百会（灸）。

刺灸法：毫针刺，用补法。留针 15～30 分钟，间歇行针 1～2 次。脾俞、胃俞、关元可用灸法，每穴灸 10～15 分钟。

其他疗法：耳针

取穴：大肠　小肠　胃　直肠下段　神门　脾　肾

操作方法：毫针刺，每次选 3～5 穴，用中等刺激，留针 10～15 分钟。

1.16　便秘

便秘是指大便秘结不通，排便间隔时间延长，或欲大便而艰涩不畅的一种病证。

本病多见于现代医学的习惯性便秘或暂时性肠蠕动功能失调之便秘，以及肛门直肠疾患所引起的便秘等。

病因病机

本病多因素体阳盛，嗜食辛辣香燥，或热病之后余热留恋，导致肠胃积热，耗伤津液以致肠道干涩燥结；或情志不畅，或久坐少动，引起气机郁滞，不能宣达，通降失常，传导失职，糟粕内停；或病后产后气血未复，气虚则运转无力，血虚则肠失润下；或因年老体衰，阳气不足，温煦无权，寒自内生，阴寒凝结，不能化气布津等而致大便秘结。

辨证

1. **热秘**　大便干结不通，数日不行，腹部痞满，按之有块作痛，面红，心烦，小便短赤，或有身热，口干口臭，舌苔黄燥，脉滑数。

2. **气秘**　大便秘而不甚干结，腹部胀痛连及两胁，嗳气频作，口苦目眩，纳少，舌苔薄腻，脉弦。

3. **虚秘**　便秘燥结难下，腹无胀痛，但觉小腹不舒，虽有便意而临厕努挣乏力，难于排出，甚者多汗，短气，疲惫，面色少华，心悸，头晕眼花，舌淡，苔薄，脉细弱无力。

4. **冷秘**　大便艰涩，不易排出，甚则脱肛，腹中或有冷痛，面色青白，手足不温，喜热怕冷，小便清长，舌淡苔白，脉沉迟。

治疗

1. **热秘**

治则：清热润燥。取阳明经穴为主。

处方：合谷　曲池　内庭　天枢　腹结　上巨虚

方义：合谷、曲池、内庭可泻阳明之热，而保津润肠；大肠之募穴天枢、下合穴上巨虚配腹结以行津液，通调大肠腑气；诸穴配伍使热邪得泄，津液得保，腑气得通，而便秘自调。

随证选穴：烦热口渴加少府、廉泉；口臭加承浆。

刺灸法：毫针刺，用泻法。留针15～20分钟，间歇行针2～3次。

2. **气秘**

治则：降气通便。取任脉、足厥阴，少阳经穴为主。

处方：中脘　天枢　行间　阳陵泉　支沟

方义：腑之会穴中脘配大肠之募穴天枢以通腑气；行间为足厥阴之荥穴配足少阳胆之合穴阳陵泉以疏肝理气解郁；支沟为手少阳之经穴用以宣通三焦气机，气机通畅，腑气通调，大便畅顺。

随证选穴：胁痛甚者加期门、日月；腹胀甚者加大横。

刺灸法：毫针刺，用泻法。留针 15～20 分钟，间歇行针 2
～3 次。

3. 虚秘

治则：补气养血。取背俞、任脉、足阳明经穴为主。

处方：脾俞　胃俞　关元　气海　足三里

方义：脾为后天之本，取脾俞配胃俞、足三里以扶助中气，
培补生化之源；关元、气海益气壮阳，以补下焦元气。诸穴合用
可使脾胃气旺，生气化血，以达补益气血，润肠通便之目的。

随证选穴：多汗加阴郄；心悸加内关。

刺灸法：毫针刺，用补法。留针 20～30 分钟，间歇行针 1
～2 次。背俞穴、气海、关元可用灸法或针灸并用，每穴灸 10～
15 分钟。

4. 冷秘

治则：补肾助阳，温腑通便。取任脉，足少阴经穴为主。

处方：神阙　气海　照海　肾俞　天枢

方义：灸神阙、气海温通下焦阳气以消阴寒；照海、肾俞补
益肾气；天枢可通调大肠腑气。诸穴配伍共奏温阳散寒，开结通
便之功效。

随证选穴：脱肛加长强、百会。

刺灸法：毫针刺，用补法。留针 20～30 分钟，间歇行针 1
～2 次。神阙、气海用灸法，每穴灸 15～20 分钟。

其他疗法：耳针

取穴：大肠　小肠　肺　脾　直肠下段　皮质下

操作方法：毫针刺，每次选 3～5 穴，强刺激，留针 15～20
分钟。或用耳穴压豆法。

1.17　脱肛

脱肛又名直肠脱垂，是指直肠下端脱出肛门之外而言。多见
于老人、小儿或久病体弱的患者。

本病与现代医学的"直肠脱垂"相类似。

病因病机

脱肛多由久痢、久泻、大病后体质虚弱，以及妇女生育过多，中气下陷，收摄无权所致；亦有因饮食不节，恣食辛辣厚味，以致脾肺湿热，其湿热下注而致。

辨证

1. 气虚下陷　　直肠脱出于肛外，一般多在便后脱出、若病久虚甚者，往往因咳嗽、行路、久立或排尿、稍用力即脱出。伴有神疲肢软，面色萎黄，头晕心悸，舌苔薄白，脉细弱。

2. 湿热下注　　直肠脱出，肛门灼热、肿痛。兼有面赤身热，口干口臭，胸脘痞闷，腹胀便结，小便短赤，舌红苔黄腻，脉濡数。

治疗

1. 气虚下陷

治则：益气升提。取督脉、足太阳经穴为主。

处方：百会　长强　大肠俞　气海　足三里

方义：百会为督脉与三阳经交会穴，气为阳，统于督脉，故灸之能升提下陷之阳气；长强为督脉之别络，位于肛门部，刺之可加强肛门的约束机能；大肠俞可补益大肠腑气；气海调补元气，配足三里益气升提，使中气恢复，升举有力，脱肛自收。

刺灸法：毫针刺，用补法。留针15～30分钟，间歇行针1～2次。百会、气海用灸法，每穴灸15～30分钟。

2. 湿热下注

治则：清泄湿热。取督脉、足太阳经穴为主。

处方：百会　长强　承山　委中　丰隆　阴陵泉

方义：取百会以升举收摄；长强、承山以疏泄肛门部湿热郁滞；委中清泄肠中之湿热；足阳明络穴丰隆与足太阴脾经合穴阴陵泉合用以健脾利湿，祛肠腑湿热。诸穴合用使腑气调畅，湿热得除，升举有力，脱肛自愈。

随证选穴：腹胀便结加天枢；因痔疾而致脱肛加二白穴。

刺灸法：毫针刺，用泻法。留针 15～20 分钟，间歇行针 2～3 次。

其他疗法

1. 耳针

取穴：直肠下段　皮质下　脾　神门

操作方法：毫针刺，中等刺激，留针 20 分钟。亦可用耳穴压豆或耳针埋藏法。

2. 挑治

在第三腰椎至第二腰椎之间，脊柱中线旁开 1～1.5 寸外纵线上，任选一点进行挑治。

1.18　黄疸

黄疸是以目黄、肤黄、尿黄为主症的疾患，其中尤以目黄为主要特征。临床甚为常见，多发于儿童及青壮年。

本病与现代医学所述的黄疸含义相同，包括肝细胞性黄疸，阻塞性黄疸，溶血性黄疸等。

病因病机

黄疸发病原因可由外感和内伤引起。凡因外感湿热之邪，内蕴于肝胆、湿郁热蒸，以致疏泄功能阻滞，胆液横溢而发黄疸为阳黄；凡因饮食不节，思虑劳伤过度，损伤脾胃，脾运失常，湿郁气滞，以致肝胆瘀积，胆汁排出不畅，外溢肌肤而渐成黄疸为阴黄。

阳黄迁延失治亦可能转为阴黄，阴黄复感外邪，亦可出现阳黄，形成虚实夹杂的证候。

辨证

1. 阳黄　　发病急，病程短。目肤色黄，鲜明如橘，发热，口渴，小便黄赤短少，大便秘结，身重腹满，胸闷呕恶，舌苔黄腻，脉弦数。若热毒内陷可见神昏、发斑、出血等重证。若湿重于热则黄疸略欠鲜明，发热较轻，脘痞便溏，口渴不甚，苔腻微黄，脉濡数。

2. 阴黄　　起病缓，病程长。目肤俱黄，其色晦暗或如烟熏，神疲身倦，畏寒纳少，恶心欲吐，口淡不渴，脘痞，大便不实，舌淡苔腻，脉沉迟。

治疗

1. 阳黄

治则：疏泄肝胆，清热化湿。取督脉、足太阳、厥阴经穴为主。

处方：至阳　腕骨　肝俞　胆俞　阳陵泉　太冲　阴陵泉
内庭

方义：至阳为督脉经气所注，可宣发督脉经气；配小肠之原穴腕骨以疏泄太阳，清化在表湿热；胆俞、肝俞配足少阳胆之合穴阳陵泉、肝之原穴太冲以疏肝利胆，清化在里之湿热；阴陵泉为足太阴之合穴，内庭为足阳明之荥穴，二穴合用能泻脾胃二经之湿热，从小便而蠲除。诸穴配伍使热退湿除，肝疏胆利，胆汁循于常道，而黄疸消退。

随证选穴：热重加大椎；腹胀便秘加天枢、大肠俞；神昏加人中、中冲、少冲；脘痞便溏加足三里。

刺灸法：毫针刺，用泻法。留针20～30分钟，间歇行针2～4次。

2. 阴黄

治则：健脾利胆，温化寒理。取足阳明、太阴，背俞穴为主。

处方：脾俞　胆俞　至阳　中脘　足三里　三阴交

方义：脾俞配腑之会中脘、足阳明胃之合穴足三里以健脾胃而化湿；胆俞以降逆气利胆汁，通利胆腑；至阳疏通阳气；三阴交补脾土，导湿下行。诸穴共奏健脾利胆，温化寒湿，以退阴黄之功。

随证选穴：神疲畏寒加气海，命门；大便溏泄加天枢、关元。

刺灸法：毫针刺，用平补平泻法。留针 20～30 分钟，间歇行针 2～3 次。

其他疗法：耳针

取穴：胆 肝 脾 胃 膈 耳迷根

操作方法：毫针刺，每次选 3～4 穴，中等刺激，留针 15～20 分钟。亦可用耳穴压豆或耳针埋藏。

1.19 胁痛

胁痛是指一侧或两侧胁肋疼痛而言，为临床常见的一种自觉症状。

本证可见于现代医学的肝、胆疾患及肋间神经痛等。

病因病机

本病多因情志郁结，或暴怒伤肝，肝气失于条达，络脉受阻，经气运行不畅；或外感湿热，或饮食不节，伤于酒食，湿热蕴结于肝胆，失于疏泄；或跌仆闪挫，胁肋络脉损伤，气滞血瘀，阻塞经络；或久病体虚，劳欲过度，精血亏损，肝脉失养而致。

辨证

1. 肝气郁结　　胁肋胀痛，走窜不定，常因情志波动而发作和加甚。伴有胸闷不舒，饮食减少，嗳气频作，易怒，少寐，舌苔薄白，脉弦。

2. 肝胆湿热　　胁痛偏于右侧，如刺如灼，急性发作时伴有恶寒发热，口苦，心烦，恶心呕吐，目赤或目黄身黄，小便黄赤，舌红，苔黄，脉弦数。

3. 瘀血停积　　胁痛如刺，痛处不移，入夜更甚，疼痛拒按，胁肋下或见痞块，舌质紫暗，脉沉涩。

4. 肝阴不足　　两胁隐隐作痛，其痛绵绵不休，口干心烦，头昏目眩，潮热，自汗，舌红少苔，脉细数。

治疗

1. 肝气郁结

治则：疏肝解郁，理气止痛。取厥阴、少阳经穴及背俞穴为主。

处方：期门　肝俞　太冲　支沟　阳陵泉

方义：期门为肝之募穴配肝俞以疏肝理气；太冲为肝之原穴配手少阳经穴支沟、足少阳合穴阳陵泉以疏肝解郁，调少阳经气。诸穴可使肝气条达，气机通畅，胁痛得愈。

随证选穴：胸闷嗳气加中脘、胃俞；少寐加大陵、神门。

刺灸法：毫针刺，用泻法。留针15～20分钟，间歇行针2～3次。

2. 肝胆湿热

治则：清热化湿，疏肝利胆。取足厥阴、手足少阳经穴为主。

处方：期门　日月　支沟　阳陵泉　丘墟　行间

方义：期门、日月是肝胆之气募集之处，泻之能疏利肝胆的气血；支沟、阳陵泉以调少阳经气，是治胁痛的成方；配胆之原丘墟，足厥阴肝之荥穴行间可和解少阳，清化肝胆湿热。诸穴合用共达清热化湿、疏肝利胆，止痛之目的。

随证选穴：热重加关冲；呕吐恶心加中脘、内关；心烦加郄门。

刺灸法：毫针刺，用泻法。留针15～20分钟，间歇行针2～3次。

3. 瘀血停积

治则：活血通络，行气止痛。取足厥阴、手足少阳经穴为主。

处方：膈俞　肝俞　期门　三阴交　太冲　支沟

方义：血之会膈俞配肝俞，三阴交以活血化瘀；期门，太冲疏肝行气，通经行瘀；支沟疏利三焦气机；使气行血行，血行则络通，而胁痛可止。

随证选穴：跌仆损伤可结合痛部取其阿是穴。

刺灸法：毫针刺，用泻法。留针 15～30 分钟，间歇行针 2～4 次。

4. 肝阴不足

治则：滋阴养血，和络定痛。取背俞、足太阴、阳明经穴为主。

处方：肝俞　肾俞　期门　太冲　足三里　三阴交

方义：肝俞、肾俞配肝之募期门、肝之原太冲以益精养血，调肝止痛；足三里、三阴交以扶脾胃后天之本，而资气血生化之源。诸穴协用可使阴血充沛，络脉得其滋养，而达止痛之目的。

随证选穴：潮热加膏肓，头晕目眩加百会，风池。

刺灸法：毫针刺，用补法。留针 20～30 分钟，间歇行针 1～2 次。

其他疗法

1. 耳针

取穴：肝　胆　神门　胸　皮质下

操作方法：毫针刺，用中等刺激，留针 20 分钟。亦可用耳针埋藏或耳穴压豆法。

2. 皮肤针

取穴：胁肋部痛点，及与痛点成水平的背俞穴上中下三个俞穴。

操作方法：轻刺激，叩至皮肤潮红为度，并加拔火罐。此法适用于劳伤胁痛。

1.20　眩晕

眩晕是目眩与头晕的总称。目眩即眼花或眼前发黑，视物模糊；头晕即感觉自身或外界景物旋转，站立不稳。二者常同时并见，故统称为"眩晕"。转者闭目即可停止；重者如坐车船，旋转不定，不能站立或伴有恶心、呕吐、汗出、甚则晕倒。

眩晕可见于现代医学的多种疾病。凡内耳性眩晕，脑动脉硬化、高血压、低血压、椎基底动脉供血不足、贫血、神经衰弱及某些脑部疾患等以眩晕为主症时，均可参考本篇辨证治疗。

病因病机

本病多因忧郁恼怒过度，使肝阴耗伤，肝阳上亢，上扰清空；或病后体虚，思虑过度，劳伤心脾，脾虚气血生化无源，脑失所养；或房劳过度，肾精亏耗，髓海空虚；或饮食肥甘，伤于脾胃，健运失司，聚湿生痰，痰浊中阻，清阳不升，浊阴不降等而致眩晕。

辨证

1. 肝阳上亢　　眩晕耳鸣，头痛且胀，每因烦劳或恼怒而加重，面红目赤，急躁易怒，失眠多梦，口苦，舌红，苔薄黄，脉弦数。

2. 气血不足　　头晕眼花，动则加剧，劳累即发，面色㿠白，精神不振，心悸失眠，唇甲不华，气短懒言，四肢无力，纳呆，舌质淡，脉细弱。

3. 肾精亏损　　眩晕健忘，腰膝酸软，遗精耳鸣，失眠多梦。偏于阳虚者则四肢不温，舌质淡，脉沉细；偏于阴虚者则五心烦热，盗汗，舌质红，脉弦细。

4. 痰湿中阻　　眩晕倦怠或头重如蒙，恶心欲吐，胸脘痞闷，口粘不渴，少食多梦，肢体麻木，舌苔白腻，脉濡滑。

治疗

1. 肝阳上亢

治则：滋阴潜阳，平肝熄风。取足厥阴、少阴经穴为主。

处方：风池　太冲　侠溪　肝俞　肾俞　太溪

方义：风池与肝之原穴太冲，足少阳之荥穴侠溪同用以平肝阳、熄肝风、兼清肝胆火热，是急则治其标之法；肝俞以滋养肝阴；肾俞、太溪以补益肾水，意在治本。诸穴配合共达滋阴潜阳、平肝熄风，以止眩晕之目的。

刺灸法：毫针刺，补泻兼施，风池、太冲、侠溪用泻法，肾俞、太溪、肝俞用补法。留针 20~30 分钟，间歇行针 3~4 次。

2. 气血不足

治则：补气益血，健脾益胃。取足太阴，足阳明经穴为主。

处方：足三里　三阴交　脾俞　肾俞　关元　百会

方义：足三里、三阴交、脾俞健补脾胃，生精化血，以扶后天之本，资生化之源；肾俞、关元以培补元气；百会升提气血。诸穴合用可使气血充盛，而眩晕遂止。

随证选穴：心悸失眠加内关、神门。

刺灸法：毫针刺，用补法。留针 15~30 分钟，间歇行针 1~3 次。脾俞、足三里、关元、肾俞可针灸并用，每穴灸 10 分钟。百会以灸为主，灸 20~30 分钟。

3. 肾精亏损

治则：补肾培元。取足少阴、任脉经穴为主。

处方：关元　肾俞　太溪　足三里

方义：关元培补元气；肾俞、太溪补肾益阴；足三里调补脾胃以生精血；肾精得充，髓海得养，而眩晕自止。

随证选穴：肾阳虚者加灸命门、百会、气海。

刺灸法：毫针刺，用补法。留针 15~30 分钟，间歇行针 1~3 次。关元、肾俞可针灸并用。

4. 痰湿中阻

治则：健脾和胃，化痰除湿。取足阳明、背俞及募穴为主。

处方：中脘　脾俞　足三里　丰隆　百会　内关

方义：胃之募中脘配脾俞、足三里、丰隆以健脾和胃，化痰除湿；百会以升清阳并疏调局部经气；内关宽胸理气，和胃止呕。诸穴合用可达调理脾胃气机，运化湿邪，升清降浊，以治眩晕之目的。

刺灸法：毫针刺，用平补平泻法，或用泻法。留针 15～20 分钟，间歇行针 2～3 次。

其他疗法

1. 耳针

取穴：肾　神门　枕　皮质下　内耳

操作方法：毫针刺，中等刺激，留针 15～30 分钟。亦可用耳穴压豆或耳针埋藏法。

2. 头针

取穴：双侧晕听区

操作方法：用中等刺激手法，留针 30～40 分钟，间歇行针 2～3 次，每次捻针 3～5 分钟。或用电针，疏密波刺激 40～60 分钟。

1.21　中风

中风是以突然昏仆，不省人事，或半身不遂，语言不利，口角歪斜为主症的一种疾病。因其起病急骤，变化多端，犹如风之善行而数变的特征相似，故类比称为中风又称"猝中"。

现代医学的脑溢血，脑血栓形成，脑栓塞，蛛网膜下腔出血，脑血管痉挛等病及其后遗症，均可参照本节辨证治疗。

病因病机

本病多因患者平素气血亏虚，心肝肾三脏阴阳失调，加以忧思恼怒，或饮酒饱食，或房室劳累，或外邪侵袭等诱因，以致肝阳暴张，气血迫走于上，痰浊蒙蔽清窍，阻滞于经络而发为中风。风阳上扰，闭塞清窍则表现为闭证；若病情危重，元气衰微，阴阳离绝者，则表现为脱证。也有仅表现经络之气阻滞而见口眼㖞斜，半身不遂者。

辨证

1. 入脏腑　　病情重，发病急，证见突然昏仆，神志不清，半身瘫痪，口㖞流涎，舌强失语。根据病因病机不同又可分为闭证和脱证。

(1) 闭证　　突然昏仆，不省人事，牙关紧闭，面赤气促，两手握固，喉中痰鸣，二便闭塞，舌红，苔黄厚或灰黑，脉弦滑有力。

(2) 脱证　　突然昏仆，不省人事，目合口开，鼻鼾息微，手撒遗尿，舌痿，脉细弱，甚则四肢逆冷，面赤如妆，脉微欲绝或浮大无根。

2. 在经络　　病情轻缓，证见半身不遂，肌肤不仁，手足麻木，口角歪斜，舌强语涩，或兼见头痛眩晕，筋脉瞤动，目赤面红，口渴咽干，多愁善怒，舌苔黄腻，脉弦或缓滑。

治疗

1. 入脏腑

(1) 闭证

治则：开窍熄风，清火豁痰。取督脉、足厥阴经及十二井穴为主。

处方：人中　十二井　劳宫　太冲　涌泉　丰隆

方义：人中为督脉急救之要穴，有开窍启闭之功；十二井穴点刺出血可清热开窍醒脑；劳宫为手厥阴心包之荥穴，泻之以清心热；太冲为肝之原穴，可降肝经逆气，平熄肝阳，通经行瘀；涌泉为足少阴之井穴，可导热下行；丰隆为足阳明之络穴，取之以宣通脾胃气机，蠲化痰浊。诸穴配伍以达平肝熄风，降火豁痰，启闭开窍之目的。

随证选穴：牙关紧闭加颊车，地仓。

刺灸法：毫针刺，用泻法。留针20～40分钟，间歇行针3～5次。井穴可用三棱针点刺出血。

(2) 脱证

治则：补益元气，回阳固脱。以取任脉穴为主。

处方：神阙（隔盐灸）　气海　关元

方义：任脉为阴脉之海，根据"孤阴不生，独阳不长"阴阳互

· 477 ·

根的原理，如元阳外出，必从阴中以救阳。关元为任脉与足三阴之交会穴，又为三焦元气所出，联系命门真阳，是阴中有阳的腧穴；气海又名丹田，为任脉之脉气所发处，系生气之海；脐为生命之根蒂，神阙位于脐中，为真气所系；故用大艾炷灸此三穴，以回垂绝之阳，使阳气来复，固卫有权，而救虚脱。

随证选穴：脉微欲绝加内关、太渊；四肢厥冷加足三里。

刺灸法：用灸法，以大艾炷灸之，不拘壮数，以汗收，肢温、脉起为度。

2. 在经络

治则：调理气血，熄风通络。取督脉和患侧阳经腧穴为主。

处方：百会　风府　人迎

半身不遂者上肢取：肩髃　曲池　外关　合谷。

下肢取：环跳　风市　阳陵泉　足三里

口眼㖞斜加取：颊车　地仓　下关　合谷　太冲

言语不利加取：哑门　廉泉

方义：督脉为阳脉之海，百会、风府以熄风通络，人迎为足阳明胃经之腧穴，阳明为多气多血之经，取之以调和周身气血，疏通上下经络；阳主动，肢体运动障碍，其病在阳，故取手足三阳经腧穴以使气血经络通畅，正气旺盛，运动功能则易于恢复；口眼㖞斜者取局部与远端穴以调经气，祛风邪；言语不利取哑门、廉泉以利舌本。

刺灸法：毫针刺，用平补平泻法。初病时可针患侧，久病则宜双侧同取。留针20～30分钟，间歇行针1～3次。

其他疗法：头针

取穴：运动区、言语区

操作方法：毫针刺，留针30～40分钟，以手捻法每10分钟捻针3～5分钟。或用电针、留针60分钟。针刺同时，鼓励患者作肢体运动，效果较好。

1.22 口眼歪斜

口眼歪斜又称面瘫。以单纯性的一侧面颊筋肉弛缓、口眼歪斜为主症。任何年龄均可发病,但以青壮年为多见。

本病相当于现代医学的周围性面神经麻痹,亦称 Bell 氏麻痹。

病因病机

本病多由络脉空虚,风寒之邪乘虚侵入阳明、少阳经脉与经筋,以致经气阻滞,经筋失养,肌肉纵缓不收而发病。

辨证

起病突然,多发于一侧。发病后病侧面部板滞不适,眼睑闭合不全,流泪,口角下垂,漱口漏水,不能蹙额、皱眉、鼓腮、闭眼、示齿和吹口哨等。部分病人有耳后、耳下疼痛或偏侧头痛,严重时可出现舌前 2/3 味觉减退或消失,听觉过敏等症,舌苔薄白,脉浮紧或浮缓。

治疗

治则:疏风通络,调和气血。取手足阳明经穴为主。

处方:风池 翳风 阳白 四白 太阳 地仓 颊车 迎香 合谷 内庭

方义:风池、翳风同属少阳经穴,可祛风止痛;太阳、阳白、四白、地仓、颊车、迎香为局部取穴,有疏风通络 调和气血的作用;合谷、内庭均为阳明经穴,可疏导阳明经气,以除头面之风邪。诸穴共用可疏风通络、调和气血,使筋肉得濡润温煦,则面瘫可愈。

随证选穴:眼睑闭合不全加攒竹、瞳子髎;人中沟歪斜加水沟;颏唇沟歪斜加承浆或夹承浆;示齿不能加巨髎;耳后疼痛加完骨、外关。

刺灸法:毫针刺,用平补平泻法,或初期用泻法,后期用补法。留针 15~20 分钟,间歇行针 1~3 次。风池、翳风针后加灸，艾条灸每穴 15～20 分钟。亦可用透刺法，阳白透鱼腰，地仓透颊车，太阳透下关。

其他疗法

1. 皮肤针

取穴：阳白　太阳　四白　地仓　颊车

操作方法：轻刺激，叩至皮肤潮红为度，隔日一次。此法适用于恢复期及其后遗症。

2. 拔罐法

取穴：颊车　下关　太阳

操作方法：毫针刺后用小型火罐拔，隔2～3日一次，亦可用皮肤针叩刺后，用小型火罐吸拔，每次拔5～10分钟。

3. 发泡灸

取穴：翳风　太阳　颊车

操作方法：将中药制成的药膏贴敷于穴位上，患部有一种热感，甚至烧灼痛，贴敷2～3小时后将药膏撕掉，此时局部皮肤轻者紫红，甚者可见有大小不等的水泡，出现水泡者，用三棱针点破使水流尽，一般无需特殊处理。

1.23　胸痹

胸痹是指胸中憋闷疼痛而言，轻者仅感胸闷如塞，重者胸痛如绞，并有短气、喘息等症。胸部为心肺两脏之所居，故本病的发生多与心肺功能失常有关。

本病主要见于现代医学的冠状动脉粥样硬化性心脏病。如慢性支气管炎、肺气肿等以胸痛为主证时，亦可参照本篇辨证治疗。

病因病机

本病多因素体心气不足，或心阳不振，寒邪侵袭，阴寒内盛，寒凝气滞，痹阻脉络；或恣食甘肥生冷，损伤脾胃，聚湿成痰，阻滞胸阳；或情志所伤，气机郁结，气滞日久，血流不畅，脉络瘀滞而致。

辨证

1. 虚寒　　胸痛彻背，心悸，胸闷短气，恶寒肢冷，受寒则甚，舌苔白滑或腻，脉沉细。

2. 痰浊　　胸闷如窒，痛引肩背，气短喘促，咳嗽，痰多粘腻色白，脘腹痞满，纳呆，肢体疲倦，舌苔白腻，脉濡缓。

3. 瘀血　　胸痛如刺，或绞痛阵发，痛彻肩背，胸闷短气，心悸，唇紫，舌质暗，脉细涩或结代。

治疗

1. 虚寒

治则：助阳散寒，行气活血。取背俞穴、手少阴、厥阴经穴为主。

处方：心俞　巨阙　厥阴俞　膻中　内关　通里

方义：心俞、巨阙为俞募配穴，可补心气。温心阳；厥阴俞、膻中亦为俞募相配，可宽中调气，以散阴寒；内关为手厥阴之络穴配手少阴之络通里，与上穴共达助阳散寒，通经活络，行气活血镇痛之目的。

随证选穴：恶寒加灸肺俞、风门；肢冷加灸气海、关元。

刺灸法：毫针刺，用补法或平补平泻法。留针 20～30 分钟，间歇行针 2～3 次。心俞；厥阴俞多用灸法或针灸并用，每穴灸 10～15 分钟。

2. 痰浊

治则：通阳祛痰化浊。取任脉、手厥阴，足阳明经穴为主。

处方：巨阙　膻中　郄门　建里　丰隆　三阴交

方义：巨阙、膻中与手厥阴心包之郄穴郄门可振奋心阳，宽胸理气止痛；建里能温中健胃，散寒祛湿；丰隆为足阳明之络配三阴交以健脾和胃、蠲化痰浊。诸穴共奏通阳祛痰化浊，活血止痛之功。

随证选穴：背痛加脾俞、心俞；气短加灸气海俞、内关。

刺灸法：毫针刺，用泻法。留针 15～30 分钟，间歇行针 2～3 次。

3. 瘀血

治则：活血化瘀止痛。取俞募穴及任脉、手少阴经穴为主。

处方：至阳　阴郄　心俞　巨阙　膈俞　膻中

方义：至阳通心气，疗心痛；阴郄为手少阴之郄，配巨阙、心俞以调气血、化瘀止痛；膈俞、膻中以行气活血。诸穴相配可使气行血行，气血调和，瘀血得通，疼痛消失。

随证选穴：唇舌紫绀加少冲、中冲点刺出血。

刺灸法：毫针刺，用泻法。留针 15～30 分钟，间歇行针 2～3 次。

其他疗法：耳针

取穴：心　小肠　神门　交感　皮质下　肺　胸

操作方法：毫针刺，每次选 3～4 穴，中等刺激，留针 20 分钟。亦可用耳穴压豆、耳针埋藏法。

1.24　惊悸

惊悸又名心悸、怔忡。以病人自感心中急剧跳动、惊慌不安，不能自主为主证。一般多呈阵发性，每因情志波动或劳累而发作和加甚。

现代医学的心肌炎、心包炎，心动过速、心动过缓等各种原因引起的心律失常及部分神经官能症等，有本病表现者，均可参考本篇辨证治疗。

病因病机

本病多因平素心气怯弱，或久病心血不足，骤遇惊恐则"心无所依，神无所归"，心神不宁；或饮食伤脾，痰饮内停，思虑烦劳，气郁化火，痰火内扰；或久患痹证，风寒湿热之邪内侵于心，心脉痹阻，气滞血瘀而致。

辨证

1. 心神不宁　　心悸，善惊易恐，烦躁不宁，多梦易醒，纳食减少，舌苔薄白，脉细数。

2. 气血不足　　心悸不安，难以自主，气短乏力，面色不华，头晕目眩，舌质淡，脉细弱或结代。

3. 痰火内动　　心悸时发时止，烦躁不宁，胸闷，头晕，失眠多梦，易惊神恍，口苦，咳嗽，咯痰粘稠，小便黄，大便不爽，舌苔黄腻，脉滑数。

4. 血脉瘀阻　　心悸持续多年，日渐加重，动则气喘，心痛时作，面色黄瘦，其者出现形寒肢冷，咳喘不能平卧，冷汗，浮肿，唇舌紫暗，脉细涩结代。

治疗

1. 心神不宁

治则：宁心安神镇惊。取手少阴、厥阴经穴为主。

处方：神门　心俞　内关　间使　巨阙

方义：神门为心之原穴，配间使、内关以宁心安神，镇惊定悸；心俞，巨阙为俞募相配以调补心气。诸穴共奏镇惊安神，宁心定悸之功效。

随症选穴：善惊加大陵。

刺灸法：毫针刺，用补法。留针15～30分钟，间歇行针1～2次。

2. 气血不足

治则：补气养血定悸。取背俞、任脉、手少阴经穴为主。

处方：心俞　巨阙　膈俞　脾俞　足三里　气海　神门　内关

方义：心俞、巨阙补心气，通心阳；膈俞为血之会，可补血以养心神；脾俞、足三里健脾胃以滋生化之源；气海益气；神门、内关以宁心安神。诸穴配伍以达补气养血，宁神定悸之目的。

随证选穴：头晕目眩加百会、风池。

刺灸法：毫针刺，用补法。留针15～30分钟，间歇行针2～3次。背俞、足三里、气海可针灸并用。

3. 痰火内动

治则：清火化痰、宁心安神。取手三阴，足阳明经穴为主。

处方：灵道　郄门　肺俞　尺泽　丰隆　阳陵泉

方义：灵道、郄门安心神止心悸；尺泽、肺俞泻肺清火；丰隆、阳陵泉清泄肝胃之火，降逆气，化痰浊。诸穴相配可清热化痰，安心宁神，而惊悸可平。

随证选穴：失眠多梦心神恍惚加厉兑；烦躁不宁加间使；便秘加大肠俞。

刺灸法：毫针刺，用泻法。留针15～20分钟，间歇行针2～3次。

4. 血脉瘀阻

治则：活血化瘀，强心定悸。取手少阴、厥阴、足太阳经穴为主。

处方：内关　曲泽　少海　膈俞　气海

方义：心包是心的宫城，故取内关配曲泽，少海以强心定悸止痛，以治其标；气海以助阳益气；膈俞以活血化瘀而治其本；标本同治以益气行血化瘀，强心定悸止痛。

刺灸法：毫针刺，用平补平泻法。留针15～30分钟，间歇行针1～2次。

其他疗法：耳针

取穴：心　交感　神门　皮质下　小肠

操作方法：毫针刺，轻刺激，留针15～20分钟。或用耳穴压豆法。

1.25　不寐

不寐即失眠。是以经常不能获得正常的睡眠为特征的一种病证。并常兼见头晕、头痛、心悸，健忘等证。不寐的临床表现不一，轻者入寐困难；或寐而多梦易惊，时寐时醒，或醒后不能再寐；严重者整夜不能入寐。

病因病机

多因忧思劳倦，损伤心脾，以致气血化源不足，不能养心安神；或房劳伤肾，肾阴亏耗，阴虚火旺，心肾不交；或饮食所伤，脾胃不和；湿盛生痰，痰郁生热，扰及心神；或因情志所伤，肝气郁结，郁而化火，肝火上扰，心神不宁等而致不寐。

辨证

1. 心脾两虚　　夜来不易入寐，寐则多梦易醒，心悸健忘，体倦神疲，面色少华，饮食无味，脘痞便溏，舌质淡，苔薄白；脉细弱。

2. 心肾不交　　心烦不寐，头晕耳鸣，口干津少，五心烦热，健忘，心悸，梦遗腰痠，舌质红，苔少，脉细数。

3. 胃气不和　　夜寐不安多梦，心中懊恼，脘腹胀满或胀痛，时有恶心或呕吐，嗳腐吞酸，大便不爽，舌苔黄腻，脉滑或弦。

4. 肝火上扰　　头晕头胀，多烦易怒，不得入眠。或伴有目赤、口苦、胁痛等，舌苔薄黄，脉弦数。

治疗

1. 心脾两虚

治则：补益心脾，养血安神。取手少阴、足太阴经穴和背俞穴为主。

处方：脾俞　心俞　隐白　神门　三阴交

方义：脾俞、心俞以补养心脾；隐白为足太阴之井穴，能治多梦易惊；神门、三阴交以益气养血安神。诸穴合用以补养心脾，益气生血，使心神得养，则睡眠自常。

随证选穴：健忘灸志室、百会。

刺灸法：毫针刺，用补法。留针15～20分钟，亦可针灸并用。

2. 心肾不交

治则：交通心肾。取背俞、手足少阴、厥阴经穴为主。

处方：心俞　肾俞　太溪　大陵　神门　照海

方义：心俞、大陵配神门以降心火，镇惊安神；肾俞配肾之原穴太溪以滋肾水；照海可益肾阴、除心热，安心神。诸穴配伍使心肾相交，水火既济，心神得宁。

随证选穴：头晕加风池；耳鸣加听宫；遗精加志室。

刺灸法：毫针刺，补泻兼施，心俞、大陵多用泻法，肾俞、太溪多用补法。留针15～30分钟，间歇行针2～3次。

3. 胃气不和

治则：健脾和胃，利湿化痰。取任脉、足阳明、太阴经穴为主。

处方：中脘　丰隆　足三里　历兑　隐白　神门

方义：胃募中脘配足阳明之络丰隆、合穴足三里以和胃安中化痰；阳明根于历兑，太阴根于隐白，二穴同用主治多梦失眠；神门宁心安神。诸穴共用可使胃和寐安。

随证选穴：懊恼、呕恶加内关。

刺灸法：毫针刺，用泻法。留针15～30分钟，间歇行针2～3次。

4. 肝火上扰

治则：清肝泻火，滋阴潜阳。取足少阳、足厥阴、手少阴经穴为主。

处方：肝俞　胆俞　行间　足窍阴　神门

方义：肝俞、行间以清肝泻火、益血养阴；胆俞、足窍阴以降胆火而除烦；神门以宁心神。诸穴可清泻肝胆之火，益阴潜阳，不寐自愈。

随证选穴：目赤加太阳。

刺灸法：毫针刺，用泻法。留针15～20分钟，间歇行针2～3次。太阳可用三棱针点刺出血。

其他疗法

1. 耳针

取穴：皮质下 交感 神门 心 脾 肾 内分泌

操作方法：毫针刺，每次选 3～5 穴，轻刺激，留针 30 分。或用耳针埋藏及耳穴压豆法。

2. 皮肤针

取穴：四神聪 安眠穴 夹脊穴

操作方法：轻刺激，叩至以皮肤微红为度，从上向下，每次叩打 2～3 遍，隔日一次。

1.26 多寐

多寐亦称"嗜睡"、"嗜卧"。以不分昼夜，时时欲睡，呼之能醒，醒后复睡为证。

现代医学的发作性睡病，神经官能症，精神病的某些患者，其临床症状与多寐类似者，均可参考本篇辨证治疗。

辨证

1. 湿盛困脾　昏昏欲睡，头蒙如裹，肢体沉重，倦怠乏力，胸痞脘闷，纳少泛恶，或见浮肿，舌苔白腻，脉濡缓。

2. 脾气不足　食后困倦嗜睡，肢体倦怠，必须少睡片刻，醒后似略常人，面色萎黄，纳少便溏，苔薄白，脉虚弱。

3. 阳气虚衰　整日嗜睡懒言，精神疲惫，畏寒肢冷，健忘，舌淡苔薄，脉沉细无力。

4. 瘀血阻滞　头昏头痛，时时欲睡，肢体困倦，记忆力减退、或有头部外伤史，舌质紫暗或有瘀斑，脉沉涩。

治疗

1. 湿盛困脾

治则：健脾祛湿醒神。取足阳阴、足太阴、督脉穴为主。

处方：中脘 丰隆 阴陵泉 百会 太阳

方义：中脘配足阳明之络穴丰隆，足太阴之合穴阴陵泉以健脾和胃利湿；百会、太阳以清脑醒神。诸穴配伍以使脾健湿祛、脑清神醒。

随证选穴：纳少泛恶加足三里、内关。

刺灸法：毫针刺，用补法或平补平泻法。留针 15～20 分钟，间歇行针 2～3 次。

2. 脾气不足

治则：健脾益气醒脑。取背俞、募穴、足太阴、足阳明经穴为主。

处方：脾俞　章门　隐白　足三里　解溪　百会

方义：脾俞、章门俞募相配以补益脾气；隐白为足太阴之井穴以益气醒脾；解溪为足阳明之经穴，五行属火，为土之母与足阳明合穴足三里同用可增健补脾胃之功，以强运化之机能；百会以醒脑提神。诸穴共用使脾气健运，运化有权，清阳得升，精神得振。

刺灸法：毫针刺，用补法。留针 20～30 分钟，间歇行针 1～2 次。脾俞、章门、足三里可针灸并用。

3. 阳气虚衰

治则：益气温阳。取背俞　足太阴　少阴经穴为主。

处方：膏肓俞　肾俞　气海　三阴交　大钟　申脉

方义：膏肓俞益气补虚；肾俞、气海以温肾壮阳；三阴交健脾益气，并可调补三阴之经气；足少阴之络穴大钟以补肾调气；申脉为阳跷脉所生，主治多眠。诸穴配伍可健补脾肾，益气壮阳，以清神志。

随证选穴：健忘加神门。

刺灸法：毫针刺，用补法。留针 15～30 分钟，间歇行针 1～2 次。膏肓俞、气海、肾俞可针灸并用，每穴灸 10～15 分钟。

4. 瘀血阻滞

治则：活血通络，醒脑提神。取背俞、阳明、厥阴经穴为主

处方：膈俞　肝俞　合谷　太冲　太阳　百会

方义：膈俞、肝俞以疏肝理气，活血化瘀；合谷升而能散，善以行气，气行血行，通经活络；太冲调肝养血，通经行瘀，配太阳、百会以开窍醒脑提神。

刺灸法：毫针刺，用泻法。留针 15～20 分钟，间歇行针 2～3 次。

1.27　健忘

健忘系指记忆力减弱，遇事易忘的一种病证。

现代医学的神经衰弱，脑动脉硬化等疾病出现健忘症状者，可参考本篇进行辨证治疗。

病因病机

本病之病因较为复杂。多因思虑过度，劳伤心脾，心脾亏损；或房事不节，肾精暗耗，肾阴不足，以致心肾不交；或年老肾衰，心气不足，神明失聪；或因痰饮瘀血，痹阻心窍等而引起健忘。

辨证

1. 心脾两虚　　遇事善忘，精神倦怠，四肢无力，心悸少寐，纳呆气短，声低语怯，面色少华，舌苔薄白或白腻，舌质淡，有齿痕，脉细弱无力。

2. 心肾不交　　遇事善忘，腰酸腿软，或有遗精，头晕耳鸣，或手足心热，心烦失眠，舌质红，苔薄白，脉细数。

3. 年老神衰　　遇事善忘，形体衰惫，神志恍惚，气短乏力，腰酸腿软，纳少尿频，心悸少寐，舌苔薄白，脉细弱无力。

4. 痰瘀痹阻　　遇事善忘，兼见语言迟缓，神思欠敏，表情呆钝，舌上有瘀点，舌苔白腻，脉滑或细涩。

治疗

1. 心脾两虚

治则：养心健脾。取背俞、任脉经穴为主。

处方：心俞　脾俞　膈俞　气海

方义：心俞、脾俞补益心脾，心气旺盛则精神充沛，思虑敏捷，脾气健运则水谷精微得以吸收输布；膈俞补血，气海补气，气血充盛，心脾得养功能正常。

刺灸法：毫针刺，用补法。留针 20～30 分钟，行针 1～2次。亦可针灸并用，每穴灸 10 分钟。

2. 心肾不交

治则：交通心肾。取背俞、手足少阴经穴为主。

处方：心俞　肾俞　太溪　劳宫　神门

方义：心俞、肾俞补心肾以交水火；太溪补肾水；劳宫泄心火；神门安神定志；肾水不亏，心火不旺，心肾相交则神清智聪。

刺灸法：毫针刺，补泻兼施。心俞、肾俞、太溪用补法，劳宫、神门用泻法。留针 15～20 分钟，间歇行针 1～2 次。

3. 年老神衰

治则：补肾、养心、健脾、益智。取背俞、足少阴经穴为主。

处方：肾俞　太溪　心俞　脾俞　四神聪

方义：肾俞配肾之原穴太溪补肾气，益肾精，生髓充脑益智；心俞、脾俞以养心脾；四神聪醒神益智为治健忘之经验穴。诸穴配伍使肾气充沛，肾精充盈，心脾之气旺盛，髓海得养，则诸症康复。

刺灸法：毫针刺，用补法。留针 20～30 分钟，间歇行针 1～2 次。肾俞、心俞、脾俞、太溪可针灸并用，或用灸法，每穴.灸 10～15 分钟。

4. 痰瘀痹阻

治则：补心气，化痰瘀。取阳明、厥阴经穴为主。

处方：丰隆　足三里　神门　大陵　三阴交　行间

方义：丰隆以清化痰浊，足三里以调理脾胃，以助豁痰降浊之效；大陵、神门化痰开窍，清心定志；三阴交调理血分配行间疏调肝脾之气，行瘀化滞。诸穴合用使痰化瘀去，气血流畅，神明有主。

刺灸法：毫针刺，用泻法。留针15~20分钟，间歇行针2~3次。

其他疗法：耳针

取穴：心　脾　肾　交感　神门　脑点

操作方法：毫针刺，每次选3~4穴，轻刺激，留针15~20分钟。或用耳穴压豆法。

1.28　癫狂

癫与狂都是精神失常的疾病。癫证是以精神抑郁，表情淡漠，沉默痴呆，语无伦次，静而少动为特征；狂证以精神亢奋，狂躁打骂，喧扰不宁，动而多怒为特征。癫属阴，狂属阳，二者在病理上有一定联系，病情亦可互相转化，故常并称为癫狂。

本病包括现代医学的精神分裂症，反应性精神病，脑器质性疾病所引起的精神障碍等。

病因病机

癫证多由忧思过度，情志抑郁以致肝失条达，脾气不运，津液凝滞为痰，痰浊上逆，精神失常而成。

狂证多因所求不遂，忿怒伤肝，不得宣泄，郁而化火，煎熬津液，结为痰火，痰火上扰，蒙闭心窍以致神志错乱而发。

辨证

1. 癫证　　发病缓慢，初起先有精神苦闷，神志呆滞，继则言语错乱，喜怒无常或终日不语，喜静多睡，不知秽洁，不思饮食，甚者妄见妄闻，舌苔薄腻，脉弦细或弦滑。

2. 狂证　　发病急速，病前亦见烦躁易怒，少睡少食，继而狂躁好动，气力倍增，高声叫骂，弃衣奔走，终日不眠，甚至毁物扛人，不避亲疏，舌苔黄腻，脉弦滑而数。

治疗

1. 癫证

治则：疏肝解郁，化痰开窍。取手少阴、厥阴、背俞穴为主。

处方：神门　大陵　心俞　肝俞　脾俞　太冲　丰隆

方义：大陵为心包之原穴，又属统治癫狂病"十三鬼穴"之一，神门是心的原穴，善治心性痴呆，二穴配用以宁心安神；心俞、脾俞、肝俞以开心窍、运脾气、疏肝郁；太冲为肝之原穴可疏肝理气解郁；膻中为气之会，配足阳明之络穴丰隆以调气化痰。诸穴共奏疏肝解郁，化痰开窍，宁心安神之效。

随证选穴：不思饮食加中脘、足三里；喜怒无常加间使；妄见加睛明；妄闻加听宫。

刺灸法：毫针刺，用平补平泻法。留针15～30分钟，间歇行针2～4次。

2. 狂证

治则：清心、豁痰、醒脑。取督脉、手厥阴经穴为主。

处方：大椎　风府　水沟　丰隆　间使　劳宫

方义：大椎为诸阳之会，配水沟能清泄阳热，醒脑开窍；风府益脑髓，宁神志；间使配丰隆清心化痰；劳宫为手厥阴心包之荥穴可清心包而泄心火，定神安志；诸穴共用可使痰火得清，神明有主，而狂躁自止。

刺灸法：毫针刺，用泻法。留针15～30分钟，间歇行针2～4次，亦可不留针。大椎可用三棱针点刺出血。

其他疗法：耳针

取穴：心　皮质下　肾　枕　额　神门　交感

操作方法：毫针刺，每次选3～4穴，癫证用轻刺激，留针15～20分钟，狂证用强刺激，多不留针。均可用耳针埋藏。

1.29 痫证

痫证是一种发作性神志失常的疾病，俗称"羊痫风"。以突然仆倒，昏不知人，口吐涎沫，两目上视，肢体抽搐，或口中如猪羊叫声，醒后如常人为主要临床特征。

本病与现代医学的癫痫基本相同，无论原发性或继发性癫痫均可参照本篇进行辨证治疗。

病因病机

本病多由惊恐郁怒，心肝气郁或饮食伤脾，脾虚生湿，以致气机郁结，郁而化火，炼湿为痰，气火挟痰横窜经络，上蒙清窍，迫使阴阳发生一时性的逆乱而发病。

辨证

1. 发作期　　发作时，常先觉头晕头痛，胸闷欠伸，旋即昏倒仆地，神志不清，面色苍白，牙关紧急，两目上视，手足抽搐，口吐涎沫，并发出类似猪羊叫声，甚至二便失禁，不久渐渐苏醒，症状消失，除感疲乏无力外，饮食起居如常，舌苔白腻，脉多弦滑。

2. 休止期　　发作后，精神萎靡，面色不华，头晕，心悸，食少，痰多，腰痠肢软，舌质淡，苔白，脉细滑。

治疗

1. 发作期

治则：化痰开窍，平肝熄风。取督脉、任脉、足厥阴经穴为主。

处方：水沟　鸠尾　大椎　间使　太冲　丰隆

方义：水沟为醒脑开窍之要穴；鸠尾为任脉之络穴，大椎为诸阳之会穴，二穴并用可协调阴阳逆乱，间使以疏通心包经气；太冲以平肝熄风、醒脑宁神；丰隆和胃降浊，清热化痰。诸穴合用以奏豁痰开窍，平肝熄风，宁神安神之功效。

随证选穴：发作昏迷不苏者加涌泉、气海。

刺灸法：毫针刺，用泻法。一般先刺人中，再针太冲、涌泉，提插捻转至神志清醒为止。或留针15～20分钟，间歇行针2～3次。

2. 休止期

治则：养心安神，健脾益肾。取手少阴、足太阴经穴为主。

处方：心俞　印堂　神门　三阴交　太溪　腰奇

方义：心俞、印堂、神门三穴合用以养心安神定志；三阴交、太溪以补脾益肾；腰奇为治疗痫证的经验效穴。

随证选穴：白昼多发作者加申脉；夜间多发作者加照海；痰多加丰隆。

刺灸法：毫针刺，用补法，或平补平泻法。留针20～30分钟，间歇行针1～2次。

按语

继发性癫痫，应重视原发病的治疗。持续发作伴有高热、昏迷等危重病例必须采取综合疗法。

1.30　郁证

郁证是由于情志忧郁，气滞不畅所引起的病证的总称。以心情抑郁，情绪不宁，胸部满闷，胁肋胀痛或易怒欲哭；或咽中如有异物梗阻等为主要症状。

现代医学的癔病，神经官能症，更年期综合症等均可参见本节辨证治疗。

病因病机

本病多因郁怒伤肝，肝失条达，气机郁结，上犯心神；或思虑伤脾，脾失健运，郁而生痰，痰气郁结，日久化火，上扰心神，以致心神不宁；或忧思过度，气机不利，营血暗耗所致。

辨证

1. 肝气郁结　精神抑郁，情绪不宁，胸闷胁痛，腹胀嗳气，不思饮食或腹痛呕吐，大便正常，舌苔薄腻，脉弦。

2. 气郁化火　　　性情急躁易怒，胸胁胀满，口苦而干，或头痛、目赤、耳鸣，或吞酸嘈杂，大便秘结，舌质红，脉弦数。

3. 痰气郁结　　　精神抑郁，胸部闷塞，咽中不适，如有物阻，咯之不出，咽之不下，但饮食吞咽不困难，舌苔薄腻，脉弦滑。

4. 阴血不足　　　无故悲伤，喜怒无常，多疑善惊，心悸烦躁，睡眠不安等，或有突发胸闷，呃逆，暴喑，抽搐等症，严重者可昏迷、僵仆，苔薄白，脉弦细。

治疗

1. 肝气郁结

治则：疏肝解郁、理气调中。取任脉、足厥阴经穴为主。

处方：膻中　肝俞　太冲　中脘　足三里　公孙

方义：膻中为气之会穴，可调理气机；肝俞、太冲以疏肝解郁；中脘、足三里和胃降逆；公孙为脾之络穴以健脾和胃。诸穴合用可使肝气条达，脾胃气机调和，诸症得平。

刺灸法：毫针刺，用平补平泻法。留针15～20分钟，间歇行针2～3次。

2. 气郁化火

治则：清肝泄火解郁，理气和中健胃。取手足少阳、足厥阴、阳明经穴为主。

处方：行间　侠溪　支沟　阳陵泉　上脘　足三里

方义：行间、侠溪为足厥阴肝及足少阳胆之荥穴，可清泄肝胆之火；支沟、阳陵泉可疏调经气，以解肝郁；上脘、足三里和胃理气。诸穴配用可达清肝泄火，理气和中，解郁宁神之目的。

刺灸法：毫针刺，用泻法。留针15～20分钟，间歇行针2～3次。

3. 痰气郁结

治则：疏肝行气，开郁化痰。取足厥阴、任脉经穴为主。

处方：天突　膻中　内关　丰隆　太冲

方义：天突降气清咽利膈；内关宽胸理气；太冲以疏肝解郁；膻中、丰隆以行气化痰。诸穴共奏疏肝行气，开郁化痰，利膈清咽之功效。

刺灸法：毫针刺，用平补平泻法。留针15～20分钟，间歇行针2～3次。

4. 阴血不足

治则：调肝养血，宁心安神。取手少阴、足厥阴经穴为主。

处方：太冲　神门　心俞　内关　三阴交　巨阙

方义：肝之原穴太冲可调肝养血，疏肝解郁；心俞配心之募巨阙，心之原神门以宁心安神；三阴交可补血育阴；内关以宽胸理气解郁。诸穴合用可使阴血得充，心神得宁，郁证得除。

随证选穴：暴喑加通里、廉泉；呃逆加天突；抽搐加合谷、阳陵泉；昏厥僵仆加水沟、涌泉。

刺灸法：毫针刺，用平补平泻法。留针15～20分钟，行针1～2次。

其他疗法：耳针

取穴：心　皮质下　枕　脑点　肝　内分泌　神门

操作方法：毫针刺，每次选3～4穴，轻刺激，留针15～20分钟。或用耳针埋藏、耳穴压豆法。

1.31　头痛

头痛系病人的一种自觉症状，可见于多种急慢性疾病中。本篇所述的头痛，是指外感或内伤杂病以头痛为主证者。如属某一疾病过程中所出现的兼证，不属本节讨论范围。

头痛可见于现代医学中感染性发热性疾病、高血压、颅内疾病，神经官能症，偏头痛等多种疾病。

病因病机

外感头痛多因风寒湿热之邪外袭，上犯经络，清阳之气受阻而致。

内伤头痛多因情志刺激，肝气郁结，郁而化火，上扰清空；或肾阴素亏，水不涵木，肝阳上亢；或饮食不节，过食肥甘，脾失健运，痰浊内生，阻遏清阳；或久病、失血之后、气血亏虚，不能上营脑髓而致。

如头痛日久，久痛入络，络脉瘀滞或跌仆损伤，脑髓受损，气血运行不畅可致瘀血头痛。

辨证

1. **外感头痛**　发病较急，头痛时作，痛连项背，痛势较剧，如锥如刺，痛有定处，舌苔薄白，脉弦紧。

2. **内伤头痛**　发病缓慢，多呈隐痛。空痛、昏痛，疲劳则剧，时作时止。

(1) 肝阳头痛　头痛眩晕，多烦易怒，睡眠不宁，面红目赤，口苦，舌红，苔薄黄，脉弦有力。

(2) 痰浊头痛　头额昏痛如裹，胸脘痞闷，恶心，甚则呕吐痰涎，便溏，舌苔白腻，脉弦滑。

(3) 气血亏虚头痛　头痛头晕，痛势绵绵，遇劳则甚，休息痛减，神疲气短，心悸健忘，食欲不振，面色少华，舌淡，苔薄白，脉细弱无力。

(4) 瘀血头痛　头痛如刺，经久不愈，痛处固定不移，视物花黑，记忆力减退，舌有紫斑，脉细涩。

治疗

1. **外感头痛**

治则：疏风通络、活血止痛。按头痛部位循经取穴为主，局部取穴为辅。

处方：风池　头维　百会　合谷

方义：取风池疏风解表止痛，以祛少阳偏头、颈项之风；头维搜风通络止痛，以治阳明头额之风；百会为厥阴肝脉之会，取之以平熄巅顶之风；头为诸阳之会，面为阳明之乡，头面有疾取合谷以蠲除头面之风。诸穴合用可达祛风疏经镇痛之效。

随证选穴：前头痛配上星、阳白、印堂；后头痛配天柱、昆仑、后溪；侧头痛配太阳、率谷、外关；头顶痛配通天、脑空、太冲。

刺灸法：毫针刺，用泻法。留针 15～20 分钟，间歇行针 2～3 次，疼痛剧烈发作时，持续行针至疼痛减轻或消失后。

2. 内伤头痛

(1) 肝阳头痛

治则：平肝降逆，熄风潜阳。取足少阳、厥阴经穴为主。

处方：风池　悬颅　太阳　行间　侠溪　太溪

方义：风池、悬颅均为足少阳之经穴，有清热熄风镇痛之作用，可平熄上亢之风阳之邪；太阳疏调局部经气；行间、侠溪为足厥阴与足少阳之荥穴，可泻肝胆之热邪；太溪补肾水以育阴潜阳。诸穴配伍共奏平肝熄风止痛之功效。

随证选穴：目赤加关冲点刺放血；心烦易怒加肝俞、间使。

刺灸法：毫针刺，用泻法，太溪穴用补法。留针 10～20 分钟，间歇行针 2～3 次。太阳亦可用三棱针点刺出血。

(2) 痰浊头痛

治则：化痰降浊，通络止痛。取任脉，足阳明经穴为主。

处方：中脘　丰隆　百会　印堂　绝骨

方义：中脘配丰隆以健运脾胃，化痰降浊，以治其本；绝骨能清三焦之湿浊之邪；百会、印堂可宣发清阳，通络止痛。诸穴配用共达化痰降浊，通络止痛之目的。

随证选穴：呕吐痰涎加内关；便溏加天枢。

刺灸法：毫针刺，用泻法。留针 15～20 分钟，间歇行针 2～3 次。

(3) 气血亏虚头痛

治则：益气养血，和络止痛。取背俞穴为主。

处方：肝俞　脾俞　肾俞　膈俞　气海　百会　足三里　三阴交

方义：肝藏血，脾统血，脑为髓海，髓生于肾，故取肝脾肾之背俞穴加膈俞、三阴交以补益气血；取足三里以助生化之源；气海以调补周身之气；百会可升阳举陷，引气血上行以养脑。诸穴可使气血充足，髓海得养，而头痛可除。

刺灸法：毫针刺，用补法。留针20～30分钟，间歇行针1～2次。

（4）瘀血头痛

治则：活血化瘀，行气定痛。取阿是穴及手阳明、足太阴经穴为主。

处方：阿是穴　合谷　三阴交　膈俞

方义：阿是穴以泻局部之瘀血，疏通局部经气；合谷升而能散，善疗头面之疾；三阴交配膈俞以活血祛瘀；诸穴配用共达化瘀定痛之目的。

随证选穴：眉棱痛加攒竹；侧头痛加太阳；后头痛加玉枕；头顶痛加四神聪。

刺灸法：毫针刺，用平补平泻或补泻兼施。合谷用补法，余穴用泻法或平补平泻法。留针15～20分钟，间歇行针2～3次。阿是穴可用三棱针点刺出血。

其他疗法

1. 耳针

取穴：皮质下　额　枕　太阳　神门　肝　脾　肾

操作方法：毫针刺，每次选3～4穴，用中等刺激，留针15～20分钟。头痛顽固者，用强刺激，或在耳背静脉放血。亦可用耳针埋藏或耳穴压豆法。

2. 皮肤针

取穴：太阳　印堂　阿是穴

操作方法：重刺激，叩至局部皮肤出血。本法适用于风袭经络的外感头痛及肝阳亢逆之头痛。

1.32 面痛

面痛指面部一定部位出现阵发性、短暂性、烧灼样剧烈疼痛而言。本病多发于一侧面部的额部、上颌部或下颌部，两侧俱痛者极少见。初起每次疼痛时间较短，间隔时间较长，久则发作次数越来越频，疼痛程度越来越重。发病年龄多在中年以后，女性患者较多。

面痛相当于现代医学的三叉神经病。

病因病机

本病多因风寒之邪袭于阳明筋脉，寒性收引，凝滞筋脉，血气痹阻；或因风热病毒侵淫面部，影响筋脉气血运行而致。亦有因肝胃实热上冲，或肾阴亏虚，虚火上炎而致面痛。

辨证

疼痛发作突然，呈阵发性、放射性、电击样剧痛，其痛如撕裂、针刺、火灼一般，数秒钟或数分钟后缓解，一日可发作数次，间隔时间不一。疼痛部位以面颊上、下颌部为多，额部较为少见。疼痛常有一起点，可因吹风、洗脸、说话、吃饭等刺激此点而诱发。

1. 风寒 面颊疼痛，面部时抽掣，眴动，遇寒发作或痛甚，得热痛减，兼有头痛，恶寒，鼻流清涕，舌苔薄白，脉弦紧。

2. 风热 面颊火灼样疼痛，面部发热，目赤流泪，烦躁，口干咽燥，苔薄黄，脉弦数。

3. 肝胃实热 面颊火灼样疼痛，烦躁易怒，口苦，目赤，眩晕，胸膈满闷，胁下胀，便秘，舌红质干，苔黄厚，脉弦数或洪数。

4. 阴虚火旺 面颊疼痛，反复发作，颧红，皮肤粗糙，头晕目眩，五心烦热，形体消瘦，舌红，苔少，脉细数。

治疗

治则：通经活络止痛。取阳明、少阳、太阳经穴为主。

处方：额部痛：攒竹　阳白　头维　率谷　中渚

上颌痛：四白　颧髎　太阳　迎香　合谷

下颌痛：承浆　颊车　下关　翳风　陷谷

(1) 风寒加风池　风府　列缺

(2) 风热加大椎　曲池

(3) 肝胃实热加行间　内庭

(4) 阴虚火旺加风池　太溪

方义：本方以近部取穴为主，远部取穴为辅，旨在疏通面部筋脉，使气血调和，以达疏经通络止痛之目的。风寒型加风池、风府、列缺以祛风散寒；风热型加大椎、曲池以祛风热；肝胃实热加行间、内庭以清热泄火；阴虚火旺型加太溪以滋补肾水，取风池以潜阳。

刺灸法：毫针刺，用泻法，阴虚火旺型加太溪应用补法。留针15~30分钟，间歇行针2~4次。亦可用电针，每次选2穴通电，疏密波，刺激约30分钟。

其他疗法：耳针

取穴：面颊　上颌　下颌　额　神门　交感　皮质下

操作方法：毫针刺，每次选3~4穴，强刺激，留针20~30分钟。或用耳针埋藏法。

1.33　痹证

痹有闭阻不通之意。凡外邪侵袭经络，气血闭阻运行不畅，引起以肢体、关节、肌肉等处疼痛、痠楚、麻木、关节肿大和屈伸不利为主要症状的病证，统称为痹证。

本病在临床上较为常见，具有渐进性或反复发作的特点。

现代医学的风湿热，风湿性关节炎，类风湿性关节炎，痛风，风湿性肌纤维炎等病，均属本证范畴。

病因病机

多由己气不固，腠理空疏，或劳累之后，汗出当风，涉水冒寒，久卧湿地等以致风寒湿邪乘虚侵入，流走脉络而致气血运行不畅发为痹证。

由于人的体质差异或感受病邪不同，其临床症候也异，若风邪偏胜者为行痹，寒邪偏胜者为痛痹，湿邪偏胜者为着痹。若素体阳气偏胜，内有蕴热，复感风寒湿邪，邪郁化热，流注经络，则发为热痹。如痹症日久，经络气血周流不畅，凝滞为瘀，阻闭经络，深入骨骱，发为顽痹。

辨证

1. 行痹　　肢体关节肌肉疼痛痠楚，游走不定，上下左右走窜疼痛，以腕、肘、膝、踝处为甚，关节运动不利，或见恶寒发热，舌苔薄腻，脉浮弦。

2. 痛痹　　肢体关节肌肉疼痛剧烈，甚者如刀割锥刺，痛有定处，得热痛减，遇寒加剧，日轻夜重，关节屈伸不利，局部不红不热，常有冷感，舌苔薄白，脉弦紧。

3. 着痹　　肢体关节肌肉痠痛沉重，痛处较为固定，肌肤麻木不仁，易受阴雨气候影响而加重，舌苔白腻，脉濡缓。

4. 热痹　　肢体关节疼痛，局部灼热红肿，痛不可近，活动受限，可涉及一个或多个关节，兼有发热、口渴、心烦、喜冷、恶热等症状，舌苔黄，脉滑数。

5. 顽痹　　痹症历时较长，反复发作，骨节僵硬变形，关节附近呈黯黑色，疼痛剧烈，停著不移，不可屈伸，或疼痛麻木，或关节红肿，兼见发热，口渴，尿短赤，或关节冰凉，寒冷季节而痛剧，得热而安，舌质紫暗有瘀斑，脉细涩。

治疗

治则：以扶正祛邪，疏通经络祛风散寒化湿为主。根据疼痛部位，局部多取阳经经穴为主，亦可采用阿是穴，并结合循经远道取穴。

处方：肩部：肩髃　肩髎　臑俞　合谷

肘部：曲池　天井　尺泽　外关

腕部：阳溪　阳池　外关　腕骨

髋部：环跳　居髎　悬钟

股部：秩边　承扶　殷门　昆仑

膝部：梁丘　血海　膝眼　阳陵泉　阴陵泉

踝部：解溪　商丘　昆仑　太溪　丘墟

腰脊背部：身柱　腰阳关　夹脊穴　大椎

(1) 行痹加风池　血海　膈俞

(2) 痛痹加关元　肾俞

(3) 着痹加脾俞　足三里　阴陵泉

(4) 热痹加大椎　曲池　委中

(5) 顽痹加脾俞　肝俞　肾俞　膈俞　大杼

方义：局部与循经远道取穴相结合，以疏通经络气血，祛风散寒化湿，扶正祛邪使营卫调和，风寒湿三气无所依附而痹病得解。行痹加风池、血海、膈俞以祛风活血通络；痛痹加关元、肾俞以温肾北阳散寒；着痹加脾俞、足三里、阴陵泉以健运脾胃而化湿；热痹加大椎、曲池、委中以疏风池热，活血通络；顽痹加背俞穴以扶正祛邪，活血化瘀，通络止痛。

刺灸法：毫针刺，用泻法或平补平泻法。留针 20～30 分钟，间歇行针 2～3 次。痛痹、着痹、顽痹多针灸并用。

其他疗法

1. 皮肤针

取穴：关节局部肿胀处、背部脊柱两侧相应的夹脊穴或背俞穴。

操作方法：中等刺激，叩至皮肤微微出血为度，刺后可局部加拔火罐，隔日一次。

2. 灸法

取穴：神阙

操作方法：切 2 分厚的姜片，在中心用针穿数孔，置于神阙穴，以中艾炷施灸，每次 5～7 壮。本法适用于痛痹、着痹、顽痹。

1.34 痿证

痿证是指肢体筋脉弛缓，手足痿软无力，伴有肌肉萎缩，甚至运动功能丧失，而成瘫痪之类的病症。因其多见于下肢，故又称痿躄。

本证常见于现代医学的多发性神经炎，急慢性脊髓炎，进行性肌萎缩，重症肌无力，周期性麻痹，肌营养不良症，癔病性瘫痪及外伤性瘫痪等。

病因病机

本病多因感受温邪热毒，上犯于肺，肺受热灼，津液耗伤，不能输精于皮毛，筋肉失于濡养；或因嗜食辛辣甘肥，脾胃积热，津液亏耗，筋肉失却滋养遂成痿证；或因久卧湿地，涉水淋雨，感受湿邪，湿留不去，郁而化热，蕴蒸阳明，以致宗筋弛缓而成；或因久病体虚，房劳过度，肝肾精血亏损，筋脉失其营养而渐成痿证；亦有因跌仆损伤，经脉受损，气血运行受阻，筋脉失养，弛缓而发为痿证。

辨证

1. 肺胃热盛　肢体突然软弱无力，兼有发热咳嗽、心烦、口渴、小便短赤，大便泄泻，舌红，苔黄脉细数或滑数。

2. 湿热浸淫　肢体困重，痿软无力，或微肿而热，兼见发热，多汗，胸脘痞满，小便混浊，舌苔黄腻，脉濡数。

3. 肝肾阴亏　两足渐见痿软，兼有腰背酸软，头晕目眩，遗精早泄，面色少华，或心悸，自汗，月经不调等，舌红少苔，脉细弱。

4. 外伤　有外伤病史，肢体麻木，痿废不用，或有大小便失禁，舌苔薄白，脉缓或涩。

治疗

治则：以通调经气，濡养筋骨为主。肺胃热盛佐以清热润肺；湿热浸淫佐以清热化湿；肝肾亏虚佐以补肝养血，益肾填精；外伤型佐以补气活血通络。取手足阳明、少阳、太阴经穴为主。

处方：上肢：肩于　曲池　外关　合谷

下肢：髀关　梁丘　足三里　阳陵泉　环跳　悬钟　解溪

(1) 肺胃热盛加尺泽　肺俞　内庭

(2) 湿热浸淫加脾俞　阴陵泉

(3) 肝肾阴亏加肝俞　肾俞　太溪

(4) 外伤加相应节段夹脊穴

方义：阳明为水谷之海，后天生化之源，至宗筋，《内经》有"治痿独取阳明"之说，故取手足阳明经穴轮换使用，清其热，而疏调经气；阳陵泉为筋之会，悬钟为髓之会，取之以濡养筋骨。配尺泽、肺俞、内庭以清池肺胃之热；脾俞、阴陵泉清利湿热；肝俞、肾俞、太溪补肝肾之阴；夹脊穴疏调局部经气，通经活络。

随证选穴：发热加大椎；多汗加合谷、复溜；小便失禁加中极、三阴交；大便失禁加大肠俞、次髎。

刺灸法：毫针刺，肺胃热盛及湿热浸淫型用泻法；肝肾阴亏型用补法；外伤型用平补平泻法。留针 15～30 分钟，间歇行针 2～3 次。

其他疗法：皮肤针

取穴：肺俞　肝俞　脾俞　胃俞　肾俞或沿手足阳明经线叩刺。

操作方法：轻刺激，叩至皮肤呈现红晕为度，隔日一次。

1.35　腰痛

腰痛又称腰脊痛。疼痛的部位或在脊中，或在一侧，或在腰脊旁，是临床常见的证候之一。

本证多见于现代医学的腰部软组织损伤，肌肉风湿，以及脊柱病变等。本节重点叙述寒湿腰痛，肾虚腰痛，外伤腰痛。其他原因引起的腰痛，可参考有关章节论治。

病因病机

多因寒湿之邪客于经络，以致腰部气血运行失畅；或久病肾虚，房劳过度，精气损耗，腰部经脉失于濡养；或因负重闪挫，跌仆撞击，经络受损，致使气滞血瘀等而发为腰痛。

腰为肾之府，督脉并于脊里，肾附其两旁，膀胱经脉挟脊络肾抵腰脊，故腰痛与肾和膀胱经的关系最为密切。

辨证

1. 寒湿腰痛　　多有感受寒湿之邪的病史，起病较急，腰脊瘘痛，或拘急强直，不可俯仰，或痛连骶、臀、股腘，疼痛时轻时重，患部有恶冷感，每逢阴雨天则加重，舌苔白腻，脉沉弱或沉迟。

2. 肾虚腰痛　　起病缓慢，腰部隐隐作痛，绵绵不已，腰腿瘘软无力，神倦肢冷，劳累则痛甚，舌淡，脉沉细。

3. 外伤腰痛　　腰部有外伤史，腰脊强痛，痛有定处，按压或身体转侧时则疼痛更甚，舌质淡红，或紫暗，脉弦或涩。

治疗

1. 寒湿腰痛

治则：散寒祛湿，温经通络。取背俞、足太阳经穴为主。

处方：肾俞　腰阳关　关元俞　次髎　委中

方义：腰为肾之府，取背俞以益肾气，腰阳关位于腰脊，可激发督脉阳气；配关元俞、次髎以调经气，通经活络止痛；委中为治腰背痛之要穴。诸穴合用共达健腰脊，除寒湿，止疼痛之目的。

刺灸法：毫针刺，用平补平泻法。留针 15～20 分钟，间歇行针 2～3 次。亦可针灸并用，每穴灸 10～15 分钟。

2. 肾虚腰痛

治则：益肾气，强腰脊。取督脉、足太阳、少阴经穴为主。

处方：肾俞　命门　志室　太溪　委中

方义：取肾俞以温补肾气；命门、志室、太溪以补肾阳，益肾精；委中通经活络，强健腰脊。诸穴共奏补肾壮阳，行气止痛之功。

刺灸法：毫针刺，用补法。留针 20～30 分钟，间歇行针 1～2 次。肾俞、命门、志室可针灸并用，每穴灸 15～20 分钟，或用温针灸。

3. 外伤腰痛

治则：通经活血，祛瘀止痛。取阿是穴和足太阳经穴为主。

处方：阿是穴　膈俞　次髎　委中　后溪

方义：阿是穴以疏调局部经气，调理局部气血；取膈俞、次髎以活血祛瘀止痛；委中为远道取穴，以通经活络；后溪为八脉交会穴之一，通于督脉，可疗腰脊痛。诸穴共用以达活血通络，祛瘀止痛之目的。

随证选穴：痛甚可加人中。

刺灸法：毫针刺，用泻法。留针 15～20 分钟，间歇行针 3～4 次。委中穴亦可用三棱针点刺出血。急性腰扭伤者人中、后溪穴进针后频频捻针，嘱患者活动腰部。阿是穴可点刺出血，然后拔火罐，使瘀血尽出。

其他疗法：耳针

取穴：腰椎　骶椎　肾　神门　皮质下

操作方法：毫针刺，强刺激，留针 20 分钟，或用耳穴压豆法。在刺激耳穴的同时，嘱患者活动腰部，作举手、弯腰、转侧等动作。

1.36　漏肩风

漏肩风又称肩凝症。患者年龄多在 50 岁左右，故又有五十肩之称。以单侧或双侧肩关节酸重疼痛，运动受限为主证。

本病现代医学称之为肩关节周围炎。

病因病机

本病多因营卫虚弱，筋骨衰颓，复因局部感受风寒，或劳累闪挫，或习惯偏侧而卧，筋脉受到长期压迫，遂致气血阻滞而成肩痛。

辨证

初病时单侧或双侧肩部痠痛，其痛多牵连上臂及项背，日轻夜重，遇冷则痛甚，得暖则减缓，晚期肩关节呈不同程度僵直，手臂上举、外旋、后伸等运动均受限制。病情迁延日久，可导致患肢肌肉萎缩。

治疗

治则：祛风散寒、活血通络。取手三阳经穴为主。

处方：肩髃　肩贞　臑臑　曲池　外关　合谷　后溪

方义：肩髃、肩贞、臑臑为局部取穴，以疏通局部经气，活血通络止痛；曲池、外关、合谷为远道取穴，疏导阳明经气，祛风散寒；后溪为手太阳小肠经之俞穴，其脉绕肩胛交肩上，取此穴能搜肩臂之风寒，通经活血止痛。诸穴配伍共达祛风散寒，活血通络止痛之目的。

随证选穴：疼痛连及项背者加天柱、秉风　曲垣。

刺灸法：毫针刺，用平补平泻法。留针 20～30 分钟，间歇行针 2～3 次。多针灸并用，肩　穴灸 20 分钟，或用温针灸。

其他疗法：耳针

取穴：肩髃肩关节　锁骨　神门　交感　皮质下

操作方法：毫针刺，每次选 3～4 穴，中等刺激，针刺时可频频捻针，嘱患者适当活动患肢，留针 20 分钟。可用耳穴压豆法。

1.37　消渴

消渴是以多饮，多食，多尿，形体消瘦或尿有甜味为特征的病证。现代医学称之为糖尿病。

病因病机

本病多因情志失调，精神烦劳，心火偏亢，消烁肺阴；或饮食不节，脾胃积热，化燥伤津；或恣情纵欲，房劳伤肾，肾精亏耗而致上、中、下三消。

辨证

1. 上消　　烦渴多饮，口干舌燥，兼见尿多、食多，舌尖红，苔薄黄，脉洪数。

2. 中消　　食量倍增，消谷善饥，嘈杂，烦热，多汗，形体消瘦，或大便干结。兼见多饮、多尿、舌苔黄燥，脉象滑数。

3. 下消　　小便频数，量多而略稠，口干舌燥，渴而多饮，头晕，目糊，颧红，虚烦，善饥而食不甚多，腰膝痠软，舌质红，脉细数。久病阴虚及阳，可兼见面色黧黑，畏寒肢冷，尿量特多，男子阳萎，女子经闭，舌质淡，苔白，脉沉细无力。

治疗

治则：清泄三焦蕴热。上消取手太阴、少阴经穴为主；中消取足阳明、太阴经穴为主；下消取足少阴、厥阴经穴为主；辅以背俞及经外奇穴。

处方：上消　少府　心俞　太渊　肺俞　胰俞

　　　　中消　内庭　三阴交　脾俞　胃俞　胰俞

　　　　下消　太溪　太冲　肝俞　肾俞　胰俞

方义：上消宜清心肺，故取手少阴心之荥穴少府配心俞以泻心火；取手太阴之俞，肺之原太渊配肺俞以补肺阴。中消宜调脾胃，清胃热，养胃阴，故取三阴交、脾俞补脾以布津液；足阳明胃经荥穴内庭以清胃热。下消宜治肝肾，故取肾之原穴太溪，肾俞以补肾纳气，太冲、肝俞以平肝降火。经外奇穴胰俞为治疗上中下三消的经验穴。

随证选穴：口干舌燥加廉泉、承浆；嘈杂善饥加中脘、内关；目糊加光明；头晕加上星；阳虚加灸命门。

刺灸法：毫针刺，补泻兼施。少府、心俞、内庭、太冲、肝俞宜用泻法；太渊、肺俞、脾俞、太溪、肾俞、胰俞宜用补法。留针20～30分钟，间歇行针2～3次。

其他疗法

1. 耳针

取穴：胰　内分泌　肾　脾　胃　肺　三焦　神门　心　肝　耳迷根

操作方法：毫针刺，每次选3～5穴，轻刺激，留针20分钟。或用耳穴压豆法。

2. 皮肤针

取穴：脊柱两侧胸7～10夹脊穴或背俞

操作方法：轻刺激，叩至皮肤微微红晕、隔日一次。

按语

本病患者正气虚弱，极易并发感染，针刺时必须注意严格消毒。

病情严重者应配合中医药物治疗。针刺治疗期间宜合理调节饮食。

1.38　脚气

脚气是以两脚软弱无力，脚胫肿满强直，或虽不肿满而缓弱麻木，步履艰难为特征的一种疾病。因病从脚起，故名脚气。

本病包括现代医学所称的维生素 B_1 缺乏所致的脚气病。此外如营养不良，多发性神经炎等，凡具有类似证候的疾患，均可参照本篇辨证治疗。

病因病机

本病多因感受水湿雨雾之气，或坐卧湿地，湿邪乘虚侵入皮肉筋脉；或饮食失调，损伤脾胃，脾胃运化失司，热壅于下焦，流注足胫，日渐肿痛而成。或因素来肝肾阴虚，湿邪易从热化，由热化燥，津血不足，遂致筋脉肌肉失养而成。

辨证

本病初起只觉两脚软弱无力，逐渐出现足胫浮肿，麻木痠痛，行动不便等证。根据临床证候，可分为湿脚气、干脚气和脚气冲心三种类型。

1. 湿脚气　足胫浮肿，脚趾疼痛麻木，其势逐渐向上蔓延，腿膝沉重痠软，步行乏力，行动不便。偏于寒湿者，则足胫怯寒喜温；偏于湿热者，则足胫灼热喜凉，或有恶寒，发热，小便短少，舌苔白腻或浮黄，脉濡数。

2. 干脚气　两足无力，腿膝麻木疼痛，时感筋肉挛急，活动欠利，足胫肌肉逐渐萎缩，甚至顽麻萎废，便秘溲黄，舌质淡红，苔薄白或少苔，脉细数。

3. 脚气冲心　足胫肿痛或萎细麻木，步行乏力，突然气急，心悸，恶心呕吐，胸中懊侬，重证则神昏烦躁，语言错乱，唇舌发绀，脉细数无力。

治疗

1. 湿脚气

治则：疏通经络、清化湿热。取足太阴、阳明、少阳经穴为主。

处方：足三里　三阴交　阳陵泉　八风

方义：湿为阴邪，其性趋下，本病为湿邪逗留下肢，壅阻经隧所致，故取足三里、三阴交以振奋脾胃气机，利太阴、阳明之湿。风能胜湿，少阳为风木之经，故取阳陵泉、八风疏风化湿以泄热，湿热既清，则筋脉和利而肿痛可消。

随证选穴：恶寒发热加合谷、大椎、外关；小便短少加阴陵泉，昆仑。

刺灸法：毫针刺，用泻法。留针20～30分钟，间歇行针2

～3 次。偏寒湿者可针灸并用，每穴灸 10～15 分钟。偏湿热者八风穴可点刺出血。

2. 干脚气

治则：益阴养血。取足阳明、太阴经穴为主。

处方：解溪　阴市　复溜　血海　照海　悬钟

方义：取解溪、阴市、血海补脾胃以资气血；照海、悬钟、复溜补肾阴以益精髓；气血精髓充沛，筋骨得以濡养，则可防痿健步。

随证选穴：筋肉挛急加承山；腰痛加委中；膝肿加膝眼、风市。

刺灸法：毫针刺，用补法。留针 15～30 分钟，间歇行针 1～2 次。

3. 脚气冲心

治则：降气泻肺、泄毒宁心。取手太阴、厥阴、手足少阴经穴为主。

处方：尺泽　膻中　劳宫　神门　足三里　涌泉

方义：取肺经合穴尺泽与气之会穴膻中以清肃宣降肺气；劳宫、神门以宁心安神；足三里和胃降浊；足少阴之井穴涌泉引湿毒下行；诸穴合用共奏降气泻肺，泄毒宁心之功效。

随证选穴：神昏加人中；虚脱灸气海、关元。

刺灸法：毫针刺，用平补平泻法。留针 15～20 分钟，间歇行针 2～3 次。

其他疗法：耳针

取穴：趾　踝　膝　脾　胃　肺　肾　神门

操作方法：毫针刺，每次选 3～4 穴，用中等刺激，留针 20 分钟。亦可用耳穴压豆法。

1.39　鼓胀

鼓胀是因腹部胀大如鼓而得名。以腹部胀大，皮色苍黄，甚则腹皮青筋暴露，四肢不肿或微肿为特征。临床上根据证候表现不同，一般分为气鼓、水鼓、血鼓三类。

本证可见于现代医学多种疾病的晚期，如肝硬化、结核性腹膜炎，腹腔内肿瘤等疾病发生腹水，而出现类似鼓胀的证候时，均可参照本篇辨证治疗。

病因病机

本病多由于酒食不节，情志所伤，劳欲过度，以及黄疸、积聚失治，使肝脾肾功能失调，导致气滞血瘀水停积于腹内而成。

亦有因感受水毒、虫积久延失治而成鼓胀者。

辨证

1. 气鼓　腹部膨隆，膜胀，肤色不变，按之陷而即起，恼怒后胀势更剧，嗳噫或转矢气则舒，腹部叩之如鼓，脘胁痞满，小便短黄，大便不爽或秘结，苔薄白，脉弦细。

2. 水鼓　腹部胀大如蛙腹，皮肤光亮，按之凹陷，移时不起，或有下肢水肿，脘腹膜胀，面色滞黄，怯寒，神倦，小便不利，大便溏薄，苔白腻，脉沉缓。

3. 血鼓　脘腹胀大坚硬，脐周青筋暴露，胁下症结，痛如针刺，皮肤甲错，面色黄滞晦暗，或见赤丝缕缕，头颈胸臂可出现血痣，潮热，口干不欲引饮，大便或见黑色，舌质紫暗，或有瘀斑，脉细弦或涩。

治疗

1. 气鼓

治则：疏肝理气，和中消胀。取足厥阴、阳明、任脉经穴为主。

处方：膻中　中脘　气海　足三里　天枢　太冲

方义：取膻中理上焦之气；中脘疏中焦之气；气海调下焦之

气；太冲疏肝解郁；足三里、天枢调肠胃之腑，以和胃消胀。诸穴配合共奏疏肝理气消胀除满之功。

随证选穴：便秘加腹结；胁痛加阳陵泉，支沟；尿黄加阴陵泉。

刺灸法：毫针刺，用泻法。留针20～30分钟，间歇行针2～3次。

2. 水鼓

治则：健脾益肾，调气行水。取背俞、足太阴、少阴、任脉经穴为主。

处方：脾俞　肾俞　水分　复溜　公孙

方义：水分是消腹水的要穴，脾主运化水湿，肾主开阖水道，故取脾俞，公孙健脾理气，以通利水湿；肾俞、复溜温补肾气以开水道。诸穴合用可使脾肾之气健旺，水湿得以气化，水道通利，而肿胀自消。

随证选穴：大便溏薄加天枢、上巨虚；怯寒灸命门、气海。

刺灸法：毫针刺，补泻兼施，脾俞、肾俞多用补法，余穴用平补平泻法。留针20～30分钟，间歇行针2～3次。水分宜用灸法，可灸15～20分钟。

3. 血鼓

治则：活血化瘀，行气利水。取募穴及任脉经穴为主。

处方：期门　章门　石门　三阴交

方义：血鼓多由胁下癥结演变而成，胁下症结多属肝脾疾患，故取肝募期门，脾募章门以通调二脏的气血；三阴交为足三阴之交会穴配三焦募穴石门有活血化瘀，行气利水，通脉散结之功效。

随证选穴：膜胀加梁门；黄疸加阳纲；潮热加太溪，膏肓俞。

刺灸法：毫针刺，用泻法。留针20～30分钟，间歇行针3～4次。

其他疗法：耳针

取穴：肝　肾　胰　大肠　艇中　小肠　三焦

操作方法：毫针刺，每次选 4～5 穴。中等刺激，留针 15～20 分钟。或用耳穴压豆法。

1.40　水肿

水肿又名水气。是指人体水液潴留，泛溢肌肤，引起头面，眼睑，四肢，腹部甚至全身水肿而言。根据病因及临床证候可分为"阳水"与"阴水"二类。

本证包括现代医学的急慢性肾炎，充血性心力衰竭，内分泌失调以及营养障碍等疾病所出现的水肿。

病因病机

阳水：多因冒雨涉水，浴后当风；或肌肤疮疖，热毒内陷，以致肺失通调，脾失输布，水湿内停，泛溢肌肤而成。

阴水：多因饮食不节，脾气虚弱或劳倦纵欲，伤及肾气。脾虚则运化无权，水湿内潴，肾虚则气化失职，开阖不利，导致水邪泛溢而成。

阳水迁延不愈，正气渐伤，则可转为阴水；阴水复感外邪，肿势增剧，亦可出现阳水证候。

辨证

1. 阳水　多为急性发作，初起面目浮肿，继则四肢及全身皆肿，按之凹陷恢复较快，皮肤光泽，阴囊肿亮，小便不利，或伴有胸中烦闷，咳嗽气粗，肢体痠楚，舌苔白滑而润，脉浮滑或浮数。

2. 阴水　　发病多由渐而起，初起足跗微肿，继则面、腹各部均渐浮肿，腰以下为甚，按之凹陷恢复较慢，皮肤晦暗，小便短少。兼有脘痞便溏，神疲怯寒，四肢倦怠，舌质淡，苔白，脉沉细或迟。

治疗

1. 阳水

治则：疏风清热，宣肺利水。取手足太阴，手阳明经穴为主。

处方：肺俞　三焦俞　偏历　阴陵泉　外关　合谷

方义：上部肿甚，治宜发散。取肺俞配偏历宣肺散寒；外关配合谷以疏风发汗清热，使在表的风湿得从汗解；三焦俞通调水道，阴陵泉健脾利水，使在里的水邪下输膀胱；表里分消，可收消肿之效。

刺灸法：毫针刺，用泻法。留针 15～20 分钟，间歇行针 2～3 次。

2. 阴水

治则：健脾温肾，助阳利水。取任脉，足阳明、少阴经穴及背俞穴为主。

处方：脾俞　肾俞　水分　气海　太溪　足三里

方义：下部肿甚，治宜分利。取脾俞配足三里健脾化湿，肾俞配太溪温补肾阳；气海以助阳化水；水分以分利水邪；气行则水行，水行则肿消。

随证选穴：脘痞加中脘；便溏加天枢。

刺灸法：毫针刺　用补法或平补平泻法。留针 15～30 分钟，间歇行针 2～3 次。可针灸并用，气海穴重灸，灸 20～30 分钟。

其他疗法：耳针

取穴：肝　脾　肾　膀胱　艇中　皮质下　肺

操作方法：毫针刺，每次选 3～4 穴，用中等刺激，留针 20 分钟。亦可用耳穴压豆法。

1.41　淋证

淋证是以小便频急，淋沥不尽，尿道涩痛，小腹拘急，痛引脐中为特征的病证。根据病机和症状的不同，临床一般分为热淋，石淋，血淋，气淋，膏淋等类型。

本病主要见于现代医学的某些泌尿系统疾病。临床上凡有尿路刺激症状，如肾盂肾炎，膀胱炎，肾结核，泌尿系统结石，急慢性前列腺炎，膀胱癌以及乳糜尿等病证，均可参考本书辨证治疗。

病因病机

凡外感湿热，或脾湿郁热下注，膀胱气化不利，小便频数热痛者为热淋；湿热蕴结，酿而成石，尿中常有砂石，堵塞尿路，刺痛难忍者为石淋；湿热聚集，伤及血分，或久病阴虚火旺，而致络脉损伤，尿中带血者为血淋；老年肾气衰惫，气化不及洲都，出尿艰涩，余沥淋漓不尽者为气淋；久病脾肾两虚，脾虚则水谷精微不能输布，肾虚则固摄无权，以致清浊不分，尿如米泔脂膏为膏淋。

辨证

1. **热淋**　起病多急，小便频数，点滴而下，尿色黄赤，灼热刺痛，急迫不爽，痛引脐中，或伴腰痛拒按；或有恶寒发热，口苦，便秘，舌质红，苔黄腻，脉濡数。

2. **石淋**　尿中时夹砂石，小便滞涩不畅，或尿不能卒出，窘迫难忍，痛引少腹，或尿时中断，或腰痛如绞，牵引少腹，连及外阴，尿中带血，苔薄白或黄，脉弦或数。

3. **血淋**　尿色红赤，或夹紫暗血块，溲频短急，灼热痛剧，滞涩不利，甚则尿道满急疼痛，牵引脐腹，舌尖红，苔薄黄，脉数有力。

4. **气淋**　少腹及会阴部痛胀不适，排尿乏力，小便断续，甚则点滴而下，尿频溲清，少气懒言，腰痠神疲，舌淡，苔薄白，脉细弱。

5. **膏淋**　小便混浊不清，呈乳糜色，置之沉淀如絮状，上有浮油如脂，或夹凝块，或混血液，尿时不畅，灼热疼痛，或腰痠膝软，头昏无力，舌质红，苔白微腻，脉濡数或细数。

治疗

治则：调理膀胱气机，清热利尿通淋。取足三阴经及背俞穴为主。

处方：膀胱俞　中极　阴陵泉　行间　太溪

（1）热淋加合谷　外关

（2）石淋加委阳　然谷

（3）血淋加血海　三阴交

（4）气淋加气海　水道

（5）膏淋加气海俞　肾俞　百会

方义：取膀胱俞配膀胱之募中极以调理膀胱气机；取足太阴经合穴阴陵泉以利小便，使气化复常，小便通利，其痛自止；因肝脉络阴器故取足厥阴肝经荥穴行间，以泻肝经之气火而镇痛；太溪为肾之原穴，取之以益肾水而清其源。诸穴合用以奏疏调气机，利尿止痛之功。

刺灸法：毫针刺，用泻法或补泻兼施。留针 15～30 分钟，间歇行针 2～3 次。

其他疗法：耳针

取穴：膀胱　肾　交感　枕　肾上腺　内分泌

操作方法：毫针刺，每次选 3～4 穴，强刺激，留针 20～30 分钟。或用耳穴压豆法。

1.42　遗精

遗精是指不因性交而精液经常性自行泄出的病证。有梦而遗精者名为"梦遗"；无梦而遗精，甚至清醒时精液流出者名为"滑精"。一般成年未婚男子或婚后久旷者偶有遗精，属生理现象，不能作为病态。

现代医学的前列腺炎，神经衰弱，精囊炎以及某些病症引起的遗精，一般可参考本节内容辨证治疗。

病因病机

梦遗多因劳神过度或恣情纵欲，心火亢盛，肾阴亏耗，心火不得下交于肾，肾水不能上济于心，心肾不交，水亏火旺，扰动精室；或因嗜食甘肥辛辣，损伤脾胃，酿湿生热，湿热下移，淫邪发梦，精室不宁而致。

滑精多系房事过频或久病伤肾，或频犯手淫，或梦遗日久，肾精内枯，肾气虚惫，气不摄精，精关不固，封藏失职而发生。

辨证

1. 梦遗　　每在睡眠时发生遗精，睡眠不安，阳事易举，遗精有一夜数次或数夜一次，或兼早泄。多伴有头昏头晕，心烦少寐，腰痠耳鸣，体倦乏力，精神不振，小便黄，舌质红，脉细数。

2. 滑精　　无梦而遗，不拘昼夜，甚则动念则精液流出，形体消瘦，面色㿠白，腰部痠冷，舌淡，苔白，脉沉细。

治疗

1. 梦遗

治则：清心降火、益阴涩精。取手足少阴经穴、背俞穴为主。

处方：心俞　神门　肾俞　太溪　关元　志室

方义：心俞配心之原穴神门以降心火，下交于肾；肾俞配肾之原穴太溪以滋肾水，上济于心；关元为足三阴与任脉之会，为人体元气之根本，用以补摄下焦元气；志室一名精室与上穴配伍以达益阴降火，交通心肾，固肾治本，固摄精关之目的。

随证选穴：体倦乏力，精神不振加足三里；头昏加百会；因湿热下注引起小便痛赤、淋漓遗精者加阴陵泉、三阴交。

刺灸法：毫针刺，补泻兼施，心俞、神门用泻法，余穴用补法。留针20～30分钟，间歇行针2～3次。

2. 滑精

治则：补肾益气，固涩精关。取足少阴、任脉经穴为主。

处方：肾俞　三阴交　关元　气海　太溪　大赫　足三里

方义：三阴交是贯通肝脾肾三经的要穴，用之以补益三阴的虚损，清泄虚火；肾俞、气海、关元、太溪可温补元阳、益气固精；大赫固摄精关；足三里健补脾胃以助生化之源。诸穴配伍共奏扶正气、补虚损，固精关之功效。

刺灸法：毫针刺，用补法。留针 20～30 分钟，间歇行针 2～3 次。亦可针灸并用。

其他疗法：耳针

取穴：精宫　内分泌　神门　心　肾

操作方法：毫针刺，轻刺激，留针 20 分钟。可用耳针埋藏或耳穴压豆法。

1.43　阳痿

阳痿又称阴痿。是指男子阴茎痿弱不起，临房时举而不坚或坚而不久的一种病症。

现代医学的性神经衰弱和某些慢性疾病表现以阳痿为主证者，可参考本篇内容辨证治疗。

病因病机

本病多因恣情纵欲，或少年误犯手淫，以致精气虚损，命门火衰；或惊恐思虑，心脾及肾气耗伤从而导致阳痿。亦有因湿热内盛，影响肝肾、宗筋弛缓而发为阳痿者。

辨证

1. 命门火衰　阴茎痿弱不举，或举而不坚，面色㿠白，形寒肢冷，头晕目眩，精神不振，腰腿痠软，小便频数，舌淡苔白，脉沉细。如兼心脾损伤者，则有心悸胆怯，失眠等证。

2. 湿热下注　阴茎痿软不能勃起，阴囊潮湿臊臭，兼见口苦或渴，小便热赤，下肢痠困，舌苔腻，脉濡数。

治疗

1. 命门火衰

治则：补肾壮阳、温补下元。取任脉，足少阴经穴为主。

处方：肾俞　命门　关元　三阴交　太溪

方义：肾俞、命门配肾之原穴太溪可补肾阳、益肾精，温下焦、固元气；三阴交补脾兼及肝肾，为治疗生殖系统病症的要穴；关元可益气填精，振奋阳气。诸穴相配可使元气振奋，精血充实，肾气作强而其病自愈。

随证选穴：心脾亏损加心俞、大陵；头晕目眩者加百会、足三里。

刺灸法：毫针刺，用补法。针关元时针尖向前阴部方向斜刺，使针感放射至前阴部。留针20～30分钟，间歇行针2～3次。关元、肾俞、命门可用灸法或针灸并用，每穴灸15～20分钟。

2. 湿热下注

治则：清热利湿。取任脉、足太阴经穴为主。

处方：中极　三阴交　阴陵泉　行间　足三里

方义：中极与脾之合穴阴陵泉及三阴交配用可利小便，清湿热；肝脉络阴器，取肝之荥穴行间以泄肝经湿热，足三里以健脾运湿，湿化则热无所恋。诸穴合用可清热除湿，以治湿热下注所致之阳痿。

刺灸法：毫针刺，用泻法。留针15～20分钟，间歇行针2～3次。

其他疗法：耳针

取穴：精宫　外生殖器　睾丸　内分泌　肾

操作方法：毫针刺，中等刺激，留针20分钟。或用耳穴压豆法。

1.44　遗尿、小便不禁

遗尿，是指在睡眠中小便自遗，醒后方知的疾病，也称尿床。多见于三岁以上的儿童及少数成年人。小便不禁，是指在清醒状态下不能控制排尿，而尿液自行排出的病证。多见于老人、妇女及病后。

本病范围包括小儿或成人遗尿，以及现代医学的神经功能紊乱和泌尿系统病变所致之小便失禁。

病因病机

本病多因素体虚弱，肾气不足，下元不固，膀胱失约；或年老气衰，房劳伤肾，下元虚冷，肾不摄水；或七情内伤，忧愁思虑伤及肺脾，肺脾气虚，上虚不能制下，膀胱约束无力；或湿热蕴结，下注膀胱所致。亦有因各种原因产生之瘀血，阻于膀胱，膀胱气化失司，不能制约而致遗尿、小便失禁。

辨证

1. 肾阳不足　　睡中遗尿，醒后方觉，或尿意频频，尿后余沥，甚则不自禁。兼见形体羸瘦，神疲怯寒，面色㿠白，腰痛肢软，舌质淡，脉沉迟无力。

2. 肺脾气虚　　尿意频急，时有尿自遗或不禁，兼见面㿠气短，精神倦怠，四肢无力，食欲不振，大便稀溏，舌质淡，脉缓或沉细。

3. 湿热下注　　小便频数，尿热，时有尿自遗，溲赤而臭或尿滴涩淋沥，腰痠低热，苔薄腻，脉细数。

4. 下焦蓄血　　小便滴沥不畅，小腹胀满隐隐作痛，可触及块状物，时有尿自遗，舌质紫暗，苔薄，脉涩或细数。

治疗

1. 肾阳不足

治则：温补肾阳。取背俞、任脉经穴为主。

处方：肾俞　膀胱俞　关元　中极　太溪　三阴交

方义：肾俞配肾之原穴太溪培补肾气以益肾阳；三阴交补益三阴，扶助元气；关元为元气之根可补元气，助气化；膀胱俞合募穴中极以振奋膀胱机能。诸穴合用可补肾气益肾阳，肾气充足，膀胱约束有权，则小便失禁与遗尿自愈。

随证选穴：睡眠深沉加百会，神门；年老体衰尿失禁者加气海、命门。

刺灸法：毫针刺，用补法。留针 20～30 分钟，间歇行针 2 ～3 次。肾俞、膀胱俞、关元多用灸法，亦可针灸并用，每穴灸 15～20 分钟。

2. 肺脾气虚

治则：补肺健脾。取任脉、手足太阴、阳明经穴为主。

处方：肺俞　太渊　脾俞　足三里　气海　三阴交

方义：肺俞配肺之原穴太渊以补益肺气，通调水道；脾俞、足三里、三阴交补脾胃，益肝肾，以助水液气化输布之功；气海温肾阳、固元气，调补下焦。诸穴配用使脾气能升，肺气能降，膀胱得以制约，小便恢复正常。

随证选穴：尿频加百会，次髎。

刺灸法：毫针刺，用补法。留针 20～30 分钟，肺俞、脾俞、足三里、气海可针灸并用。

3. 湿热下注

治则：清利湿热。取背俞、足太阴、少阴经穴为主。

处方：膀胱俞　中极　阴陵泉　足通谷　委阳　三阴交

方义：膀胱俞配中极俞募相配以疏下焦、利膀胱；阴陵泉配三阴交健脾利湿，以清下焦之湿热；委阳为三焦之下合穴，足通谷为足太阳膀胱经之荥穴，取之以清膀胱之积热；诸穴配伍，使下焦湿热祛除，湿去则膀胱自安，约束有权，小便正常。

刺灸法：毫针刺，用泻法。留针 15～20 分钟，间歇行针 2 ～3 次。

4. 下焦蓄血

治则：活血化瘀。取任脉、足太阴经穴为主

处方：中极　次髎　三阴交　气海　膈俞

方义：中极、次髎激发膀胱经气；气海配三阴交及膈俞以行气、活血、化瘀。诸穴合用使瘀血祛除，膀胱气化得复。

刺灸法：毫针刺，用泻法。留针 20～30 分钟，间歇行针 3

～4次。

其他治法: 耳针

取穴: 肾　膀胱　尿道　皮质下　交感　肺　脾

操作方法: 毫针刺, 每次选 3～4 穴, 轻刺激, 留针 15 分钟。可用耳穴压豆法。

1.45　癃闭

癃闭是以排尿困难, 少腹胀痛, 甚则小便不通为主证的一种疾病。癃, 指小便不畅, 点滴而出, 病势较缓者; 闭、指小便闭塞, 点滴不通, 病势较急者。

本证可见于各种原因所引起的尿潴留。

病因病机

本病多因年老体弱或久病体虚, 肾气不足, 命门火衰, 以致膀胱气化无权; 或下焦有热, 积于膀胱, 阻遏膀胱气化; 或跌仆损伤, 以及外科手术后, 经络瘀阻, 尿路阻塞而致小便不通。

辨证

1. 肾气不足　　小便淋沥不爽, 排出无力, 面色㿠白, 神气怯弱, 腰部酸楚, 四肢倦怠, 舌质淡, 脉沉细而尺弱。

2. 热积膀胱　　小便量少热赤或闭, 小腹胀满, 口渴不欲饮, 舌质红, 苔黄, 脉数。

3. 尿路阻塞　　小便滴沥不畅或阻塞不通, 小腹胀满疼痛, 舌有瘀点, 脉涩数。

治疗

1. 肾气不足

治则: 温阳益气、补肾利尿。取足少阴、背俞穴为主。

处方: 肾俞　三焦俞　阴谷　三阴交　气海　委阳

方义: 肾俞配足少阴肾经之合穴阴谷以振奋肾经气机, 培补肾气; 三焦俞配三焦之下合穴委阳以调理三焦气机, 通调水道; 三阴交为足三阴交会穴, 可健脾益肾、利小便; 气海可温补下焦以益元气。诸穴合用共奏补肾气、理下焦、通尿闭之功效。

随证选穴：腰部痠楚加腰阳关、命门。

刺灸法：毫针刺，用补法。留针20～30分钟，间歇行针2～3次。肾俞、三焦俞、气海多用灸法或针灸并用。

2. 热积膀胱

治则：清热利湿。取背俞、足太阴经穴为主。

处方：膀胱俞　中极　三阴交　阴陵泉

方义：膀胱俞配膀胱之募穴中极以清膀胱之积热，调整膀胱功能，疏调下焦气机；三阴交配足太阴之合穴、阴陵泉可清利下焦湿热，健脾利水。诸穴合用共达清利湿热，通利小便之目的。

刺灸法：毫针刺，用泻法。留针15～20分钟，间歇行针2～3次。

3. 尿道阻塞

治则：行瘀散结、通利小便。取膀胱俞募穴及足太阴经穴为主。

处方：膀胱俞　中极　三阴交　水泉　水道

方义：膀胱俞配中极通调膀胱气机，以利小便；三阴交活血祛瘀通络利尿；水泉为足少阴之郄配水道穴可通利小便，消肿止痛。诸穴合用共奏通经活络，疏调气机，通利小便之功用。

随证选穴：小腹胀满重加气海。

刺灸法：毫针刺，用平补平泻法或泻法。留针15～20分钟，间歇行针2～3次。

其他疗法

1. 耳针

取穴：膀胱　肾　尿道　三焦　交感　皮质下

操作方法：毫针刺，每次选3～4穴，中等刺激，留针20～30分钟。或用耳针埋藏法。

2. 电针

取穴：维道

操作方法：毫针刺，针沿皮向曲骨方向透刺约 2～3 寸，疏密波，通电 20～30 分钟。

1.46 汗证

汗证是指由于人体阴阳失调，营卫不和，腠理开阖不利而引起汗液外泄的病证。本节主要讨论自汗、盗汗两种。自汗以时时汗出，动则益甚为主证；盗汗以睡中汗出，醒来即止为特征。

汗证可见于现代医学的多种疾病。如甲状腺机能亢进，植物神经功能紊乱，低血糖，结核病，风湿热及某些传染病的发作期和恢复期等出现自汗、盗汗者，均可参见本节辨证治疗。

病因病机

导致本病的原因很多，如素体阳虚，腠理不密，风邪侵袭，以致营卫不和，卫阳不固；或饮食不节，外感湿邪，损伤脾胃，脾胃失运，湿浊中阻，蕴久化热，薰蒸肌表；或大病久病之后，阴气未复，遗热尚留；或房劳伤肾，衰耗阴精；或饮食药味，积成内热，皆伤损阴血，阴不配阳，阳气内蒸而致汗出。

辨证

1. 自汗　　醒而自汗，濈然无时，动作益甚，身冷畏寒，甚则冷汗，或兼有心悸，气短，神疲乏力，脘腹胀闷，苔白或微黄，脉虚弱无力。

2. 盗汗　　睡寝汗出，醒则汗收，面赤颧红，五心烦热，舌红少苔，脉细数。

治疗

1. 自汗

治则：补阳固表止汗。取足少阴、手阳明经穴为主。

处方：复溜　合谷　膏肓俞　肺俞　脾俞　足三里　气海

方义：合谷为手阳明大肠之原穴主气，复溜为足少阴肾之经穴主液，二穴配用以止汗；肺俞、膏肓俞补肺气，固卫表；脾俞、足三里培补脾胃之气，以资气血生化之源；气海调补元气。

诸穴共用可使元气足，卫气固，营卫调和，而汗自止。

随证选穴：心悸气短者加内关；脘腹胀闷加中脘。

刺灸法：毫针刺，补泻兼施，复溜用泻法，余穴用补法。留针15～20分钟，间歇行针1～2次。

2. 盗汗

治则：滋阴降火止汗。取手足少阴、厥阴经穴为主。

处方：太溪　阴郄　三阴交　复溜

方义：太溪为肾之原穴，用以补肾滋阴降火；三阴交以清虚热，益阴血；阴郄为手少阴之郄穴可养心阴、降心火；复溜益肾阴，除潮热。诸穴配用共达滋阴除热、降火止汗之目的。

刺灸法：毫针刺，用平补平泻法。留针15～20分钟，间歇行针1～2次。

其他刺法：耳针

取穴：肺　心　交感　肾上腺　内分泌

操作方法：毫针刺，中等刺激，留针15～20分钟，或用耳穴压豆法。

1.47　无脉证

无脉证是指寸口脉搏动减弱或消失的一种证候。亦可见于下肢的趺阳脉。

本病常见于现代医学的多发性大动脉炎，闭塞性动脉粥样硬化症，血栓闭塞性脉管炎，动脉栓塞等多种疾病。

病因病机

本病多因风寒湿邪侵犯经脉，或脾肾阳虚，气血运行不畅，血行瘀阻，以致脉搏不起。

辨证

寸口脉搏减弱或消失，兼有头昏、视力模糊、臂膊倦怠无力，麻木疼痛，感觉发凉，指端紫。严重者可见抽搐、昏迷等证。若病发下肢其症状与上肢大致相同，但见趺阳脉搏减弱或消失。

治疗

治则：调气活血，祛瘀复脉。取手太阴、足阳明经穴为主。

处方：太渊　人迎　大陵　内关　尺泽

方义：太渊为肺之原穴，又为脉之会穴，尺泽为肺之合穴，两穴合用以调肺气，活血通脉；人迎为足阳明胃经脉气所发之处，系阳明、太阳之会，阳明经脉多气多血，刺之以调气血，通脉络；大陵、内关为手厥阴心包之原穴和络穴，心包代心行令，故刺之可调血脉而化瘀。诸穴合用共达调气活血，祛瘀复脉之目的。

随证选穴：头昏加风池，百会；视力模糊加睛明；手臂麻木痠痛加曲池、合谷；病发下肢加足三里、隐白、委中、冲阳。

刺灸法：毫针刺，用平补平泻法。留针 15～20 分钟间歇行针 2～3 次。针刺手法不宜过重，以产生一定酸麻感为好，留针时间不宜过长。

其他疗法：耳针

取穴：神门　心　肾　脾　皮质下　内分泌　上肢　肾上腺

操作方法：毫针刺，每次选 4～5 穴，轻刺激，留针 10～15 分钟。一般多采用耳穴压豆法。

1.48　疟疾

疟疾是以寒战、壮热、休作有时为特征的一种传染性疾病。根据其发作间歇的时间长短不同又分为日疟、间日疟、三日疟。如久疟不愈，胁下有痞块，触之可得者称为疟母。

本病多发于夏秋季节，其他季节也有散在发病。

病因病机

多因感受疟邪及风寒暑湿之气，邪毒侵入人体，伏于半表半里，出入于营卫之间，入与阴争则寒，出与阳争则热，营卫相搏，正邪交争而发为疟疾。

辨证

寒战壮热，发作有时，先呵欠乏力，继而寒颤，寒去则内外皆热，甚则高热，神昏谵语，头痛如裂，面赤颧红，胸胁痞满，口苦口干，烦渴引饮，终则遍身出汗，热退身凉，舌苔薄腻而黄，脉弦数。

久疟不愈，时发时止无定时，面色㿠白，倦怠乏力，头目眩晕，肢体羸瘦，胁下形成痞块。

治疗

治则：通调督脉，和解少阳，祛邪截疟。取督脉、少阳经穴为主。

处方：大椎　陶道　后溪　间使　液门

方义：大椎为诸阳之会，可宣通阳气而祛表邪；配陶道能通督脉，调阴阳，为截疟之要穴。后溪属手太阳经穴，又为八脉交会穴之一，通督脉，能宣发太阳与督脉经气而驱邪外出；液门为少阳荥经穴，可和解少阳；间使为手厥阴经穴，厥阴与少阳相表里，故取间使以清心热，利三焦，和解表里。五穴合用通阳祛邪，调和营卫、表里双解，疟疾可截。

随证选穴：高热神昏谵语加十二井穴点刺；久疟加脾俞，膏肓俞；痞块加章门，痞根。

刺灸法：毫针刺，用泻法。针灸治疟，必在疟疾发作之前2～3小时进行，寒多热少者可针灸并用，热重寒轻者只针不灸。留针15～20分钟，间歇行针3～4次。大椎、陶道二穴亦可用三棱针点刺出血。久疟胁下有痞块者灸脾俞、膏肓俞、痞根，每穴灸15～20分钟，或用艾炷灸，每穴5～7壮。

其他疗法

1. 耳针

取穴：肾上腺　皮质下　内分泌　神门　肝　脾　胆　耳尖

操作方法：毫针刺，每次选3～5穴，强刺激，留针15～20分钟，耳尖采用三棱针点刺出血，均在发作前2～3小时施治。

亦可采用耳针埋藏或耳穴压豆法。

2. 拔罐法

取穴：大椎　陶道　至阳

操作方法：先用三棱针点刺出血，随即拔火罐，隔日一次。本法可以单独使用，若配合针灸应用效果更佳。

2 外科病证

2.1 红丝疔

红丝疔多发于四肢和面部，以疮形小而根深，坚硬如钉，沿一条红线迅速向上走窜为特征，因此而得名。相当于现代医学中的急性淋巴管炎。

病因病机

本病多由饮食不节，或过食肥甘，导致脏腑蕴热，毒从内发；或因手足处破损，邪毒外侵，流窜经脉，气血阻滞，邪毒留而不去，致生疔疮。

辨证

疔疮初起，形如米粒凸起于皮肤，根底坚硬如钉，自觉痒麻而微痛。继则红肿，灼热，肿势蔓延，疼痛增剧，寒战发热，恶心呕吐，不思饮食。如生于手足，常常在前臂或小腿内侧皮肤上出现一条纵行的红线，迅速向躯干方向走窜，上肢可延至于肘、腋部，下肢可延至于腘窝或腹股沟部。病变附近可见淋巴结肿大及压痛。甚者全身症状明显，壮热烦躁，神昏谵语，小便黄赤，大便秘结，舌质红绛，脉洪数。此属危重证候，中医称为"疔疮走黄"。

治疗

治则：清热解毒，凉血消肿。取督脉和手、足阳明经穴为主。

病发于上肢和头面部处方：灵台　大椎　曲池　曲泽　中冲　合谷

方义：灵台为督脉之经穴，善清胸中之热，解皮肤之疮毒；大椎为诸阳之会，阳主表主外，刺之清泄周身肌肤之邪热火毒；

曲泽、中冲清三焦之热，消肿止痛；合谷、曲池为手阳明经穴，前者升而能散，偏于行气，后者走而不守，偏于活血化瘀，二穴配伍，可调营卫气血，消散肌表之热毒。

病发于下肢处方：灵台　大椎　委中　绝骨（悬钟）

方义：灵台、大椎用意同上方；委中泻之能清热凉血，降火解毒；绝骨为足少阳之经穴，能清三焦之热，利湿降浊，消肿止痛。

随证选穴：心烦加关冲；高热神昏谵语加十宣、人中。

刺灸法：毫针刺，用泻法，持续行针 3～5 分钟，不留针。中冲、委中用三棱针点刺出血。

其他疗法：刺络拔罐

取穴：灵台

操作方法：灵台穴常规消毒后，用三棱针点刺出血，吸拔火罐。如见有红丝，沿红丝起止点常规消毒后，用三棱针从终点开始至起点，每隔 2～3 cm 点刺出血，然后拔罐。

2.2　瘰疬

瘰疬是指在耳后、颈、项部所发生的以不红、不热、不甚痛为特征的肿块，大小不一，少则一个，多则成串，累累如贯珠之状。小者名瘰，大者曰疬，故名瘰疬。相当于现代医学的颈淋巴结结核。

病因病机

本病多由情志不畅，肝气郁结，气郁化火，炼液成痰，痰火上扰，结于颈项而致；或因肺肾阴虚，肝火偏盛，火炽灼津为痰，痰随气上，结于颈项引起。痰气互结，郁久化热，热盛则肉腐成脓，破溃不收。

辨证

1.肿疡初期　　瘰疬初起，颈项部皮下肿块大小不一，结肿如豆粒，一枚或数枚不等，按之坚硬，推之能动，不热，不痛，皮色不变，一般无明显全身症状。

2.脓疡中期　　结肿日久逐渐增大，推之不易活动，稍有疼痛，局部微热，按之软而应指，皮色暗红，常伴有午后潮热、颧红、乏力等。

3.溃疡期　　常由脓疡中期得不到及时治疗发展而成。脓液稀薄如痰，夹有豆腐渣样脓块，疮口不愈合，逐渐形成窦道，脓液淋漓，长期不愈。

治疗

1、肿疡初期

治则：清热化痰，软坚散结。取手足厥阴及足少阳经穴为主。

处方：期门　内关　行间　肩井　足临泣　天井　百劳

方义：本方标本兼治，期门为足厥阴肝经之募穴，内关为手厥阴心包经之络穴，二穴相伍，可增强疏肝解郁之力，以治其本；行间为肝经之荥穴，肩井为胆经之经穴，足临泣为胆经之输穴，三穴合用，清热豁痰，消肿软坚散结，专治瘰疬；百劳、天井为治瘰疬之经验穴，配之可增强疗效。

随证选穴：项部瘰疬加翳风、颈部瘰疬加臂臑、手三里；腋下瘰疬加肘尖、阳辅。

刺灸法：毫针刺，用泻法，留针 10～15 分钟，间歇行针 2～3 次。天井、百劳小艾炷隔蒜灸各 5～7 壮。

其他疗法：火针

取穴：患处

操作方法：局部常规消毒后，将肿块捏起，用酒精灯将 26 号粗毫针烧红，与皮肤平行从肿块的一侧穿至对侧，或与皮肤呈垂直角度穿至肿核中心部，不留针，出针后用消毒敷料覆盖，每隔 7～10 天一次。

按语

针灸治疗瘰疬，主要适用于肿疡初期或脓疡中期，而溃疡期一般不宜使用。

2.3　缠腰火丹

本病是皮肤上出现成簇水泡，其痛如火燎，多缠腰而发，故名"缠腰火丹"。即现代医学中的带状疱疹。

病因病机

本病多因情志内伤，以致肝胆火盛，木旺乘土，脾胃受损，健运失职，湿热内蕴，复外感毒邪而发病。

辨证

发病之前常有全身不适，微热，乏力，纳呆等症。发病时病处常有灼痛。

病之初起，皮肤发红，继则出现密集成簇的丘状疱疹，大小不等，迅速变为水疱，三五成群，累累如珠，集聚一处或数处，带状排列，疱群之间皮肤正常。多发于身体一侧，常见于腰肋部、胸腹部，而发于面部者极为少见。

病发于腰肋部，疱疹赤红，灼热疼痛，如烧如燎，兼见口苦，头痛，眩晕，心烦易怒，或耳赤面红，尿短赤，舌红苔黄，脉弦数者，多为风火郁于肝胆之经；病发于胸腹部，疱疹色淡，灼热不甚，水疱溃破后渗出液不断，兼见乏力，纳呆，舌苔黄腻，脉滑数者，多属湿热蕴于脾胃。

治疗

1.风火

治则：泻肝利胆，清热解毒。取肝胆经穴为主。

处方：灵台　支沟　行间　足临泣　太冲　足窍阴　疹头　疹尾

方义：灵台能清胸中之热，解皮肤之疮毒，为治疗疮痒之要穴；支沟、行间、足临泣、太冲属手、足少阳和足厥阴之穴，肝胆之脉布于两胁，四穴同刺，可泻肝胆之火，理气消肿止痛；足窍阴为胆经之井穴，能清热泻火，凉血解毒；疹头、疹尾刺之能疏通局部经气，使邪毒直道而出。

随证选穴：疱疹发于头面者加合谷、内庭；热盛者加关冲。

刺灸法：毫针刺，用泻法，留针 20～30 分钟，间歇行针 3～5 次。

2.湿热

治则：清热利湿，健脾化滞。取足阳明、太阴经穴为主。

处方：局部围针　内庭　公孙　外关　侠溪　委中　足三里

方义：局部围针，防止病邪扩散；内庭为足阳明胃经之荥穴，公孙为足太阴脾经之络穴，二穴合用，共奏清热利湿解毒之功；外关为手少阳三焦经之络穴，侠溪为足少阳胆经之荥穴，取之可清热泻火解毒；委中为血中之郄穴，能清热凉血解毒；足三里为足阳明胃经之合穴，取之以健脾和胃，清热利湿。

随证选穴：纳呆加中脘；疱疹在腰以上者加膈俞；疱疹在腰以下者加血海、阳陵泉。

刺灸法：毫针刺，用泻法，留针 20～30 分钟，间歇行针 4～6 次。艾条灸足三里，每次 20 分钟。

其他疗法：耳针

取穴：肾上腺　神门　皮质下　相应部位

操作方法：毫针刺，强刺激，留针 15～20 分钟，间歇行针 3～4 次。亦可耳针埋藏或压豆。

2.4　丹毒

本病因其发病时皮肤忽然变红，色如丹涂脂染，故名丹毒。其特点是起病突然，患处皮肤红肿热痛，状如云片，边界分明，色红如丹。现代医学亦称此名。

病因病机

本病多由肝脾湿热蕴积，热邪侵及血分，或体表失于卫固，风、热、湿、火之邪毒乘隙而入，内外合邪，两热相搏，暴发于皮肤之间，不得外泄，蓄热而为丹毒。

辨证

病之初起，全身不适，恶寒发热，继则皮肤出现红斑，焮红灼热疼痛，状似云片，边缘清晰而稍突起，按之退色，松手后即复原状，常迅速向四周蔓延，中间由鲜红转为暗红，经数日后脱屑而愈。或发生水疱，破烂流水，疼痒并作。多伴有烦渴、身热、便秘、尿赤等症。

总之，本病发于半身以上者多属风热，发于半身以下者多属湿热。

治疗

1.风热

治则：疏风清热，凉血解毒。取督脉和手阳明经穴为主。

处方：灵台　大椎　中冲　曲池　合谷　曲泽

方义：灵台善清胸中之热，解皮肤之疮毒，是治疗皮肤疮疡的要穴；大椎为诸阳之会，与心包经井穴中冲配用，能疏风清热，泻火解毒；曲池主血，走而不守，合谷主气，升而能散，二者相伍，可导气直达病所速而捷；曲泽善清热凉血解毒，以泻秽气。

随证选穴：壮热加少商、商阳；头痛加太阳、印堂；心烦欲吐加内关。

刺灸法：毫针刺，用泻法，留针 15～20 分钟，间歇针 3～4次；大椎、中冲、曲泽用三棱针点刺出血。

2.湿热

治则：清热利湿，凉血解毒。取督脉与足太阳经穴为主。

处方：灵台　委中　悬钟　阴陵泉　三阴交

方义：灵台解皮肤疮疡之毒；委中清热凉血，祛风利湿，降浊解毒；绝骨为髓之大会，清三焦之热，利湿化浊；阴陵泉、三阴交健脾利湿。五穴合用，共奏清热利湿，凉血解毒之功。

随证选穴：腹泻加天枢、关元；高热加十宣、水沟（人中）。

刺灸法：毫针刺，用泻法，留针 15～20 分钟，间歇行针 3～4 次。

其他疗法

1.刺络拔罐

取穴：灵台（上半身加大椎，下半身加委中）

操作方法：常规消毒，用三棱针点刺出血后，吸拔火罐，留罐 10～15 分钟。

2.耳针

取穴：神门　肾上腺　皮质下　脾　枕

操作方法：毫针刺，强刺激，留针 10～15 分钟，间歇行针 1～2 次。亦可耳穴埋针或压豆。

2.5　湿疹

湿疹是一种常见的皮肤病，有急性和慢性之别。急性湿疹常以对称性、多形性损害，起病急骤，反复发作，局部焮红，水肿，丘疹，水疱，糜烂，瘙痒异常为主要特征，愈后结痂脱落，不留痕迹；慢性湿疹多由急性湿疹转变而来，局部皮肤增厚粗糙，暗红或带灰色，皮损呈鳞屑或苔癣样，经久不愈，常可急性发作。

病因病机

本病多由风热湿邪客于肌肤，阻遏气血，经脉不利，湿热郁遏于皮表所致；或因血虚化燥，皮肤失于濡养，而成慢性湿疹。

辨证

1.急性湿疹　　起病较急骤，常先出现红斑，继而出现丘疹，数日后形成水疱，多群集成片出现。常因搔抓而丘疹或水疱破损，引起渗出，甚者糜烂。患处皮肤焮红瘙痒异常，可伴有舌红苔厚腻，脉滑数。

2.慢性湿疹　　多由急性湿疹迁延日久，经数日或数年反复发作，耗伤阴血，血虚化燥而成。临床表现为皮肤增厚粗糙，色泽灰暗，皮纹加深，皮损边缘清晰，缠绵难愈，时休时发，可伴有舌红少苔，脉细数。

治疗

1.急性湿疹

治则：疏风清热利湿。取足阳明、太阴经穴为主。

处方：大椎　曲池　三阴交　委中　阴陵泉　灵台

方义：大椎为诸阳之会，配曲池疏表解肌，清热祛风；三阴交为肝、脾、肾三阴经之交会穴，通调足三阴而利湿热；委中清血热，祛风利湿；阴陵泉为足太阴脾经之合穴，能健脾利湿；灵台清三焦之热，解皮肤之疮毒。

随证选穴：腹痛加公孙；便秘加天枢、阳陵泉。

刺灸法：毫针刺，用泻法，留针15～20分钟，间歇行针2～3次；委中也可用三棱针点刺出血；灵台可用刺络拔罐。

2.慢性湿疹

治则：养血祛风为主，主要取足三阴经穴。

处方：太冲　三阴交　足三里　血海　膈俞　灵台

方义：太冲能调肝养血、通经行瘀；三阴交为足三阴之会穴，能补脾调肝益肾，再配足三里以资生化之源；血海、膈俞清血分之热，活血止痒；灵台解皮肌之疮毒。

刺灸法：毫针刺，用平补平泻法，留针20～30分钟，间歇行针2～3次。

其他疗法：耳针

取穴：心　肺　脾　神门　肾上腺

操作方法：毫针刺，中度刺激，留针15～20分钟；亦可耳穴埋针或压豆。

2.6　风疹

本病是皮肤出现赤色或苍白色的疹块，发作突然，痒而不痛，遇风而发，时隐时现，故名风疹或瘾疹。疹块消退后不留任何痕迹。现代医学称为荨麻疹。

病因病机

本病常因营卫不和，迎风受邪，邪客于肌腠所致。而风又常与寒、湿、热诸邪相兼侵入人体，故在病机上有风热搏于血分和风寒湿搏于气分之不同，疹块也有赤白之别。或因膏粱厚味，食鱼虾等荤腥动风之品，致风湿热毒内蕴肠胃，熏蒸于肺，内不得泄，外不得透达，郁于皮肤而发风疹。

辨证

风疹之为病，起病突然，皮肤出现疹块，痒而不痛。临证时，除了弄清诱发原因外，分别新旧，明辨疹色及兼证尤为重要，如偏于风热者，其疹块多高起皮肤，色红赤，剧痒，触之有焮热感，遇热则发，遇冷则减，或有心烦口渴，舌红苔黄厚，脉浮数；偏于风寒者，则疹色苍白，得热则缓，遇风寒则甚，或兼有恶寒发热，舌淡苔薄白，脉浮缓或浮紧；胃肠积热者，多由饮食不慎诱发或加剧，常伴有腹痛腹泻或便秘、恶心呕吐等胃肠症状，苔黄腻，脉滑数；若风疹反复发作，经久不愈，每遇劳累则发，兼见头晕、体倦乏力、面色少华、心悸气短、自汗出等，多属气血两虚。

治疗

1.风热

治则：疏风清热，活血凉血止痒。取手阳明经穴为主。

处方：合谷　曲池　大椎　灵台　风池　委中　膈俞

方义：本方取合谷、曲池、风池以解肌清热，疏风发表；膈俞、大椎、委中调和营卫、清气分而活血凉血，祛风止痒；灵台清三焦之热，解皮肤疮痒之毒邪。

刺灸法：毫针刺，用泻法，留针15～20分钟，间歇行针2～3次；大椎、委中用三棱针点刺出血。

2.风寒

治则：疏风散寒，调和营卫。取手阳明与足少阳经穴为主。

处方：风池　风门　曲池　合谷　大椎

方义：风池、风门疏风散寒；合谷升而能散，曲池走而不守，二穴共奏散寒解表，祛风止痒之功；大椎能通阳化气，与曲池同用可调和营卫。

刺灸法：毫针刺，用平补平泻，留针20～30分钟；大椎、风池、风门可用灸法，每穴灸30～40分钟。

3.胃肠积热

治则：健脾利湿，泻热清营，取手足阳明及足太阴经穴为主。

处方：曲池　足三里　血海　三阴交　灵台

方义：取曲池、足三里，乃合治六腑之意，以荡涤肠腑之热；血海为足太阴经穴，三阴交为足三阴之会穴，二穴合用，以健脾利湿，清热凉血，活血止痒；灵台为治疗疮痒的经验穴，配之疗效更佳。

刺灸法：毫针刺，用泻法，留针15～20分钟，间歇行针2～3次。

4.气血两虚

治则：补益中焦，益气养血。取足阳明与任脉经穴为主。

处方：气海　足三里　三阴交　脾俞　合谷　曲池　膈俞

方义：扶正以祛邪为治本型之根本，故取气海、足三里、三阴交、脾俞以健脾和胃，补益中气，增强气血生化之源，正足则邪自祛；合谷、曲池升而能散，走而不守，配以血之会穴膈俞以疏通周身气血，气行血活，其风自灭而痒止。

刺灸法：毫针刺，气海、足三里、三阴交、脾俞用补法，合谷、曲池、膈俞用平补平泻法，留针20～30分钟，间歇行针2～3次。亦可用艾炷直接灸足三里、脾俞，每穴7～9壮。

其他疗法：耳针

取穴：肺　肾上腺　皮质下　交感　荨麻疹区

操作方法：毫针刺，中度刺激，留针15～20分钟；亦可耳穴埋针或压豆。

2.7 白疕风

本病系一种慢性红斑鳞屑瘙痒性皮肤病，反复发作，迁延难愈。因皮疹上反复出现多层银白色干燥的鳞屑，搔之脱屑，故名白疕。现代医学称为银屑病，旧称牛皮癣。

病因病机

本病多由外感风湿热邪，蕴滞于皮肤而作。邪郁日久化热，耗伤津血，血燥生风，皮肤失荣，以致皮肤粗糙瘙痒脱屑。

辨证

病之初起多为皮肤间歇性瘙痒，继而出现扁平丘疹，丘疹逐渐融合扩大成片，或密集成群，呈现多形态红色斑丘疹。红斑表层有多层银白色鳞屑，搔之脱落。日久皮肤变得粗糙坚厚，搔之微有脱屑，阵发性剧痒难忍。若患处皮损潮红，瘙痒，脂性脱屑，舌红苔黄腻，脉濡数，多属风湿热偏胜；若病程较长，皮肤干燥肥厚，鳞屑陆续脱落，舌质红苔薄白，脉细弱，多属血虚风燥。

治疗

1.风湿热

治则：清热利湿，祛风止痒。取手阳明、足太阴经穴为主。

处方：合谷 曲池 太白 阴陵泉 风池 膈俞 人迎

方义：合谷、曲池善调气血，清阳明之热；配风池和解少阳，解肌透表，疏风散热止痒；太白、阴陵泉为足太阴脾经之原穴和合穴，能健脾利湿；膈俞为血之会穴，能活血祛风止痒；人迎为足阳明经穴，有调和气血、止痒之奇功。

随证选穴：按病变部位循经取穴。如病发于项者加少泽、委中；病发于面颊者加关冲、支沟。

刺灸法：毫针刺，用泻法，留针15～20分钟，间歇行针1～3次；曲池、阴陵泉可加灸。

2.血虚风燥

治则：补气养血，祛风润燥。取手、足阳明经穴为主。

处方：合谷　曲池　三阴交　足三里　血海　人迎

方义：合谷、曲池善清头面之风热，三阴交补益脾胃兼及肝肾，三穴合用，清热凉血，熄风润燥，为本方之主穴；三阴交配足三里，又可升阳益胃，滋阴健脾，以振生血之源；血海为足太阴脾经穴，能调血润燥；人迎，活血祛风止痒有奇能。

刺灸法：毫针刺，用平补平泻，留针15～20分钟，间歇行针2～3次；足三里、三阴交亦可用灸法。

其他疗法：耳针

取穴：肺　神门　肾上腺　肾　心　相应部位

操作方法：毫针刺，中度刺激，留针15～20分钟，间歇行针1～2次。

2.8　鹅掌风

鹅掌风即手掌部皮肤变得粗厚，硬而燥裂，有微痒，形如鹅掌，因而得名。现代医学称为手癣。

病因病机

本病多因外感毒邪，毒邪生湿，后期毒邪化热化燥，血燥生风，蕴发皮肤，皮肤失养而致。

辨证

病之初起，手掌瘙痒，继而出现皮下小水泡，自掌心延至全手掌，但不犯及手背，逐渐水泡隐没，迭起白皮，皮肤枯槁，粗糙肥厚，甚者燥裂而痒痛，日久可致皮肤皲裂，手指屈伸不利。每遇夏季则轻，逢冬则重。多发生于单侧，亦可双侧并作。

治疗

治则：搜风清热，养阴润燥。取手厥阴、足少阴经穴为主。

处方：涌泉　劳宫　人迎　间使　八邪

方义：涌泉为足少阴肾经井穴，能清热滋阴润燥，劳宫为手厥阴心包经荥穴，善清三焦之热毒，为治疗鹅掌风之要穴；人迎、间使调营卫而能解毒杀虫；八邪为经外奇穴，能搜风泄毒，为治疗鹅掌风的经验穴。

随证选穴：食欲不振加中脘、足三里；失眠加神门、内关。

刺灸法：毫针刺，用泻法，留针 20～30 分钟，间歇行针 2～3 次。

2.9　白癜风

白癜风系皮肤出现无自觉症状的白斑，以无痒痛为特征，现代医学亦称白癜风。

病因病机

本病多由风邪侵入腠理，搏结于皮肤，以致气血失和，气滞血瘀，使皮腠失于濡养所致。

辨证

临床表现分局限性和泛发性。在皮肤上出现白斑，形状大小不等，数目不定，边界清楚，斑内毛发变白，无痛痒，为局限性白癜风；若泛发至全身，终生不愈，为泛发性白癜风。白斑有的星星点点，可静止不再扩散，有的可自行消退，亦有的进展迅速，病程长短不一。

治疗

治则：调和阴阳，活血祛风。取手、足阳明及足太阴经穴为主。

处方：合谷　曲池　风池　膈俞　肝俞　太冲　三阴交　隐白　人迎

方义：合谷、曲池、风池调和营卫，清泄诸窍之热，搜周身之风邪；膈俞、肝俞、太冲益血养阴，活血祛风；三阴交健脾益肾调肝而益精血；隐白、人迎能补益脾胃之气，升诸阳。

刺灸法：毫针刺，用平补平泻，留针 15～20 分钟，间歇行针 2～3 次。

其他疗法

1.皮肤针

取穴：患处

操作方法：常规消毒后，用皮肤针轻叩，至皮肤红晕，立刻吸拔火罐。

2.耳针

取穴：肺　脾　心　神门　皮质下　肾上腺　相应部位

操作方法：毫针刺，强刺激，留针 10～15 分钟；亦可耳穴埋针或压豆。

2.10　油风

油风是指头皮部突然发生局限性斑状脱发。现代医学称为斑秃。

病因病机

本病多由肝肾亏虚，血虚不能随气上荣皮毛，毛孔开张，风邪乘虚而入，血虚风燥而发；或由肝气郁结，气机不畅，以致气滞血瘀，发失濡养而成。

辨证

本病多无自觉症状，常在无意中偶然发现。初起呈局限性圆形或不规则形斑状脱发，皮肤光亮，边界清楚，小如指甲，太如眼镜片，一至数个不等。继则损害数目与范围均可扩大，甚者头发大部或全部脱落，称为全秃。

若头发成片脱落，轻度瘙痒，伴有头晕，失眠，耳鸣，舌质淡红，苔薄白，脉细弱，多属肝肾亏虚，血虚风燥；若头发成片脱落，病程较长，或兼有面色晦暗，舌边有紫色瘀点，脉涩，多为气滞血瘀。

治疗

1.血虚

治则：养血祛风安神，补益肝肾。取手厥阴、足太阳经穴为主。

处方：内关　神门　百会　大椎　肝俞　肾俞　膈俞　合谷　三阴交

方义：内关、神门养血安神；百会、大椎清热祛风止痒；肝俞、肾俞、膈俞益肾养肝，调和气血；合谷、三阴交清上润下，调理肝脾肾，扶正祛邪，引血随气上荣于发。

随证选穴：头晕加上星；食少加足三里、中脘。

刺灸法：毫针刺，用平补平泻,留针10～15分钟，间歇行针1～2次；大椎、百会也可艾灸。

2.血瘀

治则：舒肝理气、活血化瘀。取手厥阴、足少阳经穴为主。

处方：内关　阳陵泉　膈俞　风池　百会　肝俞　人迎

方义：内关、阳陵泉舒肝理气，配膈俞活血化瘀；风池、百会疏风清热止痒；肝俞、人迎清热凉血活血，导气至病所，促进头发新生。

刺灸法：毫针刺，用泻法，留针15～20分钟；艾灸患处20～30分钟，或以患处皮肤红晕为度。

其他疗法：耳针

取穴：肺　肝　肾　肾上腺　内分泌　脑

操作方法：毫针刺，弱刺激，留针15～20分钟；或耳针埋藏或耳穴压豆均可。

2.11　粉刺

粉刺又称肺风粉刺，是在颜面胸背等处发生的丘疹结节。粉刺挤之有米粒样白色粉浆溢出，因之得名。好发于青春期男女，成年后常自愈。现代医学称为痤疮。

病因病机

本病多由肺经风热熏蒸于肌肤，或过食辛辣厚味，脾胃积热，外蕴肌肤而发；冲任不调而致肌肤疏泄功能失调，亦可引起本病。

辨证

粉刺多发生于颜面、背及前胸部。初起为散在或密集的丘疹结节，部分形成粉刺，可挤出乳白色粉质物，继发感染则形成小脓疱。形成脓疱时，面部潮红灼热，刺痒疼痛。脓疱破溃出脓，愈后遗留疤痕。

治疗

治则：疏风清热，活血散结，兼调冲任。取手、足阳明及督脉经穴为主。

处方：灵台　合谷　曲池　风池　肺俞　三阴交　太冲

方义：灵台善清胸中之热，解肌肤疮疡之毒；合谷、曲池调和气血，清泄肌肤之风热；风池和解少阳，善疗头面之风热；三阴交配太冲，调冲任，活血散瘀消结。

随证选穴：发热加大椎；痒者加关冲、委中。

刺灸法：毫针刺，用泻法，留针 15～20 分钟，间歇行针 2～3 次；灵台穴可用三棱针点刺拔罐；委中穴亦可点刺出血。

其他疗法：耳尖放血

取穴：耳尖

操作方法：于耳尖穴部位常规消毒后，左手提捏耳尖穴周围，右手持三棱针点刺，放出血液 3～5 滴，术毕用无菌干棉球按压针孔，每隔 3～5 日一次，左右交替。

2.12　扁平疣

扁平疣是发生于皮肤浅表的小赘生物，好发于手背及面部，一般无自觉症状。属现代医学中疣的范畴。

病因病机

本病因情志不舒，肝气郁结，阴虚血燥，复感邪毒，内外合邪，搏结于皮肤，以致气滞血瘀，郁于肌肤而发。

辨证

本病好发于青年人，以颜面、手背和前臂最为常见，表面光滑，略高出皮面，小如米粒，大如黄豆，呈淡黄色或正常肤色，边界清楚，或多个散在或密集分布，局部微痒或无自觉症状。有的自行消退，亦可复发。

治疗

治则：疏风清热，活血消疣。取手阳明经穴为主。

处方：合谷　曲池　风池　中渚　太冲

方义：合谷、曲池行气活血，调和营卫，善清上肢及头面之风热而疗头面诸疾；风池善除外感之风邪；中渚、太冲能泄三焦郁火，和解少阳之气，平肝降火，活血消疣。

刺灸法：毫针刺，用平补平泻，留针 20～30 分钟，间歇行针 3～4 次。或艾炷置于扁平疣上直接灸 3～5 壮。

其他疗法：火针

取穴：每次选疣 3～5 枚

操作方法：常规消毒后，用火针从疣之中心点灸至根底部。

2.13　鸡眼

鸡眼多发于足底部，其根深陷肉里，状似鸡眼，故而得名。现代医学亦称鸡眼。

病因病机

本病多由足底部或趾间部受到经常性挤压、摩擦而引起。

辨证

本病好发于足底经常受压及容易摩擦的部位，初起受压部位皮肤增厚，表面黄白色，无痛苦，继则顶起硬凸，常为圆形，其尖端根深陷向肉内，状似鸡眼，按压痛甚，影响行走。

治疗

治则：软坚化结。以局部取穴为主。

处方：鸡眼局部

刺灸法：以鸡眼为中心，毫针围刺，针刺深度以达至鸡眼的基底部为准；亦可针后加灸。

其他疗法：火针

取穴；鸡眼中心

操作方法：常规消毒后，取火针直刺鸡眼中心，深度以直达其基底部为止；或用火针于鸡眼之左右上下，各刺一针，深度同上。每隔 2～3 日一次，直至鸡眼自然脱落。

2.14　筋瘤

筋瘤为发生在关节附近筋肉上的囊状肿块，常伴有酸痛乏力。现代医学称为腱鞘囊肿。

病因病机

本病的发病原因，一般认为是局部过度劳累，外伤筋脉，或久经站立，局部气血郁滞，阴滞经脉络道所致。

辨证

本病多发于青壮年，以腕、踝关节处最为常见，肿块自指头到核桃大小不等，呈圆形或椭圆形，表面光滑，动度较小。初起时按之有囊性感，日久则囊性感不明显而表面坚实。常单个或数个同时发生，局部可有酸胀、木痛及乏力感觉。

治疗

治则：活络散结。以局部取穴为主。

处方：囊肿四周

刺灸法：局部消毒后，用 26 号粗毫针从囊肿的最高点刺入，然后再从上、下、左、右四个方向，向中心行围针刺，出针后即加挤压，挤出胶状粘液，加灸 30 分钟。

其他疗法：火针

取穴：囊肿之高点

操作方法：常规消毒后，用 24 号粗毫针在酒精灯上烧红，当顶焯刺，出针后立即挤压出囊内液体，刺后加灸 20～30 分钟，隔日一次。

2.15 脂瘤

脂瘤又称粉瘤或豆腐渣瘤，因其囊内充满豆腐渣样物质而得名。现代医学称为皮脂腺囊肿。

病因病机

本病常因痰凝气结，聚集肌肤而成。

辨证

脂瘤多发于头面、耳、项背、臀部等处。肿物位于皮肤表层内，大小不一，界限清楚，形圆质软。肿物与深部组织不粘连，但与皮肤相连，推之可动，中央有一凹陷小坑，略带黑色，用力挤之，有豆腐渣样物溢出，且有臭气。肿物生长缓慢，一般无自觉症状。

治疗

同筋瘤

2.16 乳痈

乳痈是乳房部的急性化脓性疾病。多发于产后哺乳期，尤以初产妇多见。现代医学称为急性乳腺炎。

病因病机

本病的发生，多由忧思恼怒，肝气郁结，导致肝之疏泄失司，乳汁淤滞，或饮食不节，恣食厚味，以致脾升胃降失职，积热于胃，或乳头破裂，外邪内侵，内外之邪互结，乳汁凝滞，久而化热，热盛肉腐，发为乳痈。

辨证

本病以患侧乳房红、肿、热、痛，排乳不畅，发热恶寒，全身不适，乳胀触痛拒按为主症。

1.肝郁气滞　　除主症外，兼见胸闷胁痛、腹胀、口苦咽干、心烦易怒、纳呆、舌苔薄黄、脉弦数。

2.胃经积热　　除主症外，伴有口渴欲饮、恶心纳差、口臭便秘、舌苔黄、脉洪数。

治疗

1.肝郁气滞

治则：疏肝解郁，清热化滞。取厥阴、阳明、少阳经穴为主。

处方：期门　内关　膻中　足三里　行间　肩井

方义：乳房为足阳明胃经所布，乳头归属于肝经。取肝之募穴期门与心包经之络穴内关，及气之会穴膻中，以宽胸理气，疏肝解郁；用胃腑之合穴足三里与肝经之荥穴行间，以清胃热化郁滞，消肿止痛。再配以治乳痈的经验穴肩井，其效更捷。

随证选穴：乳房壅胀加乳根；乳汁不畅加少泽；发热头痛加大椎、风池。

刺灸法：毫针刺，用泻法，留针15～20分钟，间歇行针2～3次。

2.胃经积热

治则：清热散结，消肿通乳。取阳明经穴为主。

处方：乳根　膺窗　少泽　足三里　梁丘　内庭

方义：足阳明胃经从缺盆下行乳中，故取胃经腧穴乳根、膺窗以清泻胃热，疏通乳道；取胃经之合穴足三里、郄穴梁丘、荥穴内庭，以泻热解毒，消肿散结止痛；佐以少泽，泻热通乳。诸穴相伍，共奏清热散结、消肿通乳之功。

随证选穴：乳汁壅滞加膻中、肩井；发热恶寒加大椎、合谷、风池。

刺灸法：毫针刺，用泻法，留针10～15分钟，间歇行针2～3次；少泽穴用三棱针点刺出血。

其他疗法：耳针

取穴：肝　胃　胸　耳中　内分泌　乳腺　耳尖

操作方法：毫针刺，强刺激，留针10～15分钟；耳尖穴用三棱针点刺出血。

按语

针灸治疗乳痈，主要适用于乳痈初期未成脓者。

2.17 肠痈

肠痈是热毒内聚，瘀结肠中而生痈脓，故名肠痈。临床以发热恶寒，少腹肿痞，疼痛拒按，或右腿屈而难伸为主要特征。现代医学称为阑尾炎。

病因病机

本病多由暴饮暴食，嗜食膏粱厚味，以致食滞中阻，湿热蕴结肠腑；或食后急暴奔走，伤及肠络；或因情志所伤，气机壅塞，气血瘀阻于内，瘀久化热，血败肉腐，发为肠痈。

辨证

1.瘀滞（未成脓）　　腹痛阵作，按之痛剧，腹皮微急，脘腹胀闷，嗳气纳呆，恶心欲吐，稍有发热恶寒，大便正常或秘结，舌质暗红或正常，苔薄白或薄黄，脉弦紧。

2.蕴热（脓始成而未溃）　　腹痛绞剧，腹皮绷紧，右腹下部拒按，腿屈不伸，壮热自汗，大便秘结，小便短赤，舌质红苔黄腻，脉弦滑而数。

治疗

1.瘀滞

治则：理气止痛，消肿化瘀。取定阳明、足太阴经穴为主。

处方：天枢　大肠俞　足三里　血海　地机

方义：天枢为大肠之募穴，大肠俞为背部俞穴，两者相配，即俞募配穴法，以疏通腑气，调和大肠气机；取胃经之合穴足三里，配以相表里的脾经腧穴血海，以行气活血，化滞逐瘀；取脾经之郄穴地机，理气止痛。五穴相伍，疗效卓著。

随证选穴：腹胀加腹结；发热加合谷、曲池、内庭；呕吐加内关、关冲。

刺灸法：毫针刺，用泻法，留针15～20分钟，间歇行针2

~3次。

2.蕴热

治则：清热利湿，行气导滞。取手、足阳明经穴为主。

处方：上巨虚　天枢　曲池

方义：大肠为传导之官，主传化糟粕，以通为顺。因病在肠腑，取上巨虚乃"合治内腑"之意，与大肠之募穴天枢相配，具有清热荡滞，疏通肠道气机，利湿通便的作用；曲池穴专调肠腑之气，泄热存津。

随证选穴：发热加合谷、内庭；呕吐加内关；腹胀加腹结、大肠俞；便秘加足三里、阳陵泉。

刺灸法：毫针刺，用泻法，留针15～20分钟，间歇行针3～4次。

其他疗法 耳针

取穴：阑尾　直肠下端　大肠　交感　神门

操作方法：毫针刺，强刺激，留针15分钟；亦可耳穴埋针或压豆。

按语

针灸治疗肠痈，主要适用于单纯性阑尾炎初起或脓已成而未溃者。

2.18　痔疮

痔与峙同义，即高突的意思。凡肛门内外生有小肉突起，皆称为痔。痔为肛管直肠部之常见病多发病之一，多见于成年人，故有"十人九痔"之说。现代医学亦称为痔。依发病部位不同而有内痔、外痔、混合痔之别，但以内痔最为多见。因痔核而出现肛门部肿痛、坠胀、瘙痒、出血等症，故中医又称为痔疮。

病因病机

痔多由饮食肥甘，过食辛辣，饮酒过度，燥热内生，或大便秘结，排便久蹲强努，损伤脉络，或久坐、负重、远行，及脏腑本虚，外伤风湿，内蕴热毒，导致湿热下注，结聚肛门，宿滞不散而成。

辨证

内痔初起，肛门坠胀疼痛，痔核一般较小，质柔软，色鲜红或青紫，常因大便挤压摩擦而致便中带血，甚者血出如射，轻者点滴不已。若兼见肛门灼热并有渗出，大便秘结，口渴，舌质红，脉数，多属湿热瘀滞。若患者体质素虚，或因痔疮反复发作，失血过多，而致气血亏损，症见面色萎黄，气短懒言，食少乏力，痔核经常脱出肛外而不能回纳，舌质淡，脉细弱，则属气虚下陷。

外痔主要于肛门之外产生皮瓣，逐渐增大，按之质地较硬，常因久坐、久立或摩擦而致肛部红肿疼痛，但一般不出血。

治疗

1.湿热瘀滞

治则：清热利湿，行气化瘀。取足太阳、手太阴、及手厥阴经穴为主。

处方：孔最　郄门　承山　二白　合谷　曲池

方义：孔最为肺经郄穴，肺与大肠相表里，故能清肃肺气而泄大肠之湿热，并善于行气活血止痛；郄门能清宫热利三焦，行气化瘀止痛；二白为治疗痔疮的经验穴；承山因其经脉直通于肛，故可导气直达病所，使以上诸穴之效更捷；曲池、合谷疏通大肠经气，行气活血，清大肠湿热。

随证选穴：内痔脱垂加灸十七椎、百会；痔核不消加灸商丘。

刺灸法：毫针刺，用泻法，留针 15～30 分钟，间歇行针 3～4次。

2.气虚下陷

治则：补益中气，活血消痔。取足太阳、任督二脉经穴为主。

处方：百会　气海　白环俞　承山　孔最　郄门

方义：百会能升阳举陷；气海能温肾固元气，使百会举陷之功有本基；白环俞可疏通肛门部之经气，并可振奋阳气；孔最肃降肺气，清泻肠腑之热，行气活血止痛；承山因其脉别入于肛，能疏导肛门之气机；郄门清心火，利三焦之气化，行气止痛。

刺灸法：毫针刺，用补法，留针 20～30 分钟，间歇行针 2～3 次；气海、百会可针后加灸，也可只灸不针，每次灸 30～40 分钟。

其他疗法

1.挑治法

取穴：背部反应点，即压之不变色而略突出于皮肤的褐色点；或上唇系带周围的瘀血点。

操作方法：常规消毒后，用三棱针挑断皮下纤维，或挑破上唇系带上的米粒状瘀血斑点，放出少量血液。每隔 3 天挑治一次。

2.耳针

取穴：直肠下端　大肠　痔点　皮质下　脾　肾上腺

操作方法：毫针刺，强刺激，留针 15 分钟。也可耳穴埋针或压豆。

3.激光疗法

取穴：痔核局部

操作方法：用氦－氖激光对准痔核部位，直接照射 15～20 分钟，每日 1～2 次。

2.19　落枕

落枕是指一侧项背肌肉酸痛，转动不利，活动受限为特征的一种疾患。相当于现代医学的项肌风湿痛或劳损性颈椎关节病等。

病因病机

本病多因睡眠时风寒之邪袭入经络，或因睡眠时体位不适，致使脉络受阻，气血不和，筋脉失养，拘急疼痛而发病。

辨证

多在早晨起床后，出现颈项肌肉酸痛强硬，不可左右转侧或回顾，酸楚疼痛向同侧肩臂扩散，检查时有明显压痛，但无红肿，二便正常，舌苔薄白，脉弦紧。

治疗

治则：祛风散寒，舒筋活络。取督脉及手、足太阳经穴为主。

处方：风池　大椎　天柱　肩外俞　肩井　后溪

方义：风池、大椎、天柱、肩外俞、肩井等穴，能疏通局部经气，祛风散寒；后溪为手太阳经穴，通于督脉，为八脉交会穴之一，有活络舒筋、祛风止痛之功。手太阳之脉，绕肩胛，交肩上，故取此经之穴后溪以治本病。

刺灸法：毫针刺，用平补平泻，留针 15～20 分钟，间歇行针 2～3 次。亦可灸风池、大椎各 15～20 分钟。

其他疗法

1.刺络拔罐

取穴：压痛点

操作方法：常规消毒后，用三棱针于压痛点处点刺，迅速将火罐吸拔于此外，留罐 5～10 分钟。

2.耳针

取穴：颈　枕　膀胱　反应点　皮质下　神门

操作方法：毫针刺，强刺激，留针 10～15 分钟。亦可耳穴压豆。

2.20　冻疮

冻疮是指机体局部皮肉被严寒侵袭后所引起的以局部皮肤苍白、发绀、刺痒灼痛、水肿、水疱，甚至坏死溃破等为主要特征的一种疾患。多发于手足、面部、外耳等暴露部位。属于现代医学的局部性冻伤。

病因病机

寒冷是导致冻疮的主要原因。而平素气血虚弱，身体缺乏锻炼，或在饥饿、疲劳、长时间静止不动、长时间使用止血带等情况下，再被寒邪侵袭，则更易导致气血运行不畅而瘀滞，发为冻疮。

另外，暴冻着热或暴热着冻，也能促使本病的发生。

辨证

轻证：初起受冻部位皮肤苍白，发绀，麻木冷痛，继则水肿，自觉灼痛瘙痒，或局部出现大小不等的水疱。如无感染，逐渐干枯，结痂脱落而愈，一般不遗留疤痕。

重证：初起受冻部位苍白，冷痛麻木，触觉丧失，继则暗红漫肿，水疱破后疮面呈紫色，出现腐烂或溃疡，溃后流脓流水，收口缓慢，甚则损伤肌肉筋骨，病处感觉、运动功能障碍。继发感染时，可有高热、寒战等全身症状。

治疗

1.轻证

治则：温经散寒，活血止痛。取局部穴位为主。

处方：根据病变部位选穴如下。

　　　　面部：合谷　大椎　人迎　风池　百会

　　　　手部：八邪　合谷　外关　后溪

　　　　足部：八风　太冲　足临泣　涌泉　足三里　隐白

方义：面部主要为阳明经所布，取人迎、合谷调和面部气血；大椎为诸阳之会，灸之能温经散寒；风池、百会疏通头部经气，以祛风散寒，活血止痛。手部八邪祛风散寒；合谷、后溪、外关调和手部诸阳经之经气，以温经散寒，通络活血。足部八风、涌泉能祛风温经散寒；太冲、足临泣疏经活络，理气止痛；足三里、隐白补益脾气而升诸阳。

刺灸法：毫针刺，用补法，留针20～30分钟，间歇行针2

~3次；大椎、百会、足三里、涌泉、隐白、风池可用灸法。

2.重证

治则：温经散寒，通阳化气，活血祛瘀。取任脉、督脉及足少阴经穴为主。

处方：大椎　人中　关元　气海　命门　涌泉　合谷　足三里

方义：大椎、人中、关元、气海四穴同用，可温经散寒，通阳化气；命门、涌泉补肾阳，益精血；合谷、足三里调理中焦，以资气血生化之源，祛瘀生新。

随证选穴：手背冻疮加中渚；足背冻疮加昆仑。

刺灸法：毫针刺，用补法，留针20～30分钟；大椎、关元、涌泉、足三里加灸法，每穴温灸15～20分钟。

2.21　破伤风

破伤风是指机体先有破伤，而后风毒邪气由伤口侵入所引起的以项背强直、角弓反张、口噤、言语不清、筋肉拘急、四肢颤掉、肢体疼痛、口眼㖞斜等为特征的一种疾病。现代医学亦称为破伤风。

病因病机

本病因先有机体局部破伤，风毒由伤口乘机侵袭经络，循经窜扰，引动内风，使营卫不得宣通，筋脉失于濡养而致拘急抽搐，甚则脏气逆乱而成危候。

辨证

前驱期：主要表现为乏力，头痛，多汗，烦躁，嚼骨体酸痛，或伤口有牵扯感。

发作期：可见牙关紧闭，不能进食，语言不清，苦笑面容，颈项强直，角弓反张，四肢抽搐阵作不休，高热，但神志清楚，脉沉数或弦数。若见神昏，脉沉，大汗，躁动，多属危候。

治疗

治则：平肝熄风，清热镇痉。取督脉及手、足阳明经穴为主。

处方：大椎　风府　筋缩　人中　合谷　委中　太冲　申脉

方义：中医认为，"诸暴强直，皆属于风。"阳盛则热，热极生风。治取诸阳之会大椎以及风府、筋缩，以疏通督脉，清热镇痉；取人中专调脊强反折；合谷配太冲，此为四关，意在平肝熄风，通关开窍，以解口噤、苦笑之症；委中配申脉，调理膀胱经气，以解项背强直。八穴合用，则具清热镇痉、平肝熄风之功。

随证选穴：颈项强直加后溪；牙关紧闭加下关；四肢抽搐加阳陵泉。

刺灸法：毫针刺，用泻法，留针 20～30 分钟，间歇行针 2～3 次。

其他疗法

1.刺络拔罐

取穴：大椎及大椎上、下、左、右各 1cm 处。

操作方法：以上五处，行皮肤消毒后，用三棱针重刺，直至有血流出为度，出血后迅速以大椎为中心将火罐吸拔于此处，留罐 10 分钟，以血不再流出为止。

2.耳针

取穴：肝　胸　神门　脊柱

操作方法：毫针刺，强刺激，留针 15～20 分钟；或耳穴埋针。

2.22　蛔厥

蛔厥是指由于肠道中的蛔虫上窜，钻入胆道而突然引起上腹部阵发性绞痛或钻顶样疼痛。因痛时翻滚号叫，恶心呕吐，汗出，甚至肢厥，故名蛔厥。蛔虫退出胆道则疼痛立刻缓解如常人。现代医学称为胆道蛔虫病。

病因病机

本病多由于蛔虫居于肠中，其性好动，善钻孔道，当脏寒胃热时，脏腑功能紊乱，蛔虫妄动上扰，不安其位，上窜胆道而发。

辨证

多数病人有便蛔、吐蛔史，临床上常突然发生剑突下阵发性钻顶样剧痛。病人抱腹屈膝，卧伏床上，或辗转不安，翻滚号叫，面色苍白，汗出肢厥。疼痛常向肩背或腰部放射，持续时间长短不一，短则数分钟，长则数小时。间歇期也不规则，多则一日发作数次，少则数日发作一次，蛔虫退出胆道后则疼痛缓解如常人。发作时可伴有恶心呕吐，苔白腻，脉弦数等症。

治疗

治则：疏泄肝胆，理气止痛，安蛔驱虫。取足少阳、足阳明及任脉穴为主。

处方：阳陵泉　内关　支沟　足三里　日月　胸8～10夹脊穴

方义：阳陵泉为足少阳经之合穴，日月为胆之募穴，二穴配用，能疏泄肝胆之气，以驱蛔止痛；内关通阴维脉，配支沟可调理脏腑功能而安蛔止痛；足三里可疏导胃肠之气，缓急止痛；胸8～10夹脊穴，可疏导肝胆之气，解痉挛，使驱蛔止痛之效更捷。

刺灸法：毫针刺，用泻法，留针20～30分钟，间歇行针3～4次。

其他疗法：耳针

取穴：交感　神门　肝　胆　十二指肠　胰

操作方法：毫针刺，强刺激，留针15～20分钟；或耳穴埋针或压豆。

2.23　肠梗阻

肠梗阻是指肠腔内容物不能顺利通过，淤滞梗塞于肠道而发生的以腹痛、呕吐、腹胀、矢气及大便均不通为主要特征的病证。中医称之为肠结。

病因病机

本病多因暴饮暴食，剧烈活动，或因寒邪凝滞，热邪郁闭，湿邪中阻，瘀血留滞，或因燥屎内结，蛔虫扭结聚团等因素，引起肠道痞塞，寒热结滞，以致胃肠传导阻塞，上关下格而成。

辨证

肠梗阻初起，多见阵发性剧烈腹痛，呕吐，腹胀，几日或数日大便不通，无矢气，下腹部可摸到痛性包块，舌苔黄燥，脉弦紧滑数。

治疗

治则：疏通肠腑，消积导气。取足阳明经穴为主。

处方：天枢　上巨虚　下巨虚　足三里　大肠俞　支沟　丰隆

方义：天枢为手阳明大肠经之募穴，足三里为足阳明胃经之下合穴，上巨虚为手阳明经之下合穴，下巨虚为手太阳经之下合穴，大肠俞为背俞穴，上五穴相配，共奏疏通胃肠腑气，消积导气之功；支沟配丰隆，可清热益阴，润燥通便。

刺灸法：毫针刺，用泻法，留针 20～30 分钟，间歇行针 3～4 次。

其他疗法： 耳针

取穴：大肠　小肠　胃　腹　神门　皮质下　交感

操作方法：毫针刺，用泻法，强刺激，留针 15～20 分钟；或耳穴埋针。

按语

针灸治疗仅适应于肠结初期。

3 妇科病证

3.1 月经不调

月经不调，是指月经周期、经期、经量、经色、经质的异常，或伴随月经周期出现的症状为特征的疾病。多与气候环境的改变和情绪波动等因素有关。

病因病机

经行先期：主要因气虚血失统摄，冲任失固或血热，流行散溢使血海不宁，而致月经先期而至。

经行后期：有虚有实；虚者因营血亏损或阳气虚衰心致；血源不足；实者或因气郁血滞，冲任受阻，或因寒凝血瘀，冲任不畅，而致经期后延。

经行不定期：多因肝郁气滞，或肾气虚衰，导致气血失调。常见病因如情志抑郁，或忿怒伤肝，或房室不节，生育过多，损伤肾气，冲任失调而致经行先后无定期。

辨证

1.经行先期　　月经先期而至 7 天以上，甚至经行一月两次，经量较多，色鲜红或紫红，伴有烦热，面赤口干，喜冷饮或见潮热盗汗，手足心热，舌红，苔黄或少苔，脉滑数或细数。

2.经行后期　　月经推迟来潮七天以上，月经量少，色黯或淡，质多清稀或夹有瘀血块，兼有畏寒肢冷，小腹冷痛，遇热则减，或见面色苍白，头晕目眩，小腹隐痛喜按，舌质淡，苔薄白，脉沉迟。

3.经行不定期　　月经或早或迟，不能按期来潮。经量或多或少，经色或紫或淡，经行不畅，常伴胸胁乳房胀痛，心烦易怒，或嗳气不舒，或见头晕耳鸣，腰膝酸软，舌淡，苔白，脉弦或沉弱。

治疗

1.经行先期

治则：补气养血，调养冲任。取足太阴和任脉经穴为主。

处方：隐白　三阴交　气海　足三里

方义：隐白为足太阴之根，能补益脾气升诸阳，统摄气血；三阴交能补脾兼及肝肾，调冲任，养血活血，为治疗妇科疾病要穴；足三里调脾胃，以助气血生化之源；气海固元气，温下焦，益精血，暖子宫。

刺灸法：毫针刺，用补法，留针 20 分钟。隐白灸 30 分钟。

2.经行后期

治则：行气活血，温经散寒。取任脉及足太阴经穴为主。

处方：三阴交　合谷　关元　地机　膈俞

方义：地机为足太阴脾经郄穴，配膈俞可活血通经；三阴交行气血通瘀结，益气生血，培元散寒；合谷为手阳明经穴，能行气活血；关元温下焦，暖子宫，益精血，除腹中寒冷。

刺灸法：毫针刺，用补法，留针 20～30 分钟。关元用灸法，每次灸 30～40 分钟。

3.经行不定期

治则：舒肝理气，调补冲任。取厥阴和任脉经穴为主。

处方：太冲　三阴交　中极　肝俞

方义：太冲能调肝气，通经行瘀；肝俞舒肝气，益血养阴；中极为任脉经穴，可通调冲任脉气，配三阴交可健脾兼及肝肾，使胞脉得养，冲任之脉调和。

刺灸法：毫针刺，酌情补泻。留针 15～20 分钟。

其他疗法：耳针

取穴：子宫　内分泌　肝　肾　脾　卵巢

操作方法：毫针刺，中等刺激，留针 15～20 分钟。

3.2 痛经

妇女每逢行经期间，或行经前后，出现周期性的小腹疼痛，或痛引腰骶，甚则剧痛难忍者，称为痛经。多见于青年妇女。

病因病机

主要机理是气血运行不畅，或由气虚血少，或由气滞血瘀导致冲任经脉不利，经血阻滞胞宫而作痛。

实证：本痛多因行经期受寒饮冷，或坐卧湿地，寒湿之邪客于冲任，经血凝滞胞宫；或因肝气郁结，气滞血瘀，经行受阻，不通则痛。

虚证：肝肾不足，生育过多或久病大病之后，气血双亏，血海空虚，胞脉失养，故经行腹痛。

辨证

1.寒湿凝滞　经前或经期小腹冷痛，拒按喜热，经行量少，色黯有血块，苔白腻，脉沉紧。

2.气滞血瘀　经前或经期小腹胀痛，胸胁、乳房作胀，月经量少，淋漓不畅，色紫黯有血块，血块排出后则痛减，舌质紫黯有瘀点，脉弦。

3.肝肾亏损　经期或经后小腹绵绵作痛，按之痛减，经血色淡量少质稀，兼见头晕耳鸣，腰膝酸软，舌淡红，苔薄白，脉沉细。

4.气血虚弱　经期或经后小腹隐隐作痛，按之则痛减，月经色淡质清稀，兼有全身乏力，面色苍白无华，纳少便溏，舌淡苔薄，脉细弱。

治疗

1.寒湿凝滞

治则：温经散寒，利湿化瘀。取任脉和足太阴经穴为主。

处方：气海　天枢　命门　三阴交髎次

方义：气海有肾气丸之功；天枢有天雄之热，配以命门可振阳散寒；三阴交能补脾兼及肝肾，并有利湿活血化瘀之功；次髎为治疗痛经的经验有效穴。

刺灸法：毫针刺，用补法，针后加灸，留针 20～30 分钟。

2.气滞血瘀

治则：理气活血，化瘀止痛。取任脉。足厥阴经穴为主。

处方：太冲　三阴交　合谷

方义：太冲为足厥阴经原穴，有舒肝解郁，调理气血之功；三阴交为足三阴之交会穴，配合谷以调气行血止痛。

随证选穴：胸闷胁痛加内关、阳陵泉。

刺灸法：毫针刺，用泻法。留针 15～20 分钟，不灸。

3.肝肾亏损

治则：补益肝肾，调补冲任。取任脉、背俞穴为主。

处方：肝俞　肾俞　关元　三阴交

方义：取肝俞、肾俞补益肝肾；关元属任脉穴，可补益肾气暖胞宫；三阴交补脾兼及肝肾，能补益精血，调养冲任。

随证选穴：头晕耳鸣加太溪。

刺灸法：毫针刺，用补法。留针 15～20 分钟。

4.气血虚弱

治则：益气养血。取任脉和足阳明经穴为主。

处方：关元　肾俞　足三里　三阴交

方义：关元为任脉经穴，可温补下焦，固元气暖子宫，益精血调冲任；取肾俞以补益肾气；三阴交配足三里，可补脾胃益气血，补肝肾调冲任。

刺灸法：毫针刺，用补法。留针 15～20 分钟，并可针后加灸。

其他疗法：耳针

取穴：神门　交感　子宫　内分泌　肾

操作方法：毫针刺，中等刺激，每次取 2～3 穴，留针 15～20 分钟，也可用耳穴压豆法。

3.3 闭经

闭经也称经闭，女子年过十八岁月经尚未初潮，或行经而又中断达三个月以上者，称为闭经。现代医学称前者为原发性闭经，后者为继发性闭经。

病因病机

不外虚实两方面，虚者由精血不足，血海空虚，无血可下；实者气滞血瘀，冲任受阻，经血不得下行而致经闭不行。肝肾不足，久病体弱，阴血亏耗，或脾胃虚弱，化源不足，以致冲任失养，无血以下而为经闭。或因情志抑郁，气机不畅，或外感风寒，内伤生冷，邪气客于胞宫，而致经脉郁滞，瘀血凝结，冲任受阻而闭经。

辨证

1.血虚闭经　年逾十八，尚未行经，或月经后期，经量逐渐减少乃至停闭，腰膝酸软，头晕耳鸣，或见纳少便溏，心悸怔忡，少气懒言，或五心烦热，面色少华，或两颧潮红，舌红或淡，苔少或白，脉细弱。

2.血滞闭经　月经数月不行，精神抑郁，烦燥易怒，胸胁胀满，或见小腹胀痛或冷痛，拒按，得热则痛减，舌边紫黯，脉沉弦或沉涩。

治疗

1.血虚闭经

治则：补气养血。取任脉和背俞穴为主。

处方：脾俞　肾俞　气海　足三里

方义：本方的作用为调理脾胃，补益肾气，充养冲任。脾胃为后天之本。为气血生化之源，气血之源充足，则经血自行，故取脾俞，足三里以健运脾胃；肾为先天之本，肾气胆则精血自充，故取肾俞、气海以补肾气，温固下焦。

随证选穴：纳少便溏加天枢；心悸怔忡加内关。

刺灸法：毫针刺，用补法。留针 20～30 分钟，并针后加灸，每日 1 次。

2.血滞闭经

治则：舒肝理气，温经散寒。取任脉和足太阴经穴为主。

处方：中极　合谷　肝俞　胆俞　三阴交　太冲

方义：中极为任脉经穴，能理冲任而疏调下焦；太冲能调肝养血，通经行瘀；肝俞、胆俞可舒肝理气；三阴交为足三阴经的交会穴，与合谷相配以行气调血，而达通经目的。

随证选穴：胸胁胀满加内关。

刺灸法：毫针刺，用泻法。留针 15～20 分钟，每日 1 次，属寒邪引起者，中极穴可针后加灸。

其他疗法：耳针

取穴：内分泌　子宫　肝　肾　脾　胃　神门

操作方法：毫针刺，中等刺激，每次用 3～4 穴，隔日 1 次，10 次为 1 疗程。或用耳穴压豆法。

3.4　阴挺

阴挺是胞宫不同程度的下脱，甚至脱出阴道口之外的病症，包括现代医学的子宫脱垂及阴道壁膨出。

病因病机

本病主要病机是气虚下陷与肾虚不固，致胞络损伤而不能提摄子宫。由于分娩时用力太过，或产后过早从事重体力劳动，而致脾虚气弱，中气下陷，提举无力，或因多产多育，房劳过度，肾气耗损，以致带脉失约，冲任不固，而发为阴挺。

辨证

1.气虚　　子宫下移或脱出阴道口外，劳则加剧，自觉小腹下坠，四肢乏力，少气懒言，面色少华，白带量多，质稀色白，舌淡苔薄白，脉虚弱。

2.肾虚　　子宫下脱，小腹下坠，头晕耳鸣，腰膝酸软，小便频数，夜间尤甚，舌淡红，脉沉弱。

治疗

1.气虚

治则：升阳益气，固摄胞宫。取督脉、足太阴、阳明经穴为主。

处方：百会　气海　维道　归来　足三里　三阴交

方义：百会为督脉经穴，用以升阳提气；气海、维道、归来以补气固摄胞宫；足三里、三阴交可健脾益气；诸穴相合有益气升阳，固摄胞宫的作用。

随证选穴：白带多加阴陵泉。

刺灸法：毫针刺，用补法，针后加灸，每次 20～30 分钟，每日 1 次。

2.肾虚

治则：补益肾气，固摄胞宫。取任脉、足少阴经穴为主。

处方：关元　肾俞　次髎曲泉

方义：关元、肾俞温肾阳固元气；次髎祛湿热，疗腰酸腰坠；曲泉为肝之合，以养血而利胞宫。

随证选穴：头晕耳鸣加百会。

刺灸法：毫针刺，用补法。针后加灸，每次 20～30 分钟，每日 1 次。

其他疗法：头针

取穴：双侧生殖区、足运感区。

操作方法：毫针刺，间歇捻针 15～20 分钟。

3.5　崩漏

崩漏是妇女月经周期以外的非正常性子宫出血。出血量多，来势急骤称为崩；发病较缓，出血量少淋漓不净，则称漏。两者可相互转化，交替出现，故统称崩漏。现代医学的功能性子宫出血即属本病范畴之内，是妇科常见病，以青春期和更年期妇女较为多见。

病因病机

本病主要机理是冲任损伤，不能制约经血。多因思虑伤脾，中气不足，统摄无权或肾气虚弱，冲任失固。若外感邪热或情志不舒，肝郁化火，蕴结下焦，则迫血妄行，而成崩漏。

辨证

1.脾虚　　经血突然暴下，继而淋漓不断，血色淡红，全身倦怠乏力，面色㿠白，气短懒言，纳呆便溏，舌质淡，苔薄白，脉细弱。

2.肾虚　　肾阳虚者，经血不时而下，量多或淋漓不尽，色淡质清，畏寒肢冷，面色晦黯，腰腿酸软，溲清长，舌淡苔薄白，脉沉细。心悸失眠，腰膝酸软或午后潮热，舌红少苔，脉细数为肾阴虚证。

3.血热　　经血不时突然大下如崩，或淋漓日久不净，色深红而质稠，心烦口渴，大便干结，小便黄，舌红苔黄或黄腻，脉洪数。

治疗

治则：止崩固漏，摄血培元。取任脉、足太阴经穴为主。

处方：关元　三阴交　隐白

血热者加血海　行间。脾虚者加脾俞　足三里。肾虚者加肾俞　太溪。

方义：隐白为脾经井穴，可补益脾气升诸阳，以统摄气血；关元为足三阴、冲任之会，可以调补冲任之气，温下焦固元气，暖子宫益精血，元气充实，统摄气血之功自复；三阴交为足三阴经之交会穴，有补脾统血之功，为治妇科病的要穴。血热者加血海、行间以清血热；脾虚者加脾俞、足三里以健脾益气；肾虚者加肾俞、太溪以益肾滋阴降火。

随证选穴：纳呆便溏加天枢、上巨虚；大便秘结加支沟。

刺灸法：毫针刺，血热者用泻法，只针不灸；脾虚、肾虚者用补法，针后加灸，留针 15～20 分钟。

其他疗法：耳针

取穴：子宫　内分泌　卵巢　神门　肝　肾　脾

操作方法：毫针刺，中等刺激，每次选 2～4 穴，每日或隔日 1 次，留针 30 分钟。

3.6　带下病

妇女阴道分泌物异常增多，并且色泽、质地以及气味改变者称为带下病。带下以白色的较为多见，所以又称白带，是妇科临床的常见病。

病因病机

带下病多因思虑过度，脾胃损伤，运化失职，水湿积聚，流注下焦；或因房劳多产，肾气不足，下元亏损，任带失于固约；或肝经湿热下注，而成带下。

辨证

1.脾虚　带下连绵不断，色白或淡黄，质地粘稠无臭味，面色萎黄，神疲乏力，纳少便溏，舌质淡，苔白腻，脉缓而弱。

2.肾虚　带下量多，不时而至，色白清稀，腰部酸痛，小腹发凉；小便频数清长，大便溏薄，舌淡苔白，脉沉迟。

3.湿热　带下色黄如脓或如米泔，量多而臭，阴中作痒，兼有小腹坠痛，口苦咽干，大便干结，小便短赤，舌苔黄腻，脉滑数。

治疗

1.脾虚

治则：健脾益气，利湿正带。取任脉、带脉、足太阴经穴为主。

处方：带脉　白环俞　气海　三阴交

方义：取带脉以固摄本经经气；白环俞、气海可通调任脉和膀胱之气而化湿邪。三阴交以健脾渗湿，调理肝肾。

随证选穴：纳少便溏加中脘、天枢、足三里。

刺灸法：毫针刺，用补法。留针 15～20 分钟，并可针后加灸，每日 1 次。

2.肾虚

治则：补益肾气，固摄任带。取任脉带脉和足少阴经穴为主。

处方：关元　带脉　肾俞　次髎　照海

方义：取关元、肾俞、照海温下焦固元气，暖子宫益精血，除下焦之寒冷；带脉、次髎为治疗带下病的有效穴。

随证选穴：大便稀薄加上巨虚。

刺灸法：毫针刺，用补法。留针 15～20 分钟，针后加灸，每日 1 次。

3.湿热

治则：清热、利湿、止带。取带脉和足太阴经穴为主。

处方：带脉　次髎　阴陵泉　绝骨　行间

方义：取带脉以调理本经经气；次髎清泄下焦湿热；用肝经之荥穴行间而泄肝经之郁热；泻阴陵泉以清泄脾经之湿热；绝骨可清三焦之热，祛湿降浊。

随证选穴：大便干结加支沟。

刺灸法：毫针刺，用泻法。留针 15～20 分钟，每日 1 次。

其他疗法：耳针

取穴：神门　子宫　膀胱　脾　肾

操作方法：毫针刺，中等刺激。每次选 2～3 穴，隔日 1 次，留针 15～20 分钟，或用耳穴压豆法。

3.7　妊娠恶阻

妊娠恶阻，又称妊娠呕吐。临床以恶心、呕吐，头晕、厌食或食入即吐等为主要特征，是最常见的早期妊娠反应。多在怀孕 3 个月以后逐渐消失。

病因病机

主要由冲脉之气上逆，胃失和降所致。常见有脾胃虚弱，肝胃不和两种。如脾胃素虚，孕后经血不泻，冲脉之气较盛而上逆犯胃，胃气虚则失于和降，随冲气上逆而发呕恶。或由脾虚失运，痰湿内生，阻于中焦，冲气挟痰湿上逆而发呕恶。或因孕后阴血不足，肝气偏旺犯胃，肝胃不和则胃失和降而呕恶。

辨证

1.脾胃虚弱　　受孕之后，脘腹胀满，厌食恶心，甚至食入即吐，口淡，呕吐清涎，神倦思睡，心悸气短，舌淡，苔白腻，脉缓滑无力。

2.肝胃不和　　妊娠初期，呕吐酸水或苦水，胸满胁痛，嗳气叹息，精神抑郁，头胀头晕，烦渴口苦，舌淡，苔微黄，脉弦滑。

治疗

1.脾胃虚弱

治则：健脾和胃，降逆止呕。取任脉、足阳明、足太阴经穴为主。

处方：中脘　足三里　公孙　脾俞　胃俞　内关

方义：取足三里以和胃降逆止呕，加公孙以调理脾胃气机而平冲降逆；内关宽胸理气，降逆止呕；脾俞、胃俞配中脘为俞募配穴法，可调腑气补脾胃。

刺灸法：毫针刺，用补法。留针15～20分钟。

2.肝胃不和

治则：疏肝和胃，降逆止呕。取手足厥阴，足阳明经穴为主。

处方：内关　中脘　足三里　太冲

方义：取内关可宽胸理气；太冲配足三里可平肝木补脾土，使土木不相侮；中脘和胃降逆止呕。

随证选穴：属痰浊中阻者加丰隆。

刺灸法：毫针刺，用泻法。留针 15～20 分钟，每日 1 次，妊妇精神紧张或习惯性流产者，应慎用针刺，以防流产。

其他疗法：耳针

取穴：神门 肝 胃 脾 交感

操作方法：毫针轻刺激，每日 1 次，10 次为 1 疗程，亦可用耳穴压豆法。

3.8 胎位不正

胎位不正是指妊娠 28 周后，胎儿在子宫体内的位置异常。常见于经产妇或腹壁松弛的孕妇，本身多无自觉症状。临产后容易出现并发症。因骨盆狭窄，子宫畸形等原因引起的胎位不正，不属本病的治疗范围。

治疗

处方：至阴

方义：至阴穴属足太阴膀胱经的脉气所发处，肾与膀胱相表里，两经之脉气会接于此，故温灸至阴穴能促使互为表里的两条经脉获得平衡，而使胞胎转正。

灸法：操作时须解松腰带，坐在靠背椅上或仰卧床上，以艾条灸两侧至阴穴 15～20 分钟，每天 1～2 次，至胎位转正后为止。成功率约达 80%以上，经产妇较初产妇效果更好，以妊娠 7 个月者成功率最高。

3.9 滞产

产妇临产后总产程超过 24 小时者，称为滞产。多因产力异常，或胎位异常等因素造成，如因子宫畸形，头盆不称引起的滞产，不属针灸治疗范围。

病因病机

本病多因素体虚弱，正气不足或分娩时用力过早，耗伤气血，以致宫缩无力，产力减弱，或因产前贪图安逸，临产时精神过度紧张，或感受寒邪，以致气机不利，气血瘀滞，而成滞产。

辨证

1.气血虚弱　　分娩时小腹阵阵微痛，轻度坠胀，久产不下，或下血量多色淡，面色苍白，心悸气短，神倦无力，舌淡苔薄，脉大而虚，或沉细而弱。

2.气滞血瘀　　腰腹疼痛剧烈，阵阵发作，出血量少，色黯红，产程进展缓慢，面色紫黯，精神紧张，胸脘胀闷，时欲呕恶，舌质黯红，脉象沉实，数而不均。

治疗

1.气血虚弱

治则：补养气血，益气催产。取足阳明、太阴、少阴经穴为主。

处方：气海　三阴交　复溜　至阴

方义：气海温肾阳，振奋元气；三阴交可统调三阴经气；复溜以补肾益气；至阴为足太阳膀胱经的井穴，为催产之经验要穴。

随证选穴：心悸气短加内关。

刺灸法：毫针刺，用补法。气海用灸法。

2.气滞血瘀

治则：理气、活血、催产。取手阳明、足太阴经穴为主。

处方：合谷　三阴交　至阴　独阴

方义：合谷为手阳明经原穴，三阴交为足三阴之交会穴，补合谷，泻三阴交，有补气调血下胎的作用；至阴乃足太阳经井穴，独阴为奇穴，均为催产之经验穴。四穴合用可达催产、引产的目的。

随证选穴：胸胁胀满加内关、支沟。

刺灸法：毫针刺，用泻法。

其他疗法：耳针

取穴：子宫　内分泌　皮质下　肾

操作方法：毫针刺，中等刺激。每隔 3～5 分钟捻针 1 次。

3.10　胞衣不下

胞衣不下是指胎儿娩出之后，胞衣在 30 分钟之内尚未娩出者。现代医学称为胎盘滞留。

病因病机

多因产妇体质虚弱，元气不足或产程过长，耗伤气血，或因感受寒邪，气血凝滞，导致气血运行不畅，胞宫活动力减弱，而不能促使胞衣排出。

辨证

1.气虚　　产后胞衣不下，少腹微胀，按之不痛，有块不坚，阴道流血，量多色淡，伴有面色㿠白，神疲倦怠，畏寒肢冷，舌质淡，苔薄白，脉虚弱。

2.血瘀　　产后小腹冷痛拒按，按之有块而硬，胞衣迟迟不下，阴道流血，量少色黯红，舌质黯，脉沉涩。

治疗

1.气虚

治则：补气养血。取任脉、足太阴经穴为主。

处方：关元　三阴交　独阴

方义：关元穴属任脉经穴，通于胞宫，三阴交为足三阴经的交会穴，二穴相配，针灸并用，可益气养血；独阴为经外奇穴，是治疗胞衣不下的经验效穴。

随证选穴：阴道出血较多加隐白，用灸法。

刺灸法：毫针刺，用补法，并可针后加灸。

2.血瘀

治则：活血祛瘀。取任脉、手阳明、足太阴经穴为主。

处方：中极　合谷　三阴交　肩井　独阴

方义：中极属任脉经穴，通于胞宫，泻之可活血祛瘀；补合谷，泻三阴交以行气活血，配独阴治胞衣不下；肩井为孕妇禁针穴，其性主降主坠，针之可下胞衣。

刺灸法：毫针刺，用泻法，并可针后加灸。

其他疗法：电针

取穴：合谷　三阴交

操作方法：针刺得气后，通电 30 分钟。

3.11　恶露不绝

产后胞宫内的余血浊液经阴道排出，谓之恶露。约 3 周左右干净，若产后超过 3 周恶露仍淋漓不断者，称为恶露不绝或恶露不止。

病因病机

素体虚弱，正气不足或产时气血耗伤，产后操劳过早，以致气虚下陷，冲任不固，不能摄血。或因阴液亏耗，阴虚而生内热；或外感热邪，或肝郁化热而致热扰冲任，迫血妄行；或因感受寒邪，与血相搏，瘀血阻于胞宫，冲任失畅而致恶露不绝。

辨证

1.气虚　　恶露日久不止，量多，或淋漓不绝，色淡红，质稀无臭气，小腹空坠，神疲倦怠，面色㿠白，舌淡苔薄白，脉缓弱。

2.血热　　恶露过期不止，量较多，色深红，质稠粘，臭秽，面色潮红，口燥咽干，舌质红，脉细数。

3.血瘀　　恶露淋漓，涩滞不畅，量少色紫黯有块，小腹疼痛拒按，舌紫黯，脉弦涩。

治疗

1.气虚

治则：补气摄血。取任、督、足太阴、阳明经穴。

处方：隐白　关元　足三里　三阴交

方义：隐白为足太阴之根，可补益脾气，统摄气血；关元为周身元气之所聚集之处；足三里、三阴交可补益中州，健脾统血。

随证选穴：恶露多加脾俞。

刺灸法：毫针刺，用补法。并可针后加灸，每次 20～30 分钟，每日 1 次。

2.血热

治则：养阴、清热、止血。取任脉和足三阴经穴为主。

处方：气海　血海　中都　太溪

方义：气海属任脉，通于胞宫，有理气益气之功，泻之可清下焦之热；血海属脾经，有理血调经之作用，泻之可清血中之热；中都为肝经郄穴，有疏肝清热的作用；太溪用以益肾阴，除虚热。

随证选穴：口舌干燥加照海。

刺灸法：毫针刺，用泻法。留针 15～20 分钟，每日 1 次。

3.血瘀

治则：活血化瘀。取任脉、足太阴经穴为主。

处方：中极　太冲　三阴交

方义：中极属任脉，有调理冲任，活血行瘀的作用；太冲为足厥阴肝经原穴，可调肝气养肝血，通经行瘀；三阴交为足三阴经之交会穴，有行气血，通瘀结，养血活血之功。

随证选穴：少腹冷痛加灸关元。

刺灸法：毫针刺，用泻法，留针 15～20 分钟，每日 1 次。属感受寒邪，血瘀凝滞者可针后加灸。

其他疗法：耳针

取穴：神门　交感　子宫　内分泌　脾　肝　肾　皮质下

操作方法：毫针刺，中等刺激，每日 1 次，每次选用 2～3 穴，留针 15～20 分钟。也可用耳穴压豆法。

3.12　乳少

产后乳汁甚少或全无，称为乳少。亦称缺乳和乳汁不行。

病因病机

乳汁乃气血所化，如脾胃素虚，生化之源不足，或分娩时失血过多，以致气血亏耗，不能化为乳汁。或因产后情志抑郁，肝失条达，气机不畅，经脉涩滞，乳汁运行受阻。

辨证

1.气血虚弱　　产后乳汁量少清稀，甚至全无，乳房柔软无胀感，兼见面色少华，神倦短气，纳少便溏，舌淡少苔，脉细弱。

2.肝郁气滞　　产后乳少或全无，胸胁胀满，乳房胀痛，情志抑郁，或有微热，心烦纳呆，舌苔薄黄，脉弦或弦数。

治疗

治则：气血虚弱者补养气血，肝郁气滞者疏肝解郁，佐以通乳。

处方：膻中　少泽　乳根
　　　　气血虚弱加脾俞　足三里
　　　　肝郁气滞加内关　期门

方义：取膻中以理气，气调则血行，气血和畅乳汁生化有源；乳房为足阳明经所过，故取乳根可疏通阳明经气，以使乳部脉气通畅而行乳汁；少泽为手太阳小肠经井穴，毫针浅刺，可调气行血，为通乳效穴。气血虚弱加脾俞、足三里以健脾胃而助生化之源。肝郁气滞加内关、期门以解郁宽胸理气，气行则血行，血脉畅通则乳汁可行。

随证选穴：食少便溏加关枢；胸胁胀满加阳陵泉。

刺灸法：气血虚弱者，毫针刺，用补法。脾俞、足三里、天枢并可针后加灸，每次灸 20～30 分钟；肝郁气滞者，毫针刺，用泻法，留针 15～20 分钟，每日 1 次。

其他疗法: 耳针

取穴: 胸区　内分泌　肝　脾

操作方法: 毫针刺, 中等刺激, 留针 15~20 分钟, 每日 1
次, 或用耳穴压豆法。

3.13　产后腹痛

产后以小腹疼痛为主证者, 称为产后腹痛, 亦称儿枕痛。以
经产妇较为多见, 常在产后 1~2 天出现。

病因病机

分娩时出血过多, 冲任空虚, 胞脉失养, 或血虚气衰, 以致
血行不畅, 迟滞而痛; 产后胞脉空虚, 寒邪乘虚而入, 血为寒
凝, 阻于胞脉; 或情志不畅, 肝气郁结, 气机不宣, 以致瘀血内
停, 恶露不下而腹痛。

辨证

1.血虚腹痛　　小腹隐痛喜按, 恶露量少色淡, 头晕耳鸣,
全身乏力, 大便燥结, 舌质淡红, 苔薄, 脉虚细。

2.血瘀腹痛　　产后小腹胀痛拒按, 恶露量少, 涩滞不畅,
色紫黯夹有瘀血块, 或伴胸胁胀痛, 舌质黯或有瘀点, 脉弦涩。

3.寒凝腹痛　　小腹冷痛拒按, 得热则减, 恶露量少, 有瘀
血块, 面色青白, 四肢不温, 舌质黯淡, 苔白, 脉沉紧。

治疗

1.血虚腹痛

治则: 补血益气。取任脉、足阳明、太阴经穴为主。

处方: 关元　足三里　三阴交

方义: 关元为任脉经穴, 能温下焦固元气, 暖子宫益精血,
疗腹中寒冷; 足三里、三阴交可调补脾胃, 以益生化之源。

随证选穴: 头晕加百会; 大便燥结加照海。

刺灸法: 毫针刺, 用补法, 并可针后加灸。

2.血瘀腹痛

治则：活血化瘀，通络止痛。取任脉、足太阴和背俞穴为主。

处方：中极　归来　膈俞　血海　三阴交　合谷

方义：取中极、归来以疏经通络，行气活血止痛；取血会膈俞配血海以活血化瘀；三阴交补脾兼及肝肾，调冲任而活血养血；合谷升而能散，善于行气，与上诸穴相配，使活血化瘀止痛之功更捷。

随证选穴：属气滞血瘀者加太冲。

刺灸法：毫针刺，用泻法。留针20分钟，每隔3～5分钟捻针1次。

3.寒凝腹痛

治则：温经散寒止痛。取任脉、足太阴经穴为主。

处方：关元　肾俞　三阴交

方义：关元为任脉经穴，能温下焦固元气，暖子宫益精血，疗腹中寒冷；肾俞可温肾阳以散寒；三阴交补肝肾益冲任，调气养血，活血止痛。

随证选穴：腹痛剧烈加次髎。

刺灸法：毫针刺，用补法，并针后加灸，每次灸20～30分钟，每日1次。

其他疗法：耳针

取穴：子宫　内分泌　肝　肾　神门

操作方法：毫针刺，中等刺激，留针15～20分钟，每日1次，亦可用耳穴压豆法。

3.14　子痫

妊娠后期或正位临产时，或新产后发生突然眩晕仆倒，昏不知人，四肢抽搐，全身强直，牙关紧闭、双目上视，少时自醒，醒后复发，状如癫痫发作，故称子痫，或称妊娠痫证。属现代医学之重度妊娠中毒。

病因病机

本病主要是由于素体肝肾阴虚，肝阳偏亢，孕后血聚养胎而阴血亏乏，肝失荣养，肝阳上亢，日久生风则发为子痫。

辨证

妊娠数月，时感头晕目眩，心悸气短，下肢水肿日重，面色潮红，口苦咽干，病发时突然昏倒，不省人事，四肢抽搐，牙关紧闭，双目上视或口吐白沫，间歇发作，舌红质绛，脉弦滑或弦数。

治疗

治则：滋阴养血，平肝熄风。取督脉、手、足厥阴、足少阴经穴为主。

处方：水沟　内关　风池　太冲　三阴交　照海　涌泉

方义：取水沟驱风醒神开窍；内关用以宽胸利气，宁心安神；风池、太冲可调肝养血，熄风镇惊；三阴交、照海补脾益肝肾，滋阴养血，调补冲任；涌泉补肾益精，滋阴降气。

刺灸法：毫针刺，水沟、内关、风池、太冲用泻法，三阴交、照海、涌泉用补法，留针15～20分钟。

其他疗法：耳针

耳穴：神门　肝　肾　脑点

操作方法：毫针刺，中等刺激，留针15～20分钟。

3.15 不孕

女子婚后，夫妇同居2年以上，配偶生殖功能正常，未避孕而不受孕者，称为不孕，古称无子。

病因病机

本病多因先天不足，肾气虚弱或精血亏损，冲任虚衰，胞脉失养，以致不孕；或感受寒邪，客于胞宫，寒凝血瘀，胞脉阻滞；或脾虚不运，恣食膏粱厚味，而致痰湿内生，气机不畅，胞脉受阻而不能受孕。

辨证

1.肾虚不孕　　月经失调，量少色淡，神疲乏力，头晕耳鸣，腰膝酸软，舌淡苔白，脉沉细或沉迟。

2.血虚不孕　　月经量少色淡，周期延迟，形体消瘦，面色萎黄，头晕心悸，四肢无力，舌淡少苔，脉沉细无力。

3.宫寒不孕　　月经周期正常或错后，质稀色黯或夹有血块，形寒肢冷，小腹冷痛，喜暖，小便清长，舌淡，苔白，脉沉迟。

4.痰湿不孕　　形体肥胖，经行延后，甚或经闭，带下量多，质粘稠，面色㿠白，头晕心悸，舌苔白腻，脉濡滑。

治疗

1.肾虚不孕

治则：补益肾气，调理冲任。取背俞、足太阴、少阴经穴为主。

处方：肾俞　命门　三阴交　太溪

方义：取肾俞、命门、太溪以补精血温肾阳固元气；三阴交为足三阴之交会穴，能健脾、理血、益肝肾。

随证选穴：头晕耳鸣加涌泉。

刺灸法：毫针刺，用补法，留针15～20分钟，每日1次。

2.血虚不孕

治则：补益气血，调理冲任。取任脉、足阳明、太阴经穴为主。

处方：气海　足三里　三阴交　子宫穴

方义：气海是任脉与足三阴经交会穴，能补元气温固肾阳；足三里、三阴交可调补脾胃，以助生化之源，补益肝肾，以调冲任；子宫穴为经外奇穴，是治疗不孕证的经验穴。

随证选穴：头晕、心悸加神门、内关。

刺灸法：毫针刺，用补法。留针15～20分钟，每日1次。

3.宫寒不孕

治则：温经散寒。取任督、足阳明经穴为主。

处方：关元　子宫　足三里　命门

方义：取关元温下焦固元气，暖子宫益精血，除腹中寒冷；足三里能健脾胃而助生化之源；命门可温肾阳理经血；子宫为经外奇穴，为治疗不孕证的经验穴。

随证选穴：经迟加归来。

刺灸法：毫针刺，用补法，并可针后加灸，留针 20～30 分钟，每日 1 次。

4.痰湿不孕

治则：祛湿化痰，理气调经。取任脉、足太阴、阳明经穴为主。

处方：中极　气冲　地机　丰隆　三阴交

方义：取中极、气冲以理气调经；地机可健脾祛湿；丰隆为足阳明经的络穴，有健脾利湿化痰之功；三阴交为足三阴经的交会穴，有健脾理血益肝肾和调补冲任的作用。诸穴相配可达祛湿化痰，理气调经的目的。

随证选穴：头晕心悸加内关。

刺灸法：毫针刺，用平补平泻法。留针 15～20 分钟，每日 1 次，亦可针后加灸。

其他疗法：耳针

取穴：内分泌　子宫　肾　卵巢　皮质下

操作方法：毫针刺，中等刺激，每日 1 次，每次选 2～3 穴，10 次为 1 疗程。也可用耳穴压豆法。

3.16　脏燥

本病多因情志不畅，喜怒哀思等引起，以精神抑郁，情绪不宁，哭笑无常等一系列精神症状为临床特征的疾病。相当于现代医学之癔病性情感暴发症。

病因病机

本病多因郁怒伤肝，肝失条达，气机失和而致燥扰不宁；或因素多抑郁。忧思善愁而致木郁克土，心失所养，神失所藏，则哭笑无常。

辨证

1.肝郁气滞　　精神抑郁，心烦意乱，情绪不宁，胸胁胀满，呵欠频作，不能自主，口干舌燥，大便秘结，舌红少苔，脉弦。

2.忧郁伤神　　情志不畅，精神恍惚，心神不宁；悲忧善哭，反复无常，舌淡苔白，脉细。

治疗

1.肝郁气滞

治则：疏肝理气，宁心开窍。取督脉、手、足厥阴、手少阴经穴为主。

处方：水沟　间使　神门　丰隆　太冲

方义：水沟属督脉，有开窍宁心之功；间使、神门清泄心火而安神；丰隆为胃经的络穴，能祛风化痰，通便，清肠胃之湿热；太冲可调肝养血，理气解郁。

随证选穴：大便秘结加支沟。

刺灸法：毫针刺，用泻法。留针15～20分钟，每日1次。

2.忧郁伤神

治则：疏肝解郁，养心安神。取手厥阴、少阴经穴为主。

处方：大陵　神门　三阴交　太冲　合谷　上脘

方义：取大陵、神门以宁心安神；三阴交为足三阴经交会穴，能健脾益心血补肝肾；取太冲配合谷以疏肝理气，养血解郁；取上脘以和胃宽中，理中焦，清心胃之热。

随证选穴：精神恍惚加劳宫。

刺灸法：毫针刺；用平补平泻法。留针15～20分钟，每日1次。

其他疗法：耳针

取穴：神门　心　肾　肝　枕　脑点　胃

操作方法：毫针刺，强刺激，每次取 2～3 穴，留针 15 分钟，每日 1 次，或用耳穴压豆法。

4 儿科病证

4.1 顿咳

顿咳，又称顿嗽，即现代医学之百日咳。是临床常见的小儿呼吸道传染病之一。本病以阵发性痉挛性咳嗽，咳后伴有吸气性吼声为特征。一年四季均可发病，以冬春两季多见。发病年龄以5岁以下的小儿为最多。

病因病机

本病主要是由于外感时邪，而浊痰内生，阻塞气道，肺失宣降，以致肺气上逆，发为顿咳。

辨证

1.初咳期　　本病初起，证见咳嗽、流涕、打喷嚏，或有发热、恶寒等类似上感症状。2～3天后咳声重浊，日渐增剧，吐白色泡沫样稀痰，苔薄白，脉浮。

2.痉咳期　　此期以阵发性痉咳为主要特征。咳声连作，声调高亢，咳后伴有吸气性吼声，咳痰稠粘难出，咳必作呕，呕吐乳食之后，则痉咳始得缓解。日轻夜重，反复发作，口干舌燥，便秘溲赤，或见痰中带血，鼻衄等证，苔黄，脉滑数。

3.恢复期　　痉咳症状日趋减轻，发作次数逐渐减少，精神萎靡，自汗气短，咳而无力，声音嘶哑，舌质红，苔薄净或光剥，脉细数。

治疗

1.初咳期

治则：外感时行疫邪，首犯肺卫，多见表症，故取手太阴、阳明经穴为主，以宣肺解表止咳。

处方：风门　肺俞　列缺　合谷

方义：以风门祛风解表；取肺经之络穴列缺，大肠经之原穴合谷，原络相配，宣肺止咳；取肺俞以助宣肺止咳，功效更捷。

随证选穴：恶寒无汗加大椎；喉痒咽红加少商。

刺灸法：毫针刺，用泻法，不留针，每日1次。风门、肺俞、大椎亦可针后加灸。

2.痉咳期

治则：清热泻肺，化痰止咳。故取督脉、手太阴经穴为主。

处方：大椎　身柱　尺泽　丰隆　内关

方义：取督脉经穴大椎、身柱清泄热邪；取手太阴经的合穴尺泽，足阳明经的络穴丰隆，泻肺降逆，化痰止咳；内关为手厥阴心包经的络穴，通于阴维脉，能宽胸利气，清内热。

随证选穴：身热加曲池；咯血衄血加天府、上星。

刺灸法：毫针刺，用泻法，不留针，每日1次。

3.恢复期

治则：润肺止咳，培土生金。故取手太阴和足阳明经穴为主。

处方：肺俞　脾俞　太渊　足三里　列缺　照海

方义：肺俞、脾俞、足三里健脾益肺；太渊为肺经原穴，有补肺止咳之功；列缺为手太阴肺经之络穴，通于任脉，照海为足少阴肾经之俞穴，通于阴跷脉，两穴合用，为八脉交会配穴法，能益阴润燥。

随证选穴：体弱虚损加膏肓；纳少便溏加中脘、天枢、气海；手足欠温加关元。

刺灸法：毫针刺，用补法，不留针。肺俞、脾俞、足三里亦可针后加灸，每次灸20～30分钟，每日1次。

其他疗法： 耳针

取穴：支气管　肺　神门　交感

操作方法：毫针刺，中等刺激，每次取2～3穴，两耳交替使用，每日1次；或用耳穴压豆法，该法既可单独使用，亦可同时配合运用针灸法，其效更佳。

4.2 小儿腹泻

泄泻是以大便次数增多，便质稀溏或如水样、蛋花样为其主证，是小儿最常见的一种胃肠道疾病。多发生于两岁以下的婴幼儿，一年四季均可发生，但以夏秋两季更为多见。本病类似现代医学的小儿消化不良。

病因病机

小儿脏腑娇嫩，脾胃虚弱，易受寒湿之邪侵袭；或因内伤饮食，饥饱无常，过食生冷，或因饮食不洁之食物；或先天禀赋不足，命门火衰，阴寒内盛，以致脾胃运化功能失调，水谷不化，清浊不分，则成泄泻。

辨证

1.寒湿泻　大便清稀，多有泡沫，肠鸣腹痛，身寒喜暖，口不渴，舌质淡，苔薄白，脉多沉细。

2.湿热泻　泻下稀薄，色黄而秽臭，腹痛时作，身热口渴，肛门灼热，小便短赤，舌苔黄腻，脉滑数。

3.伤食泻　脘腹胀痛，痛则欲泻，泻则痛减，大便酸臭，不欲饮食，或兼有呕吐，夜卧不安，舌苔厚腻而黄，脉滑而实。

4.阳虚泻　时泻时止或久泻不愈，食入即泻，大便稀溏如水，或蛋花样，面色㿠白，形寒肢冷，精神萎靡，寐时露睛，或见脱肛，舌淡苔白，脉微细。

治疗

1.寒湿泻

治则：温阳散寒，健脾化湿。取任脉，足阳明经穴为主。

处方：中脘　天枢　足三里　关元　神阙

方义：取腑之会穴中脘，大肠之募穴天枢以调整胃肠而和中；取胃腑的下合穴足三里，以健脾和胃化湿浊；取关元、神阙可温阳化湿。

随证选穴：腹痛重加公孙。

刺灸法：毫针刺，用平补平泻法，不留针。中脘、天枢、足三里、关元可针后加灸，神阙穴只灸不针，每次灸 20～30 分钟，每日 1 次。

2.湿热泻

治则：清热利湿，取手、足阳明经穴为主。

处方：中脘　天枢　足三里　曲池　内庭

方义：中脘为胃的募穴，天枢为大肠的募穴，两穴相使，以调整胃肠而和中，使运化有力，传导功能得复；足三里为胃经的合穴，以降胃气而化湿浊；曲池、内庭可清荡胃肠湿热。

随证选穴：热重加尺泽、委中；湿重加阴陵泉。

刺灸法：毫针刺，用泻法，不留针。委中穴可用三棱针点刺出血。

3.伤食泻

治则：消食导滞，取任脉、足阳明经穴为主。

处方：中脘　天枢　气海　足三里　里内庭

方义：取中脘、天枢、足三里调和胃肠，消食导滞；气海理气止痛；里内庭为经外奇穴，善治伤食。

随证选穴：呕吐加内关。

刺灸法：毫针刺，用泻法，不留针。

4.阳虚泻

治则：健脾温肾，取背俞、足阳明经穴为主。

处方：脾俞　肾俞　章门　中脘　足三里　百会

方义：脾俞是脾的背俞穴，章门是脾的募穴，中脘是胃的募穴，三穴合用具有振奋脾阳，健运止泻的作用；肾俞能温补肾阳；百会可升提下陷的中气，有益气止泻之功。

随证选穴：手足厥冷加关元。

刺灸法：毫针刺，用补法，不留针。脾俞、肾俞、足三里、百会、关元亦可针后加灸，每次灸 20～30 分钟，每日 1 次。

4.3 小儿疳疾

疳疾，是由喂养不当，或因多种疾病的影响，使脾胃受损，气液耗伤，临床以全身虚弱羸瘦为其主要特征。其发病年龄以5岁以下的小儿较多见。小儿疳疾包括现代医学的营养不良和维生素缺乏症等。

病因病机

本病大多由于喂养不当，饮食不节，损伤脾胃，以致脾胃运化功能失职，致使大便稀溏，水谷之精微吸收输布障碍，形体失于濡养，或因肠道寄生虫病及其他慢性疾患，而耗伤气血津液，日久则为疳疾。

辨证

形体消瘦，肌肉松弛，肌肤甲错，毛发稀疏，精神萎靡不振，面色萎黄无华，甚则青筋暴露。

脾胃虚弱者，兼见大便溏泄，完谷不化，食欲减退，睡眠不宁，舌质淡，脉细无力。

虫疾者则兼见嗜食异物，时而腹痛，睡中咬牙，舌质淡，脉弦细。

治疗

1.脾胃虚弱

治则：健脾胃，消疳积，取俞募、足太阴、阳明经穴为主。

处方：中脘　章门　脾俞　胃俞　足三里　四缝

方义：中脘为胃的募穴，章门为脾的募穴，合脾的背俞穴脾俞，胃的背俞穴胃俞，为俞募配穴法，再配胃的下合穴足三里，扶土以补中气，使后天脾胃生化之机能旺盛，则积化疳除；四缝为经外奇穴，有消积之奇功，中医认为，积为疳之母，而治疳必先去积，故取四缝消积以除疳疾。

随证选穴：腹胀便溏加下脘、天枢；四肢不温加关元；睡卧不宁加神门。

刺灸法：毫针浅刺，用补法，不留针，每日 1 次。四缝穴可用三棱针点刺后，挤出少量黄色粘液，隔日 1 次。

2.感染虫疾

治则：消积驱虫。取任脉、足阳明经穴为主。

处方：中脘　天枢　百虫窝　足三里

方义：中脘、天枢疏通胃肠积滞；足三里为阳明胃之下合穴，可扶土以补中气；百虫窝为经外奇穴，是驱虫的经验要穴。

随证选穴：腹胀加气海。

刺灸法：毫针刺，先用泻法，后用补法，不留针，每日 1 次。

其他疗法：皮肤针

取穴：脾俞　胃俞　三焦俞　华佗夹脊穴(7～17 椎)　足三里　四缝

操作方法：用中等刺激强度，叩打至皮肤充血红润为度。

4.4　小儿惊风

惊风又称惊厥，俗称抽风，是小儿时期常见的一种病症。系由多种原因及多种疾病所引起，临床以四肢抽搐，颈项强直，甚则角弓反张或意识不清等为特征。多发生于 5 岁以下的小儿，年龄越小，发病率越高。

本病可发生于任何季节，多由于高热，中枢神经系统疾病及代谢营养障碍等引起，如肺炎、细菌性痢疾、脑炎、破伤风等。因为发病有急有缓，抽搐有强有弱，其症候表现也有虚实寒热之分，故临床多将惊风分为急惊风和慢惊风两大类。

4.4.1　急惊风

病因病机

小儿形气未充，腠理不密，脏腑娇嫩，神气怯弱，最易感受时邪，由表入里，郁而化热化火，火甚生痰，热极生风；或因乳食不节，脾胃受损，痰浊内蕴，郁而化热生风；或暴受惊恐，神气逆乱，而致神昏抽搐等证。

辨证

本病来势急骤，初起壮热面赤，烦燥不安，摇头弄舌，嗜睡易惊，继则出现神志昏迷，两目上视，四肢抽搐，颈项强直，牙关紧急，呼吸急促等。

1.外感时邪　兼见发热头痛，咳嗽咽红，或见恶心呕吐，舌苔薄黄，脉浮数。

2.痰热惊风　兼见发热，腹满胀痛，呕吐纳呆，喉中痰鸣，便秘，或大便腥臭夹有脓血，苔黄腻，脉弦滑。

3.惊恐惊风　面色时青时赤，四肢欠温，夜卧不宁，惊惕频作，大便色青，脉象数乱。

治疗

1.外感惊风

治则：疏风清热，开窍镇惊。取督脉、足厥阴经和十二井穴为主。

处方：大椎　合谷　太冲　十二井穴　阳陵泉

方义：大椎为诸阳之会，可宣通一身之阳而祛表邪；合谷、太冲分别为大肠与肝之原穴，二穴合用，有清头目，醒神开窍，镇惊熄风之功效，谓之开四关，以平肝熄风；刺十二井穴出血，能泻诸经热邪；取筋会阳陵泉以舒筋止痉。

随证选穴：热重加曲池；呕吐加内关。

刺灸法：毫针刺，用泻法，不留针。大椎和十二井穴可用三棱针点刺出血。

2.痰热惊风

治则：清热豁痰，开窍熄风。取任、督、足阳明、厥阴经穴为主。

处方：水沟　中脘　丰隆　大陵　太冲

方义：水沟属督脉通于脑，有醒神开窍之功；中脘、丰隆导滞化痰，大陵能清心热以宁神；太冲为肝经原穴，有平肝熄风的作用。

随证选穴：口噤加颊车、合谷；腹胀加天枢。

刺灸法：毫针刺，用泻法，不留针。

3.惊恐惊风

治则：镇惊安神。取督脉、手足少阴经穴为主。

处方：印堂　神门　太溪　太冲

方义：印堂为奇穴，有镇惊作用；神门为心之原穴，可补心气以宁心安神；取肾经原穴太溪和肝经原穴太冲，可调肝养血，滋阴潜阳，阴阳调和，夜眠自安，惊惕自止。

随证选穴：惊风不止加颅息；昏睡不醒加水沟。

刺灸法：毫针刺，用泻法，不留针。

其他疗法：耳针

取穴：神门　交感　脑点　心　皮质下

操作方法：毫针刺，强刺激。每隔10分钟捻转一次，可留针30分钟。

4.4.2　慢惊风

病因病机

慢惊风多见于大病或久病之后，或脾胃素虚，化源不足，肾阴不足，肝血亏损，以致虚风内动；或因急惊风经治不愈而转成慢惊风。

辨证

起病缓慢，时有抽搐，患儿面色萎黄，形体消瘦，精神疲倦，昏睡露睛，四肢不温。脾胃虚弱者兼见大便稀薄，色青带绿，时有肠鸣，舌淡苔白，脉沉细无力；肝肾阴虚者兼见虚烦心热，面色潮红，舌光少苔，脉细数。

治疗

治则：补益脾肾，佐以平肝熄风。取背俞、督脉、足阳明经穴为主。

　　处方：脾俞　胃俞　肾俞　气海　足三里　太冲　百会

　　方义：脾俞、胃俞、肾俞分别为脾、胃、肾的背俞穴，有补益脾肾的作用；气海培元以助健运；足三里为阳明之合穴，是调补后天脾胃之要穴；太冲有平肝养血，镇惊熄风之效；百会有升阳醒脑之功。

　　随证选穴：大便稀薄加天枢。

　　刺灸法：毫针刺，用补法，不留针。亦可针后加灸，每次20～30分钟，每日1次。

　　其他疗法：耳针

　　取穴：神门　交感　脾　胃　肾　肝　脑点　心　皮质下。

　　操作方法：毫针刺，中等刺激，每次取3～4穴，两耳交替使用，每日1次；或用耳穴压豆法，该法既可单独使用，亦可配合运用针灸法，其效更佳。

4.5　小儿痿证

　　小儿痿证，又称小儿麻痹证、婴儿瘫。是由于感受时邪疫毒而引起的一种急性传染病。其主要临床表现为早期症状类似感冒，有发热、头痛、咽红、咳嗽，或伴有恶心呕吐，腹泻及全身肌肉疼痛。继而出现肌肉弛缓，肢体萎软瘫痪，肌肉萎缩，运动障碍等。瘫痪肢体以单侧下肢为多见，发病年龄尤以5岁以下的婴幼儿为最多，多流行于夏秋两季，相当于现代医学脊髓灰质炎后遗症。

　　病因病机

　　邪热疫毒，初犯肺胃，耗伤肺津，胃失和降，继而湿热蕴蒸阳明，邪毒流注经络，则气血运行不畅，筋脉失于濡养，宗筋弛缓不收，不能束筋骨利关节，遂成痿证。

　　辨证

　　患儿肢体软弱无力，瘫痪，以单侧下肢多见，面色少华或萎

黄。极少数病情轻者可在 1～3 个月内逐渐恢复而痊愈；而多数
患儿则肌肉萎缩，弛缓无力，运动障碍，甚者则关节畸形。

治疗

治则：养血通络，以取手足阳明经穴为主。

处方：上肢取：肩于　曲池　手三里　合谷

　　　　下肢取：环跳　髀关　伏兔　足三里　阳陵泉　三阴
　　　　交

方义：取肩于、曲池、手三里、合谷以疏调手阳明之经气，
是治痿独取阳明之法，以养血活血通络；取髀关、伏兔、足三里
也是独取阳明之法，主润宗筋，加环跳以疏调少阳之气；取筋会
阳陵泉以柔筋；三阴交为足三阴的交会穴，有养血活血之功；诸
穴相配可补气养血，强筋益髓而愈痿病。

随证选穴：腕下垂加外关，中泉；足下垂加解溪；足内翻加
绝骨，纠内翻；足外翻加照海，纠外翻。

刺灸法：毫针刺，用补法。留针 15～20 分钟，亦可针后加
灸，每日 1 次。

4.6　小儿遗尿

遗尿又称遗溺、尿床，是指 3 周岁以上的小儿，在睡眠中小
便不能自行控制而自遗，醒后方觉的一种病症。若因疲劳过度，
或精神紧张，或因睡前多饮而偶然发生遗尿者，则不属病态。

病因病机

肾为先天之本，开窍于二阴而主司二便，并与膀胱相表里；
若小儿肾气不足，则下元不固，膀胱不约，水道失制而为遗尿；
或因脾肺气虚，上虚不能制下，致使膀胱约束无力，则小便自
遗。

辨证

1.肾阳不足　　睡中遗尿，量多次频，多则一夜数次，醒后
方觉。神疲乏力，面色㿠白，下肢无力，喜暖怕冷，小便清长，

舌质淡，脉沉无力。

2.脾肺气虚　　睡中遗尿，尿频量少，精神倦怠，少气懒言，面色萎黄，食欲不振，大便稀溏，舌质淡，脉细无力。

治疗

1.肾阳不足

治则：温补肾阳，固摄小便。取任脉经穴和背俞穴为主。

处义：关元　中极　肾俞　膀胱俞　太溪

方义：取关元、肾俞、太溪补益肾气，固摄下元；取膀胱募穴中极和膀胱俞，为俞募配穴，用以振奋膀胱的制约功能。

随证选穴：尿频数加百会。

刺灸法：毫针刺，用补法。留针 15～20 分钟，亦可加灸，每日 1 次。

2.脾肺气虚

治则：补益脾肺，固摄小便。取任脉、手足太阴，足阳明经穴为主。

处方：百会　气海　太渊　足三里　三阴交

方义：取百会、气海以升阳益气；太渊补益肺气；足三里健脾益气；三阴交为足三阴经交会穴，用以调补脾肾。诸穴相配，可使脾气能升，肺气能降，则膀胱约束有权。

随证选穴：便溏加脾俞。

刺灸法：毫针刺，用补法。留针 15～20 分钟，亦可用艾条灸百会、气海、足三里、三阴交、脾俞，每日 1 次，每次 25～30 分钟。

其他疗法

1.耳针

取穴：肾　膀胱　脾　肺　脑点　皮质下　尿道区　缘中

操作方法：毫针刺，中等刺激。每次选用 2～3 穴，每日 1 次，留针 20 分钟，亦可用耳穴压豆法。

2.头针

取穴：选用两侧足运感区。

操作方法：间歇捻针，留针 15 分钟，每日 1 次。

4.7　痄腮

痄腮，是由风温邪毒引起的急性传染性疾病，临床以发热，耳下腮肿疼痛为主要特征。一年四季均可发生，春季易于流行。以 5～9 岁的儿童发病率最高，一般预后良好。现代医学称流行性腮腺炎。

病因病机

本病主要是外感风温邪毒，内袭少阳，少阳经脉失和，气血流行不畅，以致耳下腮部肿胀疼痛及发热恶寒等证。少阳与厥阴相表里，肝脉络阴器，若温毒炽盛，则可引起睾丸肿痛，内陷于手厥阴，扰乱神明，则出现高热，抽风，昏迷。

辨证

1.温毒在表　　耳下腮肿不甚，疼痛不明显，触之不坚，咀嚼不便，伴有轻微恶寒发热，全身不适等症。舌苔微黄，脉浮数。

2.热毒蕴结　　腮部焮热肿痛，坚实拒按，咀嚼困难，壮热头痛，烦燥口渴或见呕吐，大便干结，小便短赤，甚至睾丸肿疼，神昏惊厥，舌红苔黄，脉滑数。

治疗

1.温毒在表

治则：疏风解表，清热解毒。取手少阳，阳明经穴为主。

处方：翳风　颊车　外关　合谷

方义：腮部属于少阳经脉循行之处，故应以清泄少阳郁热为主。翳风为手足少阳经之会穴，能宣散局部气血壅滞；手足阳明经脉皆上循面颊，故取颊车、合谷以疏泄邪热而解毒；取外关以利少阳气机，可奏清热消肿之功。

随证选穴：热重加大椎。

刺灸法：毫针刺，用泻法。不留针，每日 1 次。大椎穴可用三棱针点刺出血。

2.热毒蕴结

治则：清热解毒，通络消肿。取手少阳、阳明经穴为主。

处方：支沟　关冲　曲池　合谷　少商　丰隆

方义：支沟、关冲可宣通三焦气血，有清热解毒消肿之功；曲池、合谷为手阳明经穴，配少商可清热解毒；丰隆为足阳明经的络穴，能清降痰火，消肿止痛。

随证选穴：高热加大椎、十二井；睾丸肿痛加太冲、曲泉；头痛加风池；惊厥神昏加水沟。

刺灸法：毫针刺，用泻法。不留针，每日 1 次。少商、大椎、十二井穴可用三棱针点刺出血。

其他疗法

1.耳针

取穴：耳尖　神门　腮腺区　面颊　耳轮$_{4\sim6}$

操作方法：毫针刺，强刺激。每次 2～3 穴，每日 1 次。亦可用耳穴压豆法。

2.灯芯灸法

取穴：角孙

操作方法：用灯芯草蘸香油，点燃后灸角孙穴，闻及“叭”的响声，立即提起，灸治 1～2 次即可，若肿势不退，次日再灸 1 次。

4.8　丹痧

丹痧又称烂喉痧，是痧毒疫疠之邪侵入口鼻而引起的急性呼吸道传染病。临床以发热，咽喉肿痛，全身伴有弥漫性猩红色皮疹，疹后脱皮为主要特征。本病相当现代医学的猩红热。多见于冬春季节，以 2～8 岁的儿童发病率最高。

病因病机

疹毒疫疬之邪侵入口鼻，蕴于肺胃，邪毒郁内化火，内蒸肺胃，上攻喉咙，故首见恶寒发热，咽喉肿痛等证；邪毒透于肌表则发为疹疹；若邪毒炽盛，内陷心肝，可出现抽风昏迷等证。

辨证

1.邪侵肺卫　　发热骤起，头痛畏寒，咽红肿痛，恶心呕吐，皮肤潮红，舌质红，苔薄黄，脉浮数有力。

2.毒在气营　　壮热不解，面赤口渴，口周苍白，咽喉肿痛，或见糜烂，皮疹密布，色红如丹，甚则紫如瘀点，融合成片。斑疹始于颈胸，继而弥漫全身，舌质红赤有刺，状如杨梅，脉数有力。

治疗

1.邪侵肺卫

治则：宣肺解表，清热利咽。取手太阴，阳明经穴为主。

处方：风池　曲池　合谷　列缺　大椎　关冲

方义：取风池、曲池、合谷以祛风清热；列缺为手太阴经络穴，有清肺热，利咽喉，疏风活络之功；关冲能清三焦之热；大椎可解肌表之风热而调和荣卫。诸穴相配，具有宣肺解表，清热利咽的作用。

随证选穴：恶心呕吐加内关。

刺灸法：毫针刺，用泻法。不留针，每日1次。大椎、关冲用三棱针点刺出血。

2.毒在气营

治则：清热，凉血。取督脉、手阳明、足太阳经穴为主。

处方：大椎　风池　曲池　合谷　内庭　委中　金津　玉液

方义：取大椎以退热；风池、曲池、合谷以祛风清热；内庭清胃肠之热而凉血；委中为血郄，可泻血分之热毒；金津、玉液能清利咽喉，生津液，除三焦之热。诸穴相配可达清热解毒，凉血利咽之功。

随证选穴：咽喉肿痛加少商。

刺灸法：毫针刺，用泻法。不留针，每日1次。大椎、委中、少商可用三棱针点刺出血。

其他疗法：耳针

取穴：神门　肺　耳尖　脾　胃

操作方法：毫针刺，中、强刺激，不留针，或用耳穴压豆法。

4.9　痴呆

小儿痴呆，属于中医的五迟、五软范畴，以发育迟缓，智力发育不全为特征。类似现代医学先天性大脑发育不全。

病因病机

本病主要由于先天禀赋不足，或后天失养，精气亏虚，不能上充于脑所致。

辨证

其主要临床症状表现为：生长发育较一般正常小儿明显迟缓，2～3岁还不能说话，智力不聪，神情滞呆、凝视、反应迟钝。并可兼见肢体软弱，筋骨不固，四肢无力，站立不稳，行走困难等。

治疗

治则：补肝肾，益精血，醒神开窍。取督脉穴为主。

处方：百会　四神聪　大椎　风府　风池　水沟　心俞　内关　三阴交　申脉　照海

方义：取百会、四神聪以益气安神醒脑；大椎、风府、风池、水沟能疏通诸阳之经气而醒神开窍；心俞、内关、三阴交能清上滋下，振心阳，益心阴，宁心安神；申脉、照海补益肝肾，填髓充精。

刺灸法：毫针刺，用补法。留针20～30分钟，每日1次。心俞、申脉、照海用灸法，每次灸30分钟，每日或隔日1次。

其他疗法：耳穴压豆

取穴：心 肾 肝 脾 神门 脑点。每次选 2～3 穴，两耳交替，3 日更换 1 次。

5 五官科病证

5.1 近视

近视，古称能近怯远症，是一种屈光不正的眼病，其主要特征是眼部外观无明显异常，而视近清楚，远视模糊。以青少年最为多见。

病因病机

本病多因阅读、书写目标太近，而且持续时间过久，或光线不足，姿式不正；或因禀赋不足及先天遗传所致。肝开窍于目，目得血而能视，若肝肾不足，气血亏损，或久视伤血，以致目失所养而远视不能及物。

辨证

近视清楚，远视模糊，可有头晕耳鸣，失眠多梦，腰膝酸软，或面色㿠白，心悸神疲，舌淡，脉细弱。

治疗

治则：调补肝肾，益气明目。

处方：承泣 睛明 风池 光明 肝俞 肾俞

方义：承泣、睛明为治目疾之常用穴，有清肝明目的作用，风池为手足少阳与阳维之会穴，有通经活络，养血明目之功；光明为胆经之络穴，用以通络明目；肝俞、肾俞有调补肝肾，益气明目的作用。

随证选穴：如脾胃虚弱者加三阴交、足三里。

刺灸法：毫针刺，用平补平泻法。眼区穴宜轻捻缓进，退针时至皮下疾出之，随即予棉球按压 1 分钟。风池，光明、肝俞、肾俞可用捻转或提插法，间歇运针。留针 15～20 分钟，每日 1次。

其他疗法: 耳针

取穴: 神门　交感　眼　目$_1$　目$_2$　肝　肾

操作方法: 毫针刺, 中等刺激。每次选 2～3 穴, 留针 30 分钟, 隔日 1 次。亦可用耳穴压豆法, 其穴同上, 两耳交替, 3～5 日更换 1 次。

5.2　目赤肿痛

目赤肿痛, 俗称"风热眼", "红眼病"等。以眼睑红肿, 白睛红赤, 羞明多泪为主要临床特征。发病急骤, 易于流行, 类似现代医学的急性结膜炎, 急性传染性角结膜炎等。

病因病机

多因风热时邪侵袭目窍, 郁而不宣, 或因肝胆火盛, 循经上扰, 内外合邪, 交攻于目。

辨证

眼睑肿痛, 白睛红赤, 畏光流泪, 目涩难开, 眵多胶粘。兼见头痛发热, 恶风, 脉浮数者多属外感风热; 兼见口苦, 烦热, 头晕, 舌红苔黄, 脉弦数者, 则多属肝胆火盛。

治疗

治则: 疏风清热, 消肿止痛。取手阳明、足厥阴经穴为主。

处方: 行间　合谷　曲池　太阳

外感风热配少商　上星

肝胆火盛配风池　侠溪

方义: 目为肝之外窍, 阳明、太阳、少阳经脉均循行于目, 行间为肝经之荥穴, 有行瘀破血, 利气消肿之功, 能清泄肝胆之热毒; 合谷为手阳明之原穴, 升而能散, 与曲池相合, 能清热散风, 为清理上焦之妙穴, 凡头、面诸窍之疾皆能治之; 太阳为经外奇穴, 点刺出血以泄热消肿止痛。外感风热配少商、上星, 以疏风清热; 肝胆火盛者配风池、侠溪, 能导肝胆之火下行。

随证选穴: 头痛加印堂。

刺灸法：毫针刺，用泻法。不留针或留针 15～20 分钟，每隔 5 分钟捻针 1 次，太阳、少商可用三棱针点刺出血少许。

其他疗法：耳针

取穴：眼　目$_1$　目$_2$　肝

操作方法：毫针刺，强刺激。留针 20 分钟，间歇运针。亦可在耳尖或耳背小静脉点刺出血。

5.3　色盲

色盲是色觉异常的一种眼病，又称视物易色症。患者主要表现为在视物时，只能辨别物体的明暗、形态，而不能辨认其为何种颜色；辨色能力减低者，则称为色弱。本病以男性较为多见，主要与先天遗传因素有关。

病因病机

多因先天不足，肝肾亏虚，精气衰退，或因目络气血不和而致目不能辨色。

辨证

患者两眼外观无异常，视力尚好，唯不能辨认其目所能及之物的某些颜色，或视赤如白，或视黄似绿，甚至仅能分辨黑白，但自己一般不易察觉，多在体检时才发现。

治疗

治则：补养肝肾。取足太阳、厥阴、少阴经穴为主。

处方：睛明　攒竹　风池　肝俞　肾俞　行间　太溪

方义：睛明、攒竹可疏通络脉，为治眼病之常用穴；风池有清头目、利五官七窍之效；肝俞有疏肝明目之功；肾俞能益肾精而养目；行间、太溪滋补肝肾，以濡养目窍。此为治本之法。

刺灸法：毫针刺，用补法。眼区穴要微捻缓进，后针，先起，留针 15～20 分钟，每日或隔日 1 次。

其他疗法：耳针

取穴：目$_1$　目$_2$　眼　肝　肾

操作方法：毫针刺，轻刺激，留针 15～20 分钟，每日 1 次。或用耳穴压豆法。

5.4 斜视

斜视又称风牵偏视，是以眼珠偏斜，转动受限，两眼不能同时正视前方为临床特征的眼病。本病主要是由于风中经络所致。相当于现代医学的麻痹性斜视等病症。

病因病机

多因脾胃不足，脉络空虚，风邪乘虚而入，目系拘急而成；或因肝肾阴亏，精血不足，目系失养所致。

辨证

一眼或双眼黑睛突然偏向内眦或外眦，转动受限，视一为二，甚至上睑下垂或口眼㖞斜。若伴发热头痛，恶心呕吐，苔白，脉浮者，多为风邪阻络；若头晕目眩，耳鸣，视物昏朦，舌淡，脉细者则为肝肾亏损。

治疗

治则：祛风通络，补益肝肾。取背俞、足厥阴肝经和手足阳明经穴为主。

处方：四白　合谷　风池　肝俞　肾俞　足三里

方义：取四白以通经活络，调气血平阴阳；合谷、风池善清头面之风邪而疗五官七窍之疾；肝俞、肾俞、足三里益气养血，调补肝肾。

随证选穴：内斜视加太阳、瞳子髎；外斜视加睛明、攒竹。

刺灸法：毫针刺，用补法，留针 15～20 分钟，每日 1 次。

其他疗法：耳穴压豆法

取穴：肝　肾　目$_1$　目$_2$，两耳交替，3 日更换 1 次。

5.5 针眼

针眼为睑缘皮脂腺的炎性疖肿，易于溃脓，以针刺破即愈，故名针眼。因疖肿形似麦粒，故又称麦粒肿。以青少年较多见，好发于上眼睑。

病因病机

多因过食辛辣，脾胃积热，上攻于目，或因外感风热，客于胞睑，致气血瘀阻，风热结聚而为疖肿。

辨证

本病初起为睑缘轻微痒痛，继而形成局部硬结，红肿，疼痛加剧，数日后出现黄白色脓点，破溃排脓后，症状迅速消失而愈。若为脾胃积热者，可伴有口臭，心烦口渴，便秘，苔黄腻，脉濡数；若为外感风热者，则可见恶寒发热，头痛等证，苔薄，脉浮数。

治疗

治则：疏风清热，解毒。取手足阳明、足太阳经穴为主。

处方：合谷　曲池　中冲　太阳

脾胃湿热加尺泽

外感风热加大椎　行间

方义：合谷升而能散，曲池走而不守，合谷配曲池，能清散头面诸窍之风热肿毒；中冲为手厥阴心包之经穴，诸痛疮痒皆属于心，刺中冲可清心火；太阳消肿止痛。脾胃湿热加尺泽，以清血祛风，利脾胃之湿热；外感风热加大椎以解毒，刺行间可泄肝胆之热毒，又能通经破瘀。

随证选穴：头痛加风池，目赤肿痛加照海。

刺灸法：毫针刺，用泻法。留针 15～20 分钟，每日 1 次。

其他疗法：耳针

取穴：眼　肝　脾　耳尖

操作方法：毫针刺，强刺激，留针 20 分钟，每日 1 次。耳尖可点刺出血。亦可用耳穴压豆法，两耳交替，3日更换1次。

5.6　眼睑下垂

本病系由多种原因引起，以上睑不能自行提起或提起不全，遮盖部分或全部瞳孔而影响视物为主要特征。

病因病机

由于先天禀赋不足，命门火衰而致眼睑松弛，提起无力；或受风邪侵袭，阻滞经络，筋脉失调；或因脾胃虚热，血气不荣，筋肉失养所致。

辨证

双眼自幼上睑下垂，终日不能抬举，视物时则仰首，皱额，抬眉，常伴有眼部其他异常者，为先天不足；发病突然，伴有眼球转动受限，或视一为二等为风邪侵袭；脾胃虚弱，中气不足，血气不荣者，则上睑下垂朝轻暮重，或休息后轻，劳累后重，可兼见精神疲乏，倦怠无力等症。

治疗

治则：疏风通络，升阳益气。取手足阳明，足太阴、少阳经穴为主。

处方：阳白　攒竹　丝竹空　申脉　照海　合谷

　　　风邪伤络加风池　外关

　　　中气不足,血气不荣加足三里　三阴交

方义：取阳白、攒竹、丝竹空为局部取穴，以调和局部气血；申脉能疏调周身之阳，照海可调补周身之阴血，两穴相配共奏调和荣卫之功，使气血上注于目而眼睑强健有力；合谷升而能散，善疗头面诸疾。风邪伤络配足少阳经风池，手少阳经外关以通经活络，疏风解表；中气不足配足阳明经的合穴足三里，足太阴经三阴交以健脾胃，补气血。

随证选穴：眩晕加百会。

刺灸法：毫针刺，用平补平泻法。刺阳白可透鱼腰，或鱼腰透丝竹空。留针 20～30 分钟，每日 1 次。足三里、百会亦可针后加灸，每次灸 20～30 分钟，每日 1 次。

其他疗法：耳穴压豆法

取穴：肝　脾　眼　交感　神门，两耳交替，3 日更换 1 次。

5.7　暴盲

暴盲是指一眼或双眼视力骤然减退，甚至失明的内障眼病，类似现代医学的视网膜中央血管阻塞，急性视神经炎，视网膜脱离等。

病因病机

多因暴怒惊恐或肝肾阴亏，以致肝阳上亢，气机逆乱，或情志抑郁，肝失条达以致气滞血瘀，脉络阻塞，脏腑之精气不能上注于目，目失涵养而致突然视物不清。

辨证

患者发病前眼睛多无不适，而一眼或双眼视力突然急剧减退甚至完全丧失，少数病人发病前眼前有火花闪烁，及眼球胀痛、压痛或转动时牵扯样疼痛等。若因肝阳上亢者，多伴有头晕耳鸣、胸胁撑胀，面赤舌绛，脉弦数；若为气滞血瘀者，则可见头目胀痛，烦燥口渴，舌紫脉涩或弦。

治疗

治则：活血、平肝、通窍、明目。以局部取穴为主。

处方：睛明　攒竹　承泣　太阳　风池　光明　合谷　太溪
　　　太冲
　　　肝阳上亢加行间
　　　气滞血瘀加膈俞

方义：取睛明、攒竹、承泣、风池、太阳疏通经气以明目；光明为足少阳之络穴，能调肝胆之气血，而疗目疾不明之要穴；合谷升散而清上焦，为疗头面诸窍之要穴；取太溪、太冲以调补肝肾，养血明目；行间为足厥阴经荥穴，有平肝泻火熄风之功；血会膈俞有活血散瘀之效。

随证选穴：目胀加关冲。

刺灸法：毫针刺，用泻法，不留针。关冲穴可用三棱针点刺出血。

5.8 迎风流泪

迎风流泪，是指眼睛无红肿、疼痛，而风吹流泪或不时泪下，迎风尤甚为特征的眼科常见病症。相当于现代医学的泪小点异位、泪小管炎、泪囊炎及沙眼、慢性结膜炎等病，以老年人多见。

病因病机

多因气血不足，肝肾两虚，目失所养，泪液不得约束而冷泪常流，或因风热邪侵袭，泪窍关闭失调，而致泪液时而外溢。

辨证

平时目无赤烂肿痛，迎风则泪出，无风则泪止，遇寒尤甚，或见不时泪出，迎风则甚。

治疗

1.肝肾两虚

治则：补益肝肾，兼祛风邪。取足太阳经穴为主。

处方：睛明　攒竹　风池　肝俞　肾俞　太溪　三阴交

方义：睛明、攒竹为局部取穴，疏通经脉以调气血和营卫，使目制约有权；风池为手少阳与阳维之会穴，为祛风之要穴，有通利五官七窍的作用；太溪、肝俞、肾俞可补益肝肾；三阴交补脾兼及肝肾。

随证选穴：目视不明加光明。

刺灸法：毫针刺，用补法，留针15～20分钟。肝俞、肾俞亦可针后加灸，每次20～30分钟，每日1次。

2.风热侵扰

治则：散风清热，疏肝明目。取足太阳、厥阴经穴为主。

处方：睛明　攒竹　合谷　风池　行间

方义：睛明、攒竹通经活络。行气活血；取合谷、风池以散风清热；足厥阴经荥穴行间，有疏肝清热之功。

随证选穴：头痛泪多加上星。

刺灸法：毫针刺，用泻法。留针15～20分钟，每日1次。

其他疗法：耳针

取穴：眼　肝　目$_1$　目$_2$

操作方法：毫针刺，强刺激。留针30分钟。亦可用耳穴压豆法，两耳交替，3日更换1次。

5.9　耳鸣、耳聋

耳鸣、耳聋是由多种原因引起的听觉异常和障碍。耳鸣的主要表现为耳中鸣响，妨碍听觉，甚至影响睡眠；耳聋是指不同程度的听力减退，甚至失听。因二者在临床上往往并见，在病因及治疗方面大致相同，故合并论述。

病因病机

本病多因暴怒惊恐，肝胆火旺，上扰清窍，或聚湿成痰，痰热郁结，阻塞气道所致；或肾精亏耗，精气不能上充于耳，均可导致耳鸣耳聋之症。

辨证

1.肝胆火旺　突然耳聋或耳鸣不止，如风贯耳，隆隆不断，按之不减，影响听力，头痛面赤，口苦咽干，心烦易怒，或夜卧不宁，两胁撑胀，大便秘结，舌红，苔黄，脉弦数。

2.痰热郁结　耳响如蝉鸣，听力减退或耳聋如塞，头昏沉重，胸闷脘满，口苦痰多，二便不畅，舌苔黄腻，脉弦滑。

3.肾精亏损　两耳鸣响，时作时止，昼轻夜甚，按之则减，多伴听力减退，头晕乏力，腰膝酸软，虚烦失眠，舌红少苔，脉细弱或细数。

治疗

1.肝胆火旺

治则：清泄胆火。取手足少阳、足厥阴肝经穴为主。

处方：翳风　听会　侠溪　中渚　行间

方义：手足少阳经脉均绕行于耳之前后，从耳后入耳中，故取手少阳之中渚、翳风，足少阳之听会以疏导少阳经气；取肝经荥穴行间，胆经荥穴侠溪，以清泄肝胆之火。亦是"病在上，下取之"和"盛则泻之"之意。

刺灸法：毫针刺，用泻法。留针15～20分钟，每日1次。

2.痰热郁结

治则：清热化痰，散郁消结。取手足少阳、阳明经穴为主。

处方：翳风　听会　侠溪　中渚　上脘　丰隆　足三里　阳陵泉

方义：取翳风、听会、侠溪、中渚疏导少阳经气；取足阳明经络穴丰隆以清热化痰；上脘配足三里、阳陵泉，以平木培土，消郁散结，清心胃之热，消上中焦之痰湿。

随证选穴：热病耳聋加偏历。

刺灸法：毫针刺，用泻法。留针15～20分钟，每日1次。

3.肾精亏损

治则：补益肾精，取手足少阳、足少阴经穴为主。

处方：翳风　听会　中渚　肾俞　命门　关元　太溪

方义：翳风、听会为近部取穴，配手少阳经穴中渚以疏导少阳经气；又因肾开窍于耳，肾虚则精气不能上注于耳，故取肾俞、命门、关元、太溪以调补肾气，使精气上输耳窍，奏止鸣复聪之效。

刺灸法：毫针刺，用补法。留针15～20分钟，肾俞、命门、关元针后加灸，每次灸20～30分钟，每日1次。

其他疗法：头针

取穴：选取两侧晕听区。

操作方法：毫针刺，间歇运针，留针 30 分钟，每日或隔日 1 次。适应于神经性耳鸣、听力下降。

5.10 聤耳

聤耳，又称脓耳、耳漏。临床表现以耳中疼痛，耳窍流脓为主要特征。类似于现代医学之急、慢性化脓性中耳炎。以儿童最多见。

病因病机

多因风热之邪侵于耳窍，引动胆火上炎，邪热结聚，热毒炽盛，而化腐成脓，或因久病脾虚，运化失职，水湿内生，痰浊不化，泛溢耳窍所致。

辨证

1.风热外侵　　起病较急，耳内胀塞疼痛，日渐加重，并有全身发热，恶寒，头痛及烦燥不安等症。数日后耳中有粘稠之脓液流出，其味恶臭，耳痛及全身症状则随之减轻。舌质红，苔黄，脉弦数。

2.脾虚湿困　　耳内流脓迁延日久，时发时愈，时轻时重，脓液清稀而臭，或兼见头晕耳鸣，听力减退等症状，舌淡，苔白，脉细弱。

治疗

1.风热外侵

治则：疏风清热，开窍。取手足少阳经穴为主。

处方：风池　完骨　耳尖　合谷　行间　关冲

方义：风池、完骨、耳尖可疏散少阳在耳窍之风热；合谷有清头面风热通诸窍之功；行间、关冲可清散肝胆三焦之火热。

随证选穴：热甚加大椎；头痛加太阳、上星。

刺灸法：毫针刺，用泻法。大椎可用三棱针点刺出血。

2.脾虚湿困

治则：健脾化湿。取手少阳、足太阴、阳明经穴为主。

处方：翳风　足三里　阴陵泉　隐白

方义：翳风为局部取穴，以通络开窍；足三里为足阳明之合穴，阴陵泉为足太阴之合穴，配隐白可补益脾气，振奋脾阳以求健脾化湿之功效。

随证选穴：头晕耳鸣加肾俞、太溪。

刺灸法：毫针刺，用补法。留针 15～20 分钟，足三里、肾俞亦可针后加灸，每次灸 20～30 分钟，每日 1 次。

其他疗法：耳针

取穴：耳尖　肾　内耳　枕　外耳　皮质下

操作方法：毫针刺，中等刺激，留针 20～30 分钟，每日或隔日 1 次。亦可用耳穴压豆法。

5.11　聋哑

聋和哑虽然是两种截然不同的症状，但哑多由聋所致，故有"哑由聋所起，治哑先治聋"，"聋是哑之因，哑为聋之果"之说，故称聋哑。临床以儿童最为多见。

病因病机

本病多由先天不足，或因感受温邪热毒，壅滞脉络，闭阻清窍，或因药物中毒所致。

辨证

以听力严重减退，甚至完全丧失，因而不会讲话为其主要特征，发音器官则无异常。

治疗

治则：通络开窍。取手足少阳经穴为主。

处方：率谷　悬颅　天冲　中渚　阳陵泉　听宫　听会　哑门

方义：率谷、悬颅、天冲、听宫、听会主要为手足少阳在耳区之经穴，其经脉皆由此入耳中出走耳前，能疏通耳部经气；中渚、阳陵泉以疏导少阳经气，使耳区诸穴通络开窍之功效更捷；

哑门能利舌咽，开窍，为治哑之要穴。

刺灸法：率谷、悬颅、天冲用平刺法透向角孙，进针 1～1.5 寸；听宫透听会用斜刺法，进针 1～1.2 寸；率谷、悬颅用电针，取疏密波，留针 40 分钟。

5.12　鼻衄

鼻衄即鼻出血，是指除外伤以外其他疾病引起的鼻腔出血。严重出血又称鼻洪或鼻大衄。

病因病机

肺气通于鼻，外感风热燥邪，首先犯肺，上壅鼻窍，灼伤脉络，或胃经素有积热，而又过食辛辣，以致胃热炽盛，循经上炎，或因年老体弱，肝肾阴亏，虚火上炎，而伤及脉络，血随火升，溢于脉外从鼻窍而出，发为鼻衄。

辨证

1.肺经蕴热　鼻中点滴出血，色鲜红，鼻腔干燥，身热口干，咳嗽痰少，舌红，苔薄白，脉浮数。

2.胃热炽盛　鼻中出血量多，色鲜红或深红，咽干口臭，烦渴喜冷饮，大便干结，小便短赤，舌红，苔黄，脉洪数。

3.肝肾阴虚　鼻衄色红，时作时止，量不多，口干少津，头晕目眩，心悸耳鸣，心烦失眠，舌红少苔，脉细数无力。

治疗

1.肺经蕴热

治则：疏风清热止血。取手太阴、阳明经穴为主。

处方：风池　迎香　合谷　少商

方义：少商点刺出血，以清泄肺热；取合谷、迎香清泄阳明，配风池以疏风。

随证选穴：热重加大椎，曲池。血出不止点刺委中出血。

刺灸法：毫针刺，用泻法。留针 15～20 分钟，少商、大椎可用三棱针点刺出血。

2.胃热炽盛

治则：清泄胃火止血。取手足阳明、督脉经穴为主。

处方：迎香　合谷　厉兑　上星

方义：迎香、合谷分属手足阳明经，能清泄阳明；厉兑为足阳明经的井穴以清泄胃火降逆气，督脉为阳脉之海，上星为督脉之穴，刺之可泄诸阳经热，使血自归经，则鼻衄可止。

随证选穴：衄血不止加隐白。

刺灸法：毫针刺，用泻法。留针15～20分钟，每隔3～5分钟捻针1次。

3.肝肾阴虚

治则：滋养肝肾，降火止血。取足少阴、厥阴经穴为主。

处方：太溪　太冲　通天　飞扬

方义：取肾之原穴太溪，肝之原穴太冲，以滋肾阴降肝火，配通天主治鼻衄；飞扬为足太阳之络穴，为主治肝肾阴虚鼻衄之要穴。

随证选穴：衄血不止加灸涌泉。

刺灸法：毫针刺，用平补平泻法。留针15～20分钟，每日1次。

其他疗法：耳针

取穴：内鼻　肺　胃　肾上腺　额

操作方法：毫针刺，中等刺激，留针20～30分钟，每日1次。亦可用耳穴压豆法。

5.13　鼻渊

鼻渊亦称脑漏，是以鼻流浊涕，鼻塞不闻香臭为其主症。因鼻流浊涕不止，如泉如渊，故名鼻渊。常伴有头额胀痛和头晕等，是鼻科的常见病多发病之一，类似现代医学之急慢性鼻窦炎。

病因病机

肺主皮毛，开窍于鼻，风寒袭表犯肺，蕴而化热，肺气失宣，而致鼻塞，郁热壅于鼻窍，则发为鼻渊；或因肝胆火盛，上犯清窍，灼伤鼻窦所致。

辨证

1.风寒化热　　恶寒发热，咳嗽痰多，头额胀痛，鼻塞多涕，嗅觉减退，舌质红，苔薄黄，脉浮数。

2.肝胆火盛　　鼻塞流涕，黄浊粘稠，腥臭难闻，眉间及颧部压痛，常见有发热，头痛，目眩口苦，急燥易怒，少眠多梦，舌红，脉弦数。

治疗

1.风寒化热

治则：祛风清热，宣肺开窍。取手太阴、阳明经穴为主。

处方：列缺　合谷　迎香　印堂

方义：鼻为肺窍，故取肺经络穴列缺以宣通肺气；散风清热；手阳明与手太阴相为表里，其脉上挟鼻孔，故取合谷、迎香以疏调手阳明经气，清泄肺热，对鼻塞，不闻香臭最为有效；印堂为督脉穴，能散郁热通鼻窍。

随证选穴：眉棱骨痛加鱼腰、照海。

刺灸法：毫针刺，用泻法。留针15～20分钟，每日1次。

2.肝胆火盛

治则：清泻肝胆，通利鼻窍。取手阳明、足厥阴、少阳经穴为主。

处方：行间　风池　上星　迎香

方义：行间为肝经的荥穴，风池为胆经与阳维之会，二穴有疏风解热，清泻肝胆的作用；取督脉的上星，手阳明经的迎香，以活血通络利鼻窍。

随证选穴：头痛加太阳。

刺灸法：毫针刺，用泻法。留针15～20分钟，每日1次。

其他疗法：耳针

取穴: 内鼻　肺　额　肾上腺　过敏者加平喘

操作方法: 毫针刺, 强刺激, 间歇运针, 留针 20～30 分钟。或用耳穴压豆法。

5.14　牙痛

牙痛是口腔疾患中常见的症状, 多因牙髓炎, 龋齿及冠周炎等病引起, 每遇热或冷等刺激而加剧, 以儿童和老年体弱者较多见。

病因病机

风火邪毒外侵, 郁阻阳明经络, 气血滞留, 郁而化火生腐, 或因过食辛辣而肠胃积热, 阳明化火, 循经上犯而发为牙痛。肾主骨, 齿为骨之余, 肾阴亏损, 牙髓空虚, 虚火上炎, 灼伤牙龈而疼痛。

辨证

1.风火牙痛　　牙齿疼痛, 齿龈红肿, 遇热痛剧, 兼见身热、恶寒、口渴等症, 舌红, 苔白, 脉浮数。

2.胃火牙痛　　齿龈红肿, 疼痛剧烈, 或出脓渗血, 头痛, 口臭, 烦渴引饮, 大便秘结, 舌苔黄厚, 脉洪数。

3.虚火牙痛　　牙痛隐隐, 时作时止, 牙齿松动, 齿龈不红不肿, 口不臭, 舌红, 少苔, 脉细。

治疗

治则: 通络止痛。风火者, 祛风泄热; 胃火者, 清胃泄火; 虚火者, 益阴降火。

处方:　合谷　下关　颊车

　　　　风火牙痛配液门　风池

　　　　胃火牙痛配内庭　劳宫

　　　　虚火牙痛配太溪　行间

方义: 合谷为治疗牙痛之效穴, 能清手阳明经之热; 下关、颊车均属胃经, 可疏通经气, 泄火止痛; 液门能清三焦之风热,引邪从表而解；风池祛风解表；内庭为足阳明之荥穴，可清阳明之实热；劳宫为手厥阴经荥穴，可清心火；取太溪以滋补肾阴而降虚火；行间则可清泻肝火。

随证选穴：龋齿痛加二间；头痛加太阳。

刺灸法：毫针刺，一般用泻法，太溪穴用补法。留针15～20分钟，每隔5分钟捻针1次。

其他疗法：耳针

取穴：上颌　下颌　神门　屏尖　牙痛点

操作方法：毫针刺，强刺激，留针20～30分钟。亦可用耳穴压豆法。

5.15　咽喉肿痛

咽喉肿痛是由多种常见的咽喉部病变引起，以局部红肿，疼痛不适为主要临床表现，常伴有发热，头痛，咳嗽等症状。本病包括现代医学的咽炎，喉炎及急慢性扁桃体炎等。

病因病机

本病是因外感风热，侵袭肺卫，结于咽喉，或因肺胃素有郁热，郁热上蒸，壅于咽喉而发病，或因肾阴不足，胃阴亏耗，津液不能滋润咽喉，虚火上炎而发病。

辨证

1.风热　　发热重，恶寒轻，头痛咳嗽，咽部红肿疼痛，舌红，苔薄黄，脉浮数。

2.实热　　壮热不退，无头痛恶寒，咽痛剧烈，面目红赤，口舌生疮，口渴引饮，大便秘结，小便短赤，舌红，苔黄燥，脉滑数。

3.虚热　　咽痛隐隐，潮热颧红，口渴不欲饮，腰膝酸软，头晕耳鸣，舌红少苔，脉细数。

治疗

1.风热

治则：疏风清热利咽。取手太阴、阳明经穴为主。

处方：风池　少商　合谷　曲池　列缺

方义：取风池以散风清热；曲池、合谷以清泄阳明邪热；少商为手太阴肺经之井穴，可泻肺中之热而利咽喉；列缺可化痰止咳，有散风清热利咽之功。

随证选穴：头痛加太阳、大椎。

刺灸法：毫针刺，用泻法。留针15～20分钟，或不留针。少商用三棱针点刺出血，每日1次。

2.实热

治则：清肺胃利咽喉。取手太阳、手足阳明经穴为主。

处方：少商　合谷　尺泽　陷谷　关冲

方义：少商系手太阴之井穴，可清泄肺热，为治喉证的主穴；尺泽为手太阳经的合穴，能泻肺经实热，取实则泻其子之意；合谷、陷谷分属手足阳明经，二穴相配以疏泄阳明之郁热；配以三焦经井穴关冲，加强清泄肺胃之热，以达消肿利咽之功。

随证选穴：便秘加支沟。

刺灸法：毫针刺，用泻法，留针15～20分钟。少商、关冲二穴用三棱针点刺出血。

3.虚热

治则：滋阴降火利咽。取手太阴、足少阴经穴为主。

处方：太溪　照海　鱼际　金津　玉液

方义：太溪为肾之原穴，照海系足少阴经和阴跷脉的交会穴，两脉均循行于喉咙，故二穴能滋阴降火，导虚火下行；鱼际为手太阴的荥穴，能清肺经之虚热而利咽；取金津、玉液以养阴液，利咽喉。

随证选穴：腰膝酸软加肾俞。

刺灸法：毫针刺，用平补平泻法。留针15～20分钟，每日1次。

其他疗法：耳针

取穴：咽喉　肺　扁桃体　耳轮$_{1\sim6}$

操作方法：毫针刺，强刺激，轮$_{1\sim6}$可用三棱针点刺出血。或用耳穴压豆法。

5.16　梅核气

梅核气系患者咽喉部的一种异常感觉，喉中似有梅核梗塞，故名梅核气。临床常以咯之不出，咽之不下为主要特征，或伴有胸膈痞闷，精神抑郁不畅等症状。以成年妇女较多见，属现代医学神经官能症范畴。

病因病机

本病多因精神刺激，情志抑郁而致肝气郁结。肝病必乘脾土，脾失健运，津液不得输布，则积湿成痰，痰气互结，阻于咽喉而发病。

辨证

患者自觉喉中有异物梗阻，咯之不出，咽之不下，此异常感觉时轻时重，常随情绪波动而变化。咽部无疼痛，饮食无妨碍，检查无异常，多见有精神抑郁，心情不畅，多猜多疑，胸胁胀满及纳呆等症状。妇女则常有月经不调。舌淡，苔白腻，脉弦。

治疗

治则：宽胸，利气，除痰。取任脉、手足厥阴经穴为主。

处方：天突　膻中　内关　行间　丰隆

方义：天突功在清咽利膈，膻中为气之会穴，有理气之功；内关为手厥阴经的络穴，有宽胸理气的作用，取行间疏肝解郁，配以足阳明胃经的络穴丰隆以祛痰，通便，理气降逆；诸穴合用，可奏宽胸利膈，理气化痰利咽喉之功效。

随证选穴；阴虚者加三阴交、太溪、照海。

气血双虚者加关元、足三里、膈俞。

刺灸法：毫针刺，用平补平泻法。留针15～20分钟，每日1次。

其他疗法：耳穴压豆法

取穴：神门　交感　咽喉　肝，左右交替，3 日更换 1 次。

6　急症

6.1　高热

　　高热是指体温骤升超过 39℃以上，以身灼热，烦渴，脉数等为主要临床特征。导致高热的原因主要可分为外感与内伤两大类。本章着重介绍外感之邪所致的高热，相当于现代医学中的急性传染性疾病的高热，急性感染性高热，及慢性疾病并发感染的高热等。

　　病因病机

　　导致高热的原因甚多。如外感风热，邪从口鼻或皮毛而入，内舍其合，使肺失清肃，卫失宣散，而致高热；或温邪侵表不解，内传气分，或内蕴营血，温邪与气血相搏，引发高热；或夏令感受暑热，暑性炎热，内扰神明，导致高热神昏；或外感时疫邪毒，郁于肌肤，内陷脏腑，邪正相争，而致高热。

　　辨证

　　1.风热犯肺　　症见高热微恶风寒，咽喉肿痛，咳嗽，吐痰色黄粘稠，口干渴，舌质红，苔薄黄，脉浮数。

　　2.温邪内蕴　　邪在气分者，症见高热不恶寒，面红目赤，口渴欲冷饮，咳嗽胸痛，腹部胀痛拒按，或大便秘结，舌质红，苔黄燥，脉洪数。邪在营血者，症见高热夜甚，烦躁不安，口干不欲饮，斑疹隐隐，或兼见神昏谵语，四肢抽搐，舌绛少津，脉细数。

　　3.暑热蒙心　　症见高热汗出，心烦不安，肌肤灼热，舌燥口干，烦渴引饮，甚则头痛，呼吸喘急，继而昏倒，不省人事，脉多沉而无力。

　　4.疫毒熏蒸　　疫毒来势凶猛，故症见高热，头目红肿热痛，咽喉肿痛，焦躁不宁，或见丹疹密布肌肤，咽喉腐烂作痛，舌红，苔黄，脉数。

治疗

1.风热犯肺

治则：疏风清热，宣肺止咳。取督脉及手太阴、阳明经穴为主。

处方：大椎　风池　少商　鱼际　合谷　曲池

方义：大椎为诸阳之会、督脉之穴，能泄热解表，风池为足少阳经穴，疏风清热力专，二穴相伍，宣散风热之邪；少商为手太阴井穴，鱼际为手太阴荥穴，井荥相配，清热宣肺利咽；合谷、曲池为手阳明经穴，合谷升而能散，曲池走而不守，二穴配用，可调和气血，疏散表邪，宣肺清热。

随证选穴：头痛加太阳；咳嗽甚者加列缺、肺俞。

刺灸法：毫针刺，用泻法，留针10～15分钟，间歇行针2～3次；少商可用三棱针点刺出血。

2.温邪内蕴

（1）气分证

治则：清热解毒驱邪。取督脉及手、足阳明经穴为主。

处方：大椎　尺泽　合谷　关冲　内庭

方义：取大椎以泄热解表；尺泽配合谷，可清泄肌表蕴积之热邪，助大椎而斡旋营卫，清里达表；关冲为三焦经井穴，可清泄气分之热，疏通三焦气机；内庭为足阳明荥穴，能清泄胃腑之热。五穴配用，可荡涤内外之蕴热秽邪。

（2）营血证

治则：清热透营，凉血解毒。取手厥阴、足太阳经穴为主。

处方：曲泽　委中　中冲　少冲　曲池　太冲

方义：本证因温邪侵入营血，故取手厥阴经穴曲泽与足太阳经穴委中（又名血中之郄穴），以清泄血分之热毒；因心主血脉，故取心包经井穴中冲与心经井穴少冲，以泻心火，清血热；

曲池为手阳明经合穴，能调和气血；太冲为足厥阴经原穴，善清热凉血。诸穴相伍，共奏清热透营、凉血解毒之功。

随证选穴：神昏谵语加十宣、人中；鼻衄加上星；咯血加孔最；便血加二白；四肢抽搐加筋缩、阳陵泉。

刺灸法：毫针刺，用泻法，留针15～20分钟，间歇行针2～3次；曲泽、委中、中冲、少冲用三棱针点刺出血。

3.暑热蒙心

治则：祛暑泄热，开窍启闭。取督脉、手厥阴经穴为主。

处方：大椎　上星　曲泽　人中　十宣　合谷　劳宫　内关　巨阙　膻中

方义：大椎为诸阳之会，与上星同用能祛暑解表；曲泽为手厥阴之合穴，点刺放血可清心泄热祛暑；人中、十宣、合谷透劳宫，可泄热醒神，开窍启闭；内关、巨阙、膻中能宽胸理气，宁神定志。

刺灸法：毫针刺，用泻法，留针20～30分钟，间歇行针5～6次；曲泽、十宣用三棱针点刺放血。

4.疫毒熏蒸

治则：清热解毒。取阳明经穴为主。

处方：曲池　少商　少泽　商阳　中冲　合谷　风池　外关　委中

方义：少商、少泽、商阳、中冲分别为肺经、小肠经、大肠经、心包经之井穴，四穴相配，可表里双解，清卫透营；曲池、合谷清热散风，消散头面诸窍之风热疫毒；风池、外关宣通三焦气机，疏风清热，消肿止痛；委中为血之郄穴，点刺能清热凉血解毒。

随证选穴：咽喉肿痛加列缺；头痛加天柱。

刺灸法：毫针刺，用泻法，留针15～20分钟，间歇行针3～4次；委中用三棱针点刺出血。

其他疗法：耳针

取穴：耳尖　肾上腺　皮质下　三焦　肺　胃

操作方法：毫针刺，强刺激，留针 10～15 分钟，间歇行针 1～2 次。

6.2　厥证

厥证是一个证候，可见于多种疾病之中，以突然昏倒，不省人事，四肢厥冷为主要特征。轻者昏厥时间较短，逐渐自行苏醒，醒后无后遗症；重者可一厥不醒而致死亡。现代医学中的休克、中暑、低血糖昏迷及精神性疾病等出现的昏厥，均可参考本病辨证论治。

病因病机

厥证的病机，主要是由于气机突然逆乱，升降失调，阴阳之气不相顺接所致。但气机逆乱又有虚实之分：气盛有余者，气逆上冲，血随气逆，或挟食挟痰，壅塞于上，以致清窍被蒙，发生厥证；气虚不足者，清阳不升，气陷于下，血不上达，以致精明失养，也可发生厥证。此外，在热性病过程中，阴盛阳衰，或阳郁于里，或气郁不达，或瘀血阻滞等，均可导致阴阳之气不相顺接而发生厥证。

气厥　　因恼怒惊骇，情志过极，以致气机逆乱，上壅心胸，蒙闭清窍，而致昏倒；或因素体元气虚弱，偶遇劳累过度，或悲恐之时，以致阳气消乏，气虚下陷，清阳不升，造成突然昏厥。

血厥　　肝阳素旺，又加暴怒，以致血随气逆，气血并壅于上，闭塞清窍，昏倒无知；或因失血过多，气随血脱，亦可发生昏厥。

痰厥　　形盛气弱之人，嗜食肥甘，脾胃受伤，运化失常，聚湿生痰，痰浊内阻，气机不利，又逢恼怒气逆，痰随气升，上蒙清窍，以致突然眩仆而厥。

食厥　　饮食不节，食滞内停，传化失常，气机受阻，以致窒闷而厥。多见于儿童。而成人在饱食之后，骤逢恼怒，气逆挟食，食填脘腹，上下痞隔，气机受阻，清窍，亦可致昏厥。

寒厥　　素体元阳亏损，不能温通经脉，寒邪直中于里，发生昏厥。

热厥　　邪热过盛，阳郁于里不能外达，而致热厥。

辨证

厥证的临床表现主要是突然昏倒，不省人事，四肢厥冷，面色苍白，属于危象。而厥证的发生，常有明显的诱因，故在辨证过程中了解病史极为重要，并须分辨虚、实、寒、热、气、血、痰、食。

气厥

　　(1) 实证：偶因恼怒，突然昏倒，不省人事，口噤拳握，呼吸气粗，四肢厥冷，舌苔薄白，脉沉弦。

　　(2) 虚证：素体虚弱，疲劳惊恐，而致眩晕昏仆，面色苍白，呼吸微弱，汗出肢冷，舌质淡，脉沉微。

血厥

　　(1) 实证：暴怒之后，突然昏倒，不省人事，牙关紧闭，面赤唇紫，舌质红，脉多沉弦。

　　(2) 虚证：多因失血过多，突然昏厥，面色苍白，唇口无华，四肢震颤，目陷口张，自汗肤冷，呼吸微弱，舌质淡，脉细数无力。

痰厥　　突然昏厥，喉中痰鸣，或呕吐涎沫，呼吸气粗，苔白腻，脉沉滑。

食厥　　饱食之后，骤加恼怒，突然昏厥，气息窒塞，脘腹胀满，舌苔厚腻，脉滑实。

寒厥　　面青肢冷如冰，踡躯而卧，口不渴，下利清谷，舌淡苔白，脉沉细。

热厥　　病初身热头痛，烦渴躁妄，胸腹灼热，尿赤便秘，继则神志昏愦，四肢厥冷，舌红苔黄燥，脉沉数有力。

治疗

1.实证

治则：苏厥开窍。取督脉、手厥阴经穴为主。

处方：人中　中冲　内关　足三里　涌泉

方义：人中为督脉经穴，督脉入络于脑，总督诸阳，刺之醒脑开窍；中冲、内关为手厥阴经井穴与络穴，用之苏厥开窍启闭；足三里为胃经之合穴，涌泉为肾经之井穴，二穴同灸，温阳救逆。

随证选穴；气厥加太冲；血厥加行间；寒厥加神阙、命门；热厥加十二井穴；痰厥加天突、巨阙、丰隆；食厥加中脘。

刺灸法：毫针刺，用泻法，留针 20～30 分钟，间歇行针 4～6 次；足三里、涌泉艾条温和灸 20～30 分钟；中冲用三棱针点刺出血。

2.虚证

治则：回阳救逆。取任、督脉穴为主。

处方：人中　内关　百会　气海　合谷　足三里

方义：人中可开关窍，醒神苏厥；内关能宽胸理气，强心救逆；百会为督脉经穴，督脉总督一身之阳；气海为任脉经穴，任脉总领一身之阴；百会能升阳醒神，气海可回阳固脱，二穴相配，可调整阴阳；合谷、足三里为手、足阳明经穴，阳明经多气多血，取二穴可补中益气，调和气血，扶正固本。

随证选穴：气厥加膻中；血厥加太冲、三阴交；寒厥加神阙；热厥加十宣。

刺灸法：毫针刺，用补法。百会、气海加灸，留针 20～30 分钟，间歇行针 4～6 次；神阙用隔盐灸。

其他疗法：耳针

取穴：心　脑　神门　皮质下　肾上腺　交感

操作方法：毫针刺，强刺激，留针 10～15 分钟。

6.3 脱证

脱证是以亡阴亡阳为其病机的内科急症。临床上以面色苍白、四肢厥冷、汗出气短、神情淡漠、血压下降，甚至昏不知人，唇面发绀，脉微欲绝等为主要特征。相当于现代医学的感染性休克、失血性休克、心源性休克、过敏性休克以及药物（或食物）中毒性休克等范畴。

病因病机

脱证多由素体羸弱，久病不愈，或突然大汗、大吐、大下、大失血之后，元气耗竭。阴亡则阳无所依附而脱失，阳亡则阴无以化生而消亡，以致阴阳不相维系，阴阳离决而发。

辨证

1.阴脱　　多见于热性病中。面唇苍白，发热烦躁，心悸多汗，汗出粘而热，口渴欲饮，尿少色黄，其则昏迷，脉细数或沉微欲绝。

2.阳脱　　多由亡阴之后演变而成。面色晦暗，大汗淋漓，汗清稀而凉，口不渴，身冷如冰，下利清谷，尿少或遗尿，神情淡漠，其则昏不知人，舌淡苔白，脉微欲绝。

3.阴阳俱脱　　神志昏迷，目呆口张，瞳孔散大，喉中痰鸣，气少息促，汗出如油，舌卷囊缩，周身俱冷，二便失禁，脉微欲绝。

治疗

治则：回阳固脱，调和阴阳。取任、督脉穴为主。

处方：人中　素髎　关元　神阙　涌泉　足三里　内关

方义：人中、素髎可醒脑振阳升血压；神阙、关元回阳固脱救逆；涌泉为肾经井穴，能益阴敛阳，清脑醒神；足三里益气助阳，固表止汗；内关可强心升血压。

随证选穴：多汗加合谷、复溜；痰多加丰隆；脉微欲绝加太渊。

刺灸法：毫针刺，用补法，留针 30～40 分钟，间歇行针 5～8 次；关元、神阙用灸法。以病情好转为度。

按语：脱证是由多种原因所引起的危重病候，病情复杂而变化迅速，故临证时应严密观察，分秒必争，积极进行综合救治药物与针灸、中医与西医综合治疗最为适宜。在救治脱证中，如药物治疗配合针灸，不仅奏效快，而且可使本来单用药物救治不活的病人，化凶为吉。

6.4 中暑

中暑是指在酷暑炎热之夏季，烈日之下长时间的停留和工作，暑热内袭或夹湿伤人，逼汗出而伤阴，骤然发为高热、汗出、嗜睡、神昏、躁扰抽搐等症的一种危急病证。现代医学亦称为中暑。

病因病机

中暑多因素体虚弱，暑热或暑湿秽浊之气侵袭人体，以致邪热郁蒸，正气耗伤，蒙闭清窍，经络之气厥逆不通所致.

辨证

中暑的临床分型，主要根据病情的程度不同，而分为轻型和重型两种。轻证主要表现为头痛，头晕，胸闷，恶心，口渴，汗出，高热，烦躁不安，全身疲乏酸痛；重证除上述症状外，还可见汗多肢冷，面色苍白，心慌气短，甚则神志不清，猝然昏迷，四肢抽搐等症。

治疗

1.中暑轻型

治则：清泄暑热，佐以和胃。取督脉与足阳明经穴为主。

处方：大椎　曲泽　合谷　太阳　足三里　内关

方义：大椎为诸阳之会，能清泄一身暑热之邪；曲泽能清心热，除心烦，通心窍；合谷配太阳，可清头面诸窍之热而医头痛头晕；足三里配内关以和胃止呕，强心安神。

刺灸法：毫针刺，用泻法，留针 5～10 分钟，间歇行针 1～2 次；大椎、曲泽、太阳用三棱针点刺出血。

2.中暑重型

治则：清泄暑热，开窍固脱。取督脉与足太阳经穴为主。

处方：人中　大椎　曲泽　委中　十二井穴　承山　内关
关元　神阙

方义：人中可开关窍，镇惊醒神；大椎可清泄一身暑热之邪；曲泽配委中，能清心热，除心烦，通心窍，解痉挛；十二井穴清暑热，开关窍而醒神；承山解痉挛，止抽搐；内关和胃止呕，强心升血压；关元、神阙固元气而复虚脱。

刺灸法：毫针刺，用泻法，留针 10～15 分钟，间歇行针 1～2 次；关元、神阙用灸法，每次灸 30～40 分钟；大椎、曲泽、委中、十二井穴用三棱针点刺出血。

其他疗法：刮痧

取穴：曲泽　委中　脊椎两侧的背俞穴大杼～三焦俞

操作方法：每刮一处，先用水湿润皮肤，右手持刮具，边蘸水边刮，直至皮肤起紫红色痧点为度。

7 其他病证

7.1 坐骨神经痛

坐骨神经痛是指沿坐骨神经通路及其分布区的疼痛，即在臀部、大小腿后外侧部和足外侧的放散性或持续性的疼痛。

本病根据病因可分为原发性和继发性二类。原发性坐骨神经痛即坐骨神经炎，主要由感染或寒冷刺激而引起。继发性坐骨神经痛为邻近组织的病变刺激、压迫、或破坏该神经所致，故又称症状性坐骨神经痛。临床上以继发性坐骨神经痛为多见，原发性较为少见。

临床表现

原发性坐骨神经痛起病急，疼痛重，多由臀部、髋部向下扩散至足部，疼痛呈持续性钝痛，并有发作性加剧。发作性疼痛可为烧灼样和刀割样，遇寒则疼甚，得温则减。坐骨神经通路各点常有明显压痛，直腿抬高试验阳性，病变初期踝反射可能增强，后期一般减弱，无明显肌肉萎缩。

继发性坐骨神经痛起病较缓，能查到原发病，临床常见为腰椎病变所引起的根性坐骨神经痛，疼痛呈放射性，常因咳嗽、喷嚏和并气用力时加剧，腰椎棘突和横突压痛明显，而坐骨神经通路各点压痛较轻微，直腿抬高试验也呈阳性，颏胸试验和颈静脉压迫试验阳性，踝反射多减弱，严重者可消失，病久者可见肌肉萎缩。

治疗

1.原发性坐骨神经痛

处方：环跳　风市　阳陵泉　昆仑　承山

刺灸法：毫针刺，用泻法。留针 15～20 分钟，间歇行针 1～2 次。

2.继发性坐骨神经痛

处方：腰4、5夹脊　大肠俞　关元俞　秩边　委中　阳陵泉　绝骨　昆仑

刺灸法：毫针刺，用平补平泻法。留针15～20分钟，间歇行针1～2次。

其他疗法

1.耳针

取穴：坐骨　臀　神门　交感　皮质下　腰椎

操作方法：毫针刺，用中度刺激，留针20分钟。亦可用耳穴压豆法。

2.电针

取穴：腰4、5夹脊　秩边　阳陵泉　环跳

操作方法：每次选2穴，针刺后，接电疗机，用疏密波，每次通电刺激20分钟。

7.2　枕神经痛

枕神经痛是枕区和上颈部的疼痛。多因感染性疾病及枕部损伤和第一至第四颈椎的病变等引起。

临床表现

枕区及上颈部疼痛，常因头颈部的动作、喷嚏、咳嗽等而诱发。发作时病人常保持头部不动。疼痛多为持续性，亦可阵发性加剧，但在发作间歇期仍可有钝痛。检查时可找到枕神经的压痛点。枕大神经压痛点位于乳突与第一颈椎后面中点连线的中点（风池穴），枕小神经压痛点位于胸锁乳突肌附着点的后上缘（翳明穴）。当按压这些部位时，病人感到剧烈的疼痛，疼痛可沿神经分布扩散。枕部的皮肤常有感觉过敏及营养障碍。

治疗

处方：风池　天柱　脑空　完骨　后溪　昆仑

刺灸法：毫针刺，用泻法。留针15～30分钟，间歇行针2

~3次。

其他疗法：耳针

取穴：神门　皮质下　枕　颈

操作方法：毫针刺，中度刺激，留针15～20分钟。亦可用耳穴压豆法。

7.3　面肌痉挛

面肌痉挛是指阵发性半侧面肌不规则抽搐而言。多见于中年以上的女性。

临床表现

症状开始仅有眼轮匝肌间歇性抽搐，逐渐发展至面部其他肌肉，严重的口角也会一起抽动。抽搐的程度轻重不等，可因疲倦、精神紧张、自主运动而加剧，入睡后抽搐即停止。个别病人可伴有头痛、病侧耳鸣。神经系统检查无阳性体征。

治疗

处方：太阳　四白　地仓　迎香　下关　合谷　太冲

刺灸法：毫针刺，用泻法。留针15～30分钟，间歇行针2～3次。亦可用电针，疏密波，通电15～20分钟。

其他疗法：耳针

取穴：交感　神门　肝　太阳　面颊　皮质下

操作方法：毫针刺，每次选3～4穴，强刺激，留针20分钟。或用耳针埋藏及耳穴压豆法。

7.4　多发性神经炎

多发性神经炎又名周围神经炎。是一种以对称性四肢远端运动、感觉、植物神经障碍为主要特征的疾病。本病多由感染、中毒、代谢障碍，或变态反应等原因而引起，其中以感染和中毒最为常见。

临床表现

本病初起即表现四肢远端手指、足趾麻木或刺痛，或有蚁行感，以后病情进一步发展面呈现典型的对称性手套或袜套样感觉障碍，同时四肢运动无力，肌肉萎缩出现悬垂腕或下垂足，腱反射减退或消失，肢体远端皮肤发冷，多汗或无汗。由于致病原因不同，而临床表现的运动、感觉和植物神经障碍各异。

治疗

处方：肩髃　曲池　外关　合谷　八邪　大椎　陶道　足三里　阳陵泉　三阴交　解溪　八风

刺灸法：毫针刺，初期宜用泻法，后期宜用补法或平补平泻。留针20～40分钟，间歇行针2～4次。并可针灸并用。

7.5　桡神经麻痹

桡神经麻痹是指桡神经损伤后，其支配的骨骼肌运动功能减退或丧失。主要表现为腕下垂，不能做仰掌和提腕动作。导致本病的原因很多，如腕肘扭挫伤，肱骨骨折，或睡眠时以手臂代枕，手术时上肢长期外展，上肢放置止血带不当，以及铅中毒、酒精中毒等均可导致桡神经麻痹。

临床表现

主要表现为腕下垂，所有伸指肌及拇指外展功能丧失，第一、二掌骨背面皮肤感觉消失。桡神经深支损伤时，则出现患肢所有伸指肌及拇指外展肌功能丧失，而桡侧伸腕长肌功能存在，但无感觉障碍。

治疗

处方：曲池　手三里　外关　阳溪　阳池　合谷

刺灸法：毫针刺，用平补平泻法。留针20～30分钟，间歇行针2～3次。可针灸并用，亦可用电针，选曲池、外关，通电20分钟。

7.6 尺神经麻痹

尺神经麻痹是指尺神经损伤后，其支配的骨骼肌运动功能减弱或丧失。手指以爪形畸形为特征，并伴有所支配区的感觉障碍。本病多因外伤或长期以肘支撑劳动损伤尺神经引起。

临床表现

手向桡侧偏斜，拇指处于外展状态，手指基底节过伸，末节屈曲，小鱼际平坦，骨间肌萎缩凹陷，手指分开合并受限制，小指动作丧失，各精细动作丧失，形成鹰爪手。手背尺侧、小鱼际、小指和无名指尺侧一半感觉丧失。

治疗

处方：小海　支正　外关　阳谷　中渚　八邪

刺灸法：毫针刺，用平补平泻法。留针20～30分钟，间歇行针2～3次。亦可用电针，少海、支正通电20分。

7.7 腓总神经麻痹

腓总神经麻痹是指腓总神经损伤后，其支配的骨骼肌运动功能减弱或丧失，出现足下垂及神经分布区的感觉障碍的一种病症。本病多因外伤，腓骨头骨折，或下肢以石膏固定时腓骨头处保护不当受到挤压所致，或久蹲后缺血致使腓总神经受损。

临床表现

足下垂，病人不能伸足、提足、扬趾及伸足外翻，足呈马蹄内翻状，行走时足尖下垂，为了避免足趾触地跌倒，用力提高下肢，使髋关节、膝关节过度屈曲，类似马步或鸡步，或称跨阈步态。小腿外侧和足背皮肤感觉减退或消失，胫骨前肌可见萎缩。

治疗

处方：足三里　阳陵泉　条口　悬钟　解溪　申脉　照海

刺灸法：毫针刺，用平补平泻法。留针20～30分钟，间歇行针2～3次。可用电针，阳陵泉、悬钟通电20分钟。

7.8 股外侧皮神经炎

股外侧皮神经炎又名感觉异常性股痛。以股外侧下 2／3 部位出现蚁行、麻木、针刺样感觉异常为特征。多见于肥胖中年男性，也常见于妊娠期妇女。

临床表现

自觉大腿前外侧下 2／3 处有蚁行感，或针刺、麻木样感觉异常，亦可出现疼痛，在行走或站立时加重。检查可在股外侧发现大小不等的感觉迟钝区或感觉缺失区，有时可发现有压痛点。

治疗

处方：局部围刺，风市　阳陵泉　三阴交

刺灸法：毫针刺，用平补平泻法。留针 15～30 分钟，间歇行针 2～3 次。局部围刺是以毫针沿感觉迟钝区皮下围刺。亦可用灸法，局部以艾条温和灸 20～30 分钟。

其他疗法：皮肤针

取穴：病变局部

操作方法：轻刺激，叩至皮肤潮红而不出血为度，每日或隔日一次。

7.9 颈椎病

颈椎病是颈椎骨关节病变（如增生性颈椎炎、颈椎间盘脱出等），压迫神经根和脊髓，而引起以头、颈、臂、手及前胸等部位的麻木、疼痛，伴有进行性肢体感觉及运动功能障碍的一种临床常见病。此病多见于成年人，好发于 40～60 岁之间，男性多于女性。

临床表现

颈项疼痛，常放射至肩、前臂、手指及前胸，往往头部活动或叩击头顶时疼痛更为明显，颈项僵硬，活动受限，相应区域的皮肤可出现感觉障碍，腱反射减弱。若病变累及脊髓则出现下肢麻木、沉重、肌张力增高，肌力减退，并出现病理反射，严重者可出现不完全性痉挛性瘫痪。部分病人常有头痛、头胀、当颈部过伸或转动时出现眩晕发作，甚至昏厥。

治疗

处方：风池　颈部夹脊　秉风　肩髃　曲池　外关　合谷后溪

下肢瘫痪者取：腰部夹脊穴　足三里　阳陵泉

刺灸法：毫针刺，用平补平泻法。留针20～30分钟，间歇行针2～3次。

其他疗法：皮肤针

取穴：颈部夹脊

操作方法：轻刺激，叩至皮肤潮红为度，隔日一次。

7.10　雷诺氏病

雷诺氏病系由肢端小血管痉挛性或功能性闭塞引起的局部缺血现象。病人如暴露于冷空气中或因情绪激动，即可发生肢端皮肤色泽的间歇性苍白及紫绀改变，伴有指（趾）的疼痛。本病易发于青年女性。

临床表现

每当环境温度降低或情绪激动时，两侧手指或足趾、鼻端、外耳突然变白，僵冷，皮肤出冷汗，常伴有蚁走感，麻木感或疼痛感，渐即转入青紫，或呈蜡状，经过一段时间后，皮肤又潮红、变暖，恢复正常。晚期有时症状呈持续地出现，手指（足趾）疼痛加剧，且有指（趾）端营养障碍，出现指（趾）甲裂纹、小溃疡，但很少坏死，即使发生坏死也仅限于皮肤。

治疗

处方：上肢：曲池　太渊　内关　合谷　后溪

　　　　下肢：足三里　三阴交　太溪　冲阳　太冲

刺灸法：毫针刺，用补法，留针15～20分钟，间歇行针2

～3次。亦可针灸并用。

其他疗法：耳针

取穴：神门　交感　心　肺　内分泌　肾上腺　皮质下　趾指

操作方法：毫针刺，每次选3～4穴，轻刺激，留针15～20分钟。或用耳穴压豆法。

7.11　红斑性肢痛症

红斑性肢痛症是一血管性疾病，其特征为阵发性肢端皮肤温度升高，皮肤潮红，肿胀，产生剧烈灼热痛，尤以足底、足趾为著，环境温度增高时，则灼痛加剧。此病多见于青年男女，其原因尚未肯定。

临床表现

缓慢起病，但也可突然发生。初起为局限性肢体远端（足底或手掌）的发作性、烧灼样疼痛，患处皮肤发红、发热、肿胀、出汗，局部血管博动增强，以后疼痛可扩及整个肢体。多数在晚间发作，每阵发作历时几分钟至数小时。各阵发作间局部仍有麻木疼痛感。可引起血管扩张或充血的各种因素，如局部加热、温暖的环境、运动、站立、甚至肢体的下垂，均可导致疼痛的加剧。休息、冷敷、将患肢抬高或裸露在被外可减轻疼痛。患处多汗，皮肤感觉灵敏，病人不愿穿袜或戴手套，屡次发作后，可发生肢端皮肤与指甲变厚或溃硬，偶见皮肤坏死，但一般无感觉及运动障碍。

治疗

处方：上肢：曲池　外关　合谷　劳宫　人迎

下肢：足三里　三阴交　行间　内庭　涌泉　人迎

刺灸法：毫针刺，用泻法。留针15～30分钟、间歇行针3～5次。

其他疗法：耳针

取穴：交感　神门　皮质下　内分泌　指　趾　踝　肾上腺

操作方法：毫针刺，每次选 3～5 穴，中等刺激，留针 15～20 分钟。或用耳穴压豆法。

77.12　单纯性甲状腺肿

单纯性甲状腺肿是一种因缺碘而引起的代偿性甲状腺肿大。由于碘的缺少，甲状腺素的合成减少，降低了血液中甲状腺素的浓度，致使垂体分泌更多的促甲状腺激素，引起甲状腺细胞增生和肥大，形成甲状腺肿大。本病多见于女性，其发病可以是地区性的，但也可是无地区性而散在发生。

临床表现

甲状腺肿多为弥漫性，也有呈结节性肿大。皮色如常，不觉疼痛，按之皮宽而质较软，一般无全身症状。地方性甲状腺肿，有时可高度肿大，环绕颈前，压迫邻近器官，导致呼吸不畅，咳嗽，吞咽不利，声音嘶哑等；散在性甲状腺肿，肿大程度较轻，质软光滑，常为对称性，可以随吞咽动作而上下移动，日久则质地逐渐偏硬，或出现结节。实验室检查：基础代谢率及血浆蛋白结合碘一般均属正常。

治疗

处方：人迎　水突　合谷　曲池　颈$_{3～5}$夹脊　风池

刺灸法：毫针刺，用泻法或补泻兼施，留针 15～30 分钟，间歇行针 2～3 次。

其他疗法：耳针

取穴：内分泌　神门　甲状腺　颈

操作方法：毫针刺，中等刺激，留针 20 分钟。亦可用耳穴压豆法。

7.13　甲状腺机能亢进

甲状腺机能亢进简称甲亢。系甲状腺素分泌过盛所致的常见内分泌疾病。临床上除见甲状腺肿大外，常伴有心悸、多汗、手颤、多食、消瘦和烦躁等证。本病多见于女性，可发于任何年龄，但以青、中年发病率为高。其发病原因多是病人受到严重精神创伤，以及发育、月经、妊娠，感染疾病等因素，引起大脑皮层机能紊乱，产生病理性兴奋，导致甲状腺机能亢进与腺体增生、肥大而成。

临床表现

前颈部呈轻度或中度弥漫性、对称性肿大，少数可见单叶或结节性肿大，局部可触及震颤和听到杂音，性情急躁，精神紧张而易激动，失眠，心动过速，怕热、多汗，两手平举时可见手指微颤，低热，食欲亢进，形体消瘦，月经过多等。有的出现突眼征。实验室检查：基础代谢升高，血浆蛋白结合碘测定超过正常范围。

治疗

处方：人迎　间使　三阴交　太冲　合谷　颈$_{3\sim5}$夹脊

刺灸法：毫针刺，补泻兼施。留针 15～20 分钟，间歇行针 2～3 次。

随证选穴：多汗加阴郄、复溜；失眠加神门、安眠；心动过速加内关、通里。

其他疗法：耳针

取穴：神门　皮质下　内分泌　甲状腺　平喘　心肺

操作方法：毫针刺，每次选 3～4 穴，留针 15 分钟。或用耳穴压豆法。

7.14　震颤麻痹

震颤麻痹又称帕金森病，是发生于中年以上的中枢神经系统变性疾病。以震颤、肌肉强直和运动减少为主要临床特征。

临床表现

起病缓慢，逐渐增剧。震颤最先见于肢体远端，通常从一侧上肢的远端（手指）开始，然后，逐渐扩展到同侧下肢及对侧上下肢，手指的节律性震颤呈搓丸样，称"搓丸样动作"。震颤多于肢体静止时发生，随意运动时减轻，情绪激动时加重，睡眠时完全消失。并见肌肉强直，肌张力增高，关节被动运动时感有均匀阻力，加上震颤因素似齿轮转动样，称"齿轮样强直"。病人常出现特殊姿态，头部前倾，躯干俯屈，上肘肘关节屈曲，腕关节伸直，前臂内收，下肢之髋及膝关节略为弯曲。行走呈急速小步，向前冲去，越走越快，不能即时止步或转弯，称"慌张步态"。一切运动显见缓慢、减少，面部缺乏表情，呈现"面具脸"。手不能作精细动作，书写困难，所写的字越写越小，称"写字过小症"。说话缓慢单调，严重者出现吞咽困难。

治疗

处方：人迎　扶突　合谷　太冲　阳陵泉

刺灸法：毫针刺，用平补平泻法。留针 15～20 分钟，间歇行针 2～3 次。

其他疗法：头针

取穴：运动区　舞蹈震颤控制区

操作方法：毫针刺，留针 30～40 分钟，间歇行针 3～5 次。或用电针，疏密波，通电 60 分钟。

7.15　小舞蹈病

小舞蹈病又称风湿性舞蹈病。临床特征为不规则的不自主运动，伴有自主运动障碍，肌力减弱和情绪改变。多见于儿童和青少年，女性较多。其病因除风湿病可引起外，其他如猩红热、白喉、脑炎、甲状腺机能减退等也可引起。

临床表现

早期症状常不明显，表现为患孩比平时不安宁，注意散漫，学业退步，肢体动作笨拙，字迹歪斜和手中所持的物体经常失落等，过一定时期后出现不自主地、快速而不规则地舞蹈样动作。起于一侧，逐渐发展蔓延至对侧，面部往往表现出无意义而又频繁的皱眉、眨眼、呶嘴、吐舌、缩鼻等动作，并可随情绪紧张而加剧，严重时还能影响语言、咀嚼和睡眠。肌力减弱、肌张力普遍降低。腱反射减弱，甚者消失。

治疗

处方：大椎　风池　肝俞　内关　合谷　阳陵泉　三阴交　足三里　太冲

刺灸法：毫针刺，用平补平泻法。留针 20～40 分钟，间歇行针 3～4 次。

其他疗法

1.耳针

取穴：心　肝　脾　肾　交感　神门　皮质下　枕　脑点　相应病区压痛点

操作方法：毫针刺，每次选 4～5 穴，中等刺激，留针 15～20 分钟。亦可用耳针埋藏或耳穴压豆法。

2.头针

取穴：舞蹈震颤控制区　运动区

操作方法：毫针刺，留针 30～40 分钟，间歇行针 3～5 次。或用电针，疏密波，通电 60 分钟。

7.16　白细胞减少症

当周围血液白细胞计数持续低于每立方毫米 4 000 以下时，称为白细胞减少症。本病主要由于中性粒细胞的缺少，临床所见原因有不明性和继发性二种，以前者为多见。

临床表现

原因不明性白细胞减少症患者可无症状，或出现容易疲劳，全身乏力，低热、盗汗以及失眠等神经官能症表现，多呈慢性良性过程，即使患病多年，也大多无明显恶化现象，白细胞多在3000～4000之间，分类计数粒细胞百分率正常或轻度降低，有时波动较大。血红蛋白量或血小板数大多正常或稍降低。

继发性白细胞减少症的临床表现决定于原发疾病。

治疗

处方：大椎　肝俞　脾俞　膏肓俞　膈俞　曲池　足三里三阴交　肾俞

刺灸法：毫针刺，用补法。留针15～30分钟，间歇行针2～3次。大椎、膏肓俞、脾俞、足三里可用灸法或针灸并用，每穴灸10～15分钟。

按语：继发性白细胞减少症应以治疗原发病为主，配合针灸治疗。

7.17　肥胖症

肥胖症是人体内脂肪贮存过多，如体重超过标准体重的15～20%即为肥胖。临床上肥胖症可分为单纯性和继发性两类。单纯性肥胖多因过食肥腻及甜食物，摄入量超过机体热能的消耗而致脂肪积聚。形体虽胖，但无明显内分泌功能障碍症状。继发性肥胖可因间脑、垂体、皮质醇分泌过多等继发，常伴有相应的神经、内分泌功能失调的症状。

临床表现

患者有不同程度的肥胖，可见颈，小腹和臀部脂肪明显积聚。轻者无其他症状，显著者出现一定的代谢失调现象。如畏热、多汗、易感疲乏无力，头晕头痛，心悸、腹胀等。

治疗

处方：人迎　胰俞　足三里　水分　复溜

刺灸法：毫针刺，用平补平泻法。留针 15～30 分钟，间歇行针 2～3 次。

其他疗法

1.耳针

取穴：交感　神门　胃　口　内分泌　皮质下　饥点　三焦

操作方法：毫针刺，每次选 3～4 穴，中等刺激，留针 15～20 分钟。临床多用耳针埋藏法或耳穴压豆法。

2.皮肤针

取穴：胸$_{7～12}$夹脊

操作方法：在应用体针的同时，用皮肤针轻叩夹脊穴，叩至皮肤潮红为度，隔日 1 次。

按语

1.针灸治疗单纯性肥胖症疗效较好，继发性肥胖症必须同时结合其病因进行综合治疗。

2.在针灸治疗的同时，应配合其他辅助治疗，主要是控制饮食与坚持体育锻炼，控制盐、蛋白、脂肪、糖类的饮食，多食蔬菜。

7.18　晕车、晕船

晕车、晕船是指在乘车船或飞机时，由于不规则颠簸，过度刺激内耳前庭，使前庭神经机能紊乱，或因精神紧张，视觉作用，嗅闻不良气味而出现头晕、呕吐等症状。

临床表现

轻者恶心、呕吐、头晕、眼昏花；重者突然晕倒，面色苍白，四肢发凉，出冷汗。

治疗

处方：内关　足三里　百会　风池

刺灸法：毫针刺，用平补平泻法。留针 20～30 分钟，亦可达 40～60 分钟，间歇行针 3～5 次。

其他疗法: 耳针

取穴: 神门　交感　枕　胃　肾上腺　皮质下

操作方法: 多用耳针埋藏或耳穴压豆法, 每隔 10～20 分钟按揉一次, 每次每穴按 10～20 下。

按语

习惯晕车、晕船者, 于乘车船之前可先刺内关、足三里预防。或行耳针埋藏、耳穴压豆。对危重病人应及时采用药物抢救。

7.19　针刺戒烟

针刺戒烟是指通过针刺, 使吸烟成瘾者对吸入和喷出的烟草雾产生一种恶嗅感, 从而使已吸烟成瘾癖者达到戒烟的目的。

临床表现

吸烟成瘾, 当中断吸烟后可出现全身软弱无力, 烦躁不安, 呵欠连作, 感觉迟钝等证。

治疗

处方: 人迎　足三里　太冲　合谷

刺灸法: 毫针刺, 用泻法。留针 20～30 分钟、间歇行针 2～3 次。足三里、太冲可用电针, 疏密波, 通电刺激 15～20 分钟。

其他疗法: 耳针

取穴: 交感　神门　肺　气管　胃　口　内分泌

操作方法: 毫针刺, 每次选 3～4 穴, 强刺激, 留针 15～20 分钟。可用耳针埋藏法。

按语

针刺戒烟疗效一般产生在针后 2～3 天, 表现为吸烟量明显减少或停止吸烟, 口腔味觉改变, 烟呈枯焦草味, 吸烟念头下降。戒烟期间适当增加饮食营养, 或适当内服宁心安神的中药及维生素类药物。

THE ENGLISH–CHINESE ENCYCLOPEDIA OF PRACTICAL TCM

(Booklist)

英汉实用中医药大全

（书目）

VOLUME	TITLE	书名
1	ESSENTIALS OF TRADITIONAL CHINESE MEDICINE	中医学基础
2	THE CHINESE MATERIA MEDICA	中药学
3	PHARMACOLOGY OF TRADITIONAL CHINESE MEDICAL FORMULAE	方剂学
4	SIMPLE AND PROVEN PRESCRIPTION	单验方
5	COMMONLY USED CHINESE PATENT MEDICINES	常用中成药
6	THERAPY OF ACUPUNCTURE AND MOXIBUSTION	针灸疗法
7	*TUINA* THERAPY	推拿疗法
8	MEDICAL *QIGONG*	医学气功
9	MAINTAINING YOUR HEALTH	自我保健
10	INTERNAL MEDICINE	内科学

（京）112 号

The English—Chinese

Encyclopedia of Practical TCM

Chief Editor   Xu Xiangcai

6

**THERAPEUTICS OF ACUPUNCTURE
AND MOXIBUSTION**

Euglish   Chief Editor   Yu Changzheng

Chinese   Chief Editor   Liu Yutan

英汉实用中医药大全

主编   徐象才

6

针灸治疗学

中文   英文

主编   刘玉檀   俞昌正

*

高等教育出版社出版

高等教育出版社激光照排技术部排版

新华书店总店北京科技发行所发行

国防工业出版社 印刷厂印装

*

开本 850×1168 1／32   印张 21   字数 540 000

1991年10月第1版 1991年10月第1次印刷

印数 0001— 7 175

ISBN7-04-003617-7／R·13

定价 10.85 元